DATE DUE FOR RETURN

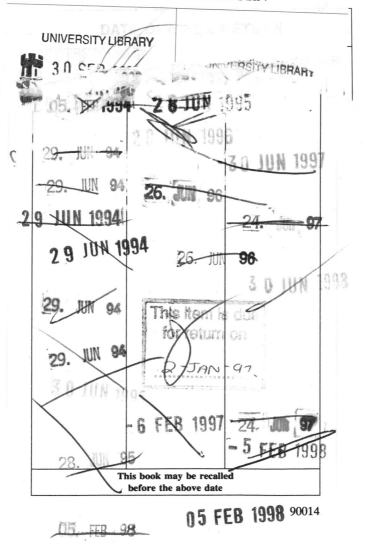

UNIVERSITY LIBRARY

30 SEP

05. JUL 1994   2 6 JUN 1995

UNIVERSITY LIBRARY

29. JUN 94   2 8 JUN 1996

30 JUN 1997

29. JUN 94   26. JUN 96

29 JUN 1994   24. JUN 07

2 9 JUN 1994   26. JUN 96

3 0 JUN 1998

29. JUN 94

This item is due
for return on

29. JUN 94

2 JAN 97

3 0 JUN

-6 FEB 1997   24. JUN 97

28. JUN 95   -5 FEB 1998

**This book may be recalled
before the above date**

05. FEB 98   **05 FEB 1998** 90014

MODERN MEDICINAL CHEMISTRY

MODERN MEDICINAL CHEMISTRY

JOHN B. TAYLOR, B.Sc., D.I.C., Ph.D.,
Senior Vice President, Central Research,
Rhône-Poulenc Rorer,
Dagenham Research Centre, Essex

and

PETER D. KENNEWELL, B.A., M.A., Ph.D.,
Scientific Adjoint to the Immunology Group,
Roussel Laboratories Limited,
Swindon, Wiltshire

ELLIS HORWOOD
NEW YORK   LONDON   TORONTO   SYDNEY   TOKYO   SINGAPORE

First published 1993 by
Ellis Horwood Limited
Market Cross House, Cooper Street
Chichester
West Sussex, PO19 1EB
A division of
Simon & Schuster International Group

Printed and Bound in Great Britain by
Hartnolls Limited, Bodmin, Cornwall.

Library of Congress Cataloging-in-Publication Data

Available from the publisher

10000132189

British Library Cataloguing in Publication Data

A catalogue record for this book is available from the British Library

ISBN   0-13-590399-8   (pbk)

1 2 3 4 5   97 96 95 94 93

Table of contents

Authors' preface

This work is intended to update our previous book *Introductory Medicinal Chemistry* which was published in 1981. The intervening 12 years have seen such major changes in the science of medicinal chemistry that it is no longer unjustified hyperbole to claim that the day of truly rational drug design is here. Much of this advance has been due to the enormous progress made in computer technology, both hardware and software, and in molecular biology although significant developments in organic chemistry, biochemistry, pharmacy and physiology have also played their parts. The greater size of this volume and notably inclusion of the chapter on 'Drug discovery' underline scientific progress during the intervening period.

A further development has been the number of universities in the United Kingdom which now routinely offer courses in medicinal chemistry as part of their honours degree syllabus. It is hoped that this work will offer students a basic introduction which will complement many of these courses.

The format of the book follows the general lines of its predecessor, commencing with a general introduction to the subject and then systematically following the entry, distribution, action and elimination of a drug in the body. A complete section is then devoted to drug design methodology.

The ideas and concepts discussed in this book have been refined over many years in stimulating discussions with our many colleagues in Roussel Laboratories and Rhône-Poulenc Rorer. In addition Yvonne Raindle and Susan Hughes are warmly thanked for their invaluable secretarial help. We are deeply grateful to our families for their support and patience during the preparation of this text which is therefore dedicated to them.

April 1993

P. D. Kennewell
J. B. Taylor

1

Introduction

> Medicinal chemistry remains a challenging science, which provides profound satisfaction to its practitioners. It intrigues those of us who like to solve problems posed by Nature. It verges increasingly on biochemistry and on all the physical, genetic and chemical riddles in animal physiology which bear on medicine. Medicinal chemists have a chance to participate in the fundamentals of prevention, therapy and understanding of diseases and thereby to contribute to a healthier and happier life.

Thus wrote Alfred Burger, one of the great figures of medicinal chemistry in the opening chapter of *Comprehensive Medicinal Chemistry*. Burger's life and career has encompassed much of development of the subject in the 20th century (he was a co-founder of the *Journal of Medicinal Chemistry*), and this statement sums up his belief in the value of the subject. It is a view which is very much shared by the authors who hope that this work will encourage others to take up this science.

1.1 DEFINITIONS

Medicinal chemistry is the study of those chemicals which have potential beneficial effects on disordered living systems. At its heart is chemistry, notably organic chemistry, but no medicinal chemist is interested solely in the chemical properties of the molecules under investigation. The whole "raison d'être" for the synthesis of any new compound lies in its anticipated biological activity or, unfortunately as happens all too frequently, in its lack of activity. Modern drug design is a multidisciplinary activity in which the combined expertise of the chemist, biologist, biochemist, pharmacologist, theoretical and computational chemist, together with many others, take part. Indeed, it often appears to chemists that their role in the discovery of a new therapeutic agent, commencing as it must at the very beginning of the discovery process, is often neglected or forgotten by the time that the molecule enters clinical use.

The process of drug design comprises two important and distinct processes, namely the discovery of a new molecule as a lead structure which shows some elements of the desired biological activity, and an optimisation process whereby this lead structure is modified until the desired pharmacological profile for the required therapeutic agent has been obtained. These two processes use a number of different techniques and scientific inputs and will be discussed in greater detail in Chapter 5. Modern science is evolving at ever increasing rates, and this is especially true of medicinal chemistry situated as it is at the interface of chemistry and biology. Thus when the first edition of the book was written drug design was concerned essentially with the techniques of Hansch and others to determine, from large groups of synthesised molecules, the essential chemical properties needed for the biological activity. The use of this knowledge enabled the design and synthesis of further structures with better activities to be carried out. Most significantly, the design of new lead structures *de novo* was, with perhaps the notable exception of captopril, still a dream. Today enormous advances in theoretical understanding and computer technology are making such design the reality.

The many other disciplines associated with medicinal chemistry in drug discovery are mentioned in the following sections.

1.1.1   Pharmacology
This science is the study of the effects of pharmaca, or biologically active chemical substances, on the intact animal organism. Pharmacology is not restricted to therapeutic agents or drugs, because it also applies to all active agents such as fungicides, insecticides, and toxins which can affect the physiology of the living animal. Essential requirements for the discovery of any new therapeutic agent for man or other animal (veterinary use) are the understanding of drug action and the design of test procedures. These two elements will allow experimental drugs to be designed and evaluated against a disease-simulating process in animal models or in isolated tissue preparations which, in turn, can be correlated to the human disease or disorder. There are of course many inherent problems in this process, notably the questionable extrapolation of such simulated conditions in animal experiments (usually small rodents) to the clinical situation, and the inevitable imprecision of such experiments because of the inherent biological variation. Biological variation is an inevitable consequence of the ultimate interspecies physiological divergence.

1.1.2   Clinical pharmacology
The study of the effect of drugs on both healthy volunteers and patients is the responsibility of the clinical pharmacologist, who is a medically qualified person. Such studies take place when a new compound has a sufficiently interesting pharmacological profile and no overt toxicity. In fact the level of dosing of a compound permitted for a volunteer is strictly related to the amount of toxicological data which has been generated. As more data are acquired the dosing regimen can be increased until a safety margin has been defined where no adverse effects on healthy individuals have been demonstrated and patients suffering from the target disease can now be treated.

1.1.3   Molecular pharmacology
This is the study of the pharmacological action of drugs at the molecular level which attempts to define the site of action of the drug, the receptor, or possibly the specific enzyme with which it interferes. The objective of such studies is to elucidate the precise sequence of chemical and biological events resulting from the drug–receptor interaction. Such biochemical studies are much less susceptible to the problem of biological variability found in whole animals, and much more consistent structure activity relationships can thus be determined. How receptors can be identified in small fragments of tissues and how the ability of compounds to bind these receptors can be measured will be discussed in Chapter 4. Such measurements are not complicated by other factors in the transit of the drug from its point of entry into the body to its ultimate site of action in the living animal.

1.1.4   Microbiology
The study of microorganisms, their growth and the effects of chemicals on them, is the province of microbiology. Because many diseases which infect man are the result of bacterial infection, the design of agents to destroy or at least limit the growth of bacteria *in vivo* is an important aspect of medicinal chemistry. Microorganisms themselves are an important source of novel chemotherapeutic agents which often have novel and highly complex structures.

1.1.5   Biochemistry
Biochemistry is the study of the chemical processes occurring within all cells which constitute the living organism. Studying modifications or disregulation of these chemical processes particularly in the disease state, is frequently a valuable approach to the design of a new therapy. Conversely, during detailed investigation of a new drug substance the biochemist will ensure that the drug causes no untoward changes in all essential physiological functions or homeostatic processes.

1.1.6   Physiology and medicine
Whilst biochemistry is concerned with the chemical reactions within the cells, the way in which these cells are grouped together to produce specific organs and the functioning of these organs in the body provide the field of study known as physiology. The comparison between healthy and diseased organs can provide information as to the nature of the disease process, and if this can also be related to biochemical changes in the tissues and cells this information can be used as a rational approach to the design of new drugs intended to alleviate the condition. Truly rational approaches to drug design must be based on an appreciation of the bodily dysfunctions occurring in an identified disease state with the aim of subsequent correction of the malfunction selectively by chemical means.

Medicine itself is the study of the effects of diseases on the body (diagnosis), and their cure or prevention by selected processes such as vaccination, drug treatment and surgery, or merely allowing the disease to run its natural course whilst alleviating the manifested symptoms (pain, swelling, etc.). In most, if not all situations, it is certain that medicines discovered by the medicinal chemist will be employed.

1.1.7   Pharmacy

The clinician does not usually administer a pure homogeneous compound itself but a complex formulation, of which the biologically active constituent is but a part. Pharmacy is the study of the formulation of active chemical entities, or active principles, into an appropriate dosage form. The drug composition is the vehicle selected which is most appropriate for the administration of a desired therapy; such formulations are usually tablets, capsules, syrups, powders, suppositories or aerosols. In general, the tablet form is preferred for routine prescription because this format is usually the simplest to manufacture, transport, handle and ingest, and is frequently the most suitable form for long-term storage. The active principle constitutes only a small proportion of the whole tablet whose bulk is mainly composed of fillers and binders which hold the tablet together, and dispersants which help to break up the tablet efficiently in the gastrointestinal tract of the patient. The pharmacist must produce a compressible mixture with high flow properties giving a hard tablet which can withstand shock, shaking and mishandling and which will, nevertheless, rapidly disintegrate to release the active constituent after being swallowed.

1.1.8   Molecular biology

The study of the structure and function of nucleic acids, deoxyribonucleic acid (DNA) and ribonucleic acid (RNA) and their derived proteins comprises the subject of molecular biology. This has rapidly evolved over the last few years with the use of the insights gained through investigations into the actions of the genetic material by using formidable techniques capable, inter alia, of producing proteins not previously readily available. This has had two major consequences for drug research. On the one hand the isolation of proteins involved in a number of physiological processes has enabled these processes to be much better characterised and understood with attractive potential targets for therapeutic intervention in important illnesses being identified. On the other hand, a number of these proteins are attractive therapeutic agents in their own right. The first of these proteins are now beginning to reach the clinician, though this process is perhaps taking longer, and costing more, than some of its early protagonists had envisaged.

It cannot be doubted, however, that molecular biology has already contributed much to modern medicinal chemistry and will continue to contribute greatly in future. It is, perhaps, less obvious whether the greater contribution to mankind will come from the protein products themselves or indirectly from the fundamental understandings arising from these investigations.

The majority of effective drugs used in medicine today are relatively low molecular weight organic compounds. Whilst many inorganic ions play a crucial role in nerve conduction, in cell activation and as complexes in enzymes, haemoglobin etc., by far the greatest interest of practising medicinal chemists lies in organic chemistry, their primary expertise. The powerful separation techniques and structure determination methodology now available give them the ability to isolate and identify microgram quantities of active agents from natural sources. Modern synthetic methods make it possible to contemplate the synthesis of almost any characterised structure which may be desired. Such a powerful combination of resources provides the medicinal chemist with considerable opportunities to design and construct any appropriate molecules required for the understanding of drug action and for the development of improved medicines. The medicinal chemist should make very significant contributions to the new "generation" medications of the next decade.

1.2   DRUG DEVELOPMENT

1.2.1   Historical development

Mankind has always been afflicted by disease and ailments and it is likely that he has attempted to control these afflictions from time immemorial by treating himself with herbs, berries and other substances gathered from his environment. Documentary evidence for the existence of such activities is of course dependent upon the survival of appropriate records. The earliest such report appears on a Sumerian clay tablet from 2100 BC which lists a number of recipes but unfortunately does not indicate their usage. A more complete listing of remedies is given in the Ebers papyrus of Ancient Egypt (ca 1500 BC) which includes some 800 recipes and also a number of ritual incantations calling on divine intervention to help control the course of the disease. The Egyptians apparently had a significant effect on the Greeks. Homer in the *Odyssey* tells that "the fertile soil of Egypt is most rich in herbs, many of which are wholesome in solution although many are poisonous, and in medical knowledge the Egyptian leaves the rest of the world behind". In their turn the Greeks also influenced the subsequent development of Western medicine as will be discussed later.

During this period, of 2000–3000 years ago, significant efforts to combat diseases were being made in two other great civilisations namely those of India and China. In contrast to Europe, significant elements of these early investigations remain today. Thus the Indians created the system of Ayurvedic medicine, a general philosophical approach to maintenance of good health and long life and to the treatment of disease. Drugs, diet and other regimes are part of a holistic view of man in the universe, and the growth and popularity of this philosophy is such that today some 50–75% of the population of India relies on Ayurvedic and related traditional medicines. Of a number of drugs which have been isolated from traditional Indian plants, the best known is perhaps the antihypertensive and tranquillising agent reserpine (1).

In China, the first written medical text was "Huang Di Nei Jing" (Emperor's Canon of Internal Medicine) compiled around 300 BC which provided a comprehensive theory for both diagnosis and treatment. This served as the philosophical concept for further development, elaboration and proliferation of the diverging schools of Chinese medicine during the following two millennia. Since then some 10 000 medical works have been published, amongst them *Shen Nong ben cao Jing* (Shen Nong's canon of materia medica) which appeared in the centuries around the birth of Christ and described other characteristics, processing, classification and physiological and pharmaceutical effects of 365 entries (252 from plants, 67 from animals and 46 related to minerals). In its time this led to the first official Pharmacopoeia, Tang ben cao (AD 657–9) a cooperative work in 53 volumes of 20 medical officers in the Tang Dynasty and then the renowned comprehensive classic materia written by Li Shizher

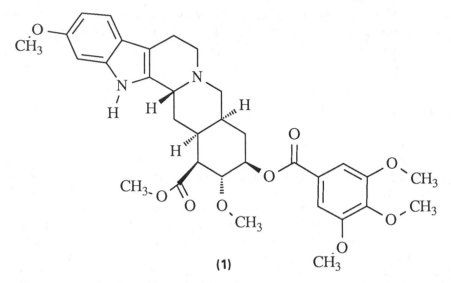

(1)

Den can gang mu of 1596. This took the authors 30 years to complete and contained 1892 entries, including 57% from plants, 23 from the zoological domain and 14 from minerals. These were included in 11 000 prescriptions. This great and long tradition of medicine is still in use in China both as a treatment *per se* and as a rich source of interesting leads for therapeutically active agents, amongst these being quingaosu (artemisimine, **2**) an antimalarial.

Returning to the evolution of Western therapy, the links between Egypt and Greece have already been mentioned. The Greeks adopted many Egyptian remedies and often tried to rationalise their use in terms of their "humoral" theories of disease. These held that an excess or deficiency of any of the four humours, blood, phlegm, black and yellow bile resulted in illness and the affect of herbal remedies was to reduce this imbalance. The leading proponent of this theory was Galen (129–199) whose work *On the art of healing* influenced, negatively, the development of medical science in Europe until the end of the Middle Ages. The leading antagonist was Dioscorides who urged his contemporaries to concentrate on what actually happens when drugs were administered rather than idly speculating on what might be the reason for their activities. His monumental five volume *De materia medica* discussed over 600 plants, 35 animal products and 90 minerals, and it influenced Arab and European medical evolution alike. Amongst the many products cited in his works are almond oil, aloes, belladonna, cinnamon, ginger, marjoram, thyme and wormwood.

The theories and findings of these ancient civilisations were propagated and bequeathed to Europe by Muslim conquerors of the former Roman Empire who also added to the pharmacopoeia the use of metallic salts. Indeed the first use of careful quality control was introduced by Abuleasis in the late 10th century as part of his description of the preparation of mineral salts for therapeutic use.

As the Renaissance replaced the dark ages and Europe moved into a more scientific, investigational phase, travelling Jewish physicians introduced the ideas of Dioscorides and Galen into medicinal usage. Initially there was a great upsurge in the medical

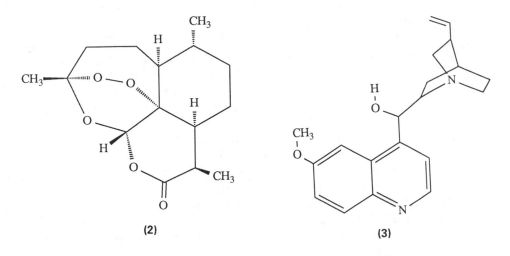

(2)   (3)

use of herbs, but Paracelsus in the early 16th century strongly urged the use of chemical remedies, particularly those of antimony, gold and mercury.

One of the greatest herbal remedies of all was introduced into Europe in the 17th century by Jesuit missionaries who accompanied the Spanish conquistadors on their exploration of Central and South America. This was an extract of the cinchona bark obtained from South American Indians who had long used it as an agent against chills and fevers. It soon became the favoured medicine for fevers, chills, and malaria in Europe. Two centuries later in 1820 its active principle, quinine (**3**), was isolated. Nevertheless, in spite of the large number of organic drugs of botanical origin which appeared from the New World during the 16th and 17th centuries, the more rapid scientific progress which was then being made in inorganic chemistry meant that inorganic drugs of mineral origin were still being favoured.

In England in the 18th century, Withering introduced the use of an extract of foxglove plant for the treatment of dropsy, a heart condition characterised by excessive accumulation of liquid in the lower limbs of the afflicted. He used this extract on the personal recommendation of country folk who had been using the elixir for untold years, a fine example of an enquiring medical practitioner following up and developing a lead from the folk culture of his day. The active ingredient digitalis is still extensively used today for controlling threatened heart failure and is still obtained from foxgloves by extraction.

By the 18th century the situation in Europe was one of acceptance that illness could be controlled by a mixture of herbs and powders although physicians were well aware of the limitations of these natural products. With the founding of organic chemistry as a science and the demystifying of natural products by Wohler's synthesis of urea from inorganic salts in 1828, the scene was set for a systemic investigation into the active ingredients contained in therapeutic herbs. In addition the synthetic potential of organic chemistry promised the preparation of hitherto unknown materials. That this promise has been amply borne out is illustrated in Table 1.1 which lists some of the more significant chemical discoveries of the last two centuries.

Table 1.1.   Some important developments in medicinal chemistry

1805	Serturner isolated morphine (**4**, R = H) in an impure form. The correct structure was determined in 1923 by Gulland and Robinson.
1819	Runge isolated quinine (**3**) from cinchona bark.
1820	Pelletier and Caventon isolated colchicine (**5**) from the crocus for use in gout.
1829	Leroux isolated salicin from willow bark.
1832	Robiquet isolated codeine (**4**, R = Me).
1842	Ether first used as an anaesthetic by Long.
1844	Wells used nitrous oxide in dentistry.
1847	Simpson used chloroform as anaesthetic.
1848	Merck isolated papaverine (**6**) from mother liquors remaining after extracting morphine from opium. The spasmolytic activity was found by Macht in 1917.
1864	Jobst and Hesse isolated physostigime (**7**) from Calabar bean.
1867	Lister pioneered the use of phenol as an antiseptic in surgery.
1868	Liebreich discovered the sleep-producing properties of chloral hydrate.
1841, 1869	Attempts to isolate the active principle of foxglove. This was shown to be digoxin (**8**) by Smith in 1930.
1874	Maclagan used salicin in rheumatic fever.
1876	Stricker showed that salicylic acid was an analgesic. In 1898 Hoffman prepared acetylsalicylic acid (**9**), aspirin.

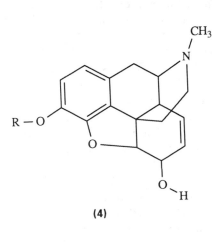

(4)

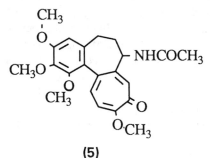

(5)

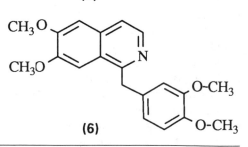

(6)

continued

Table 1.1.   *Continued*

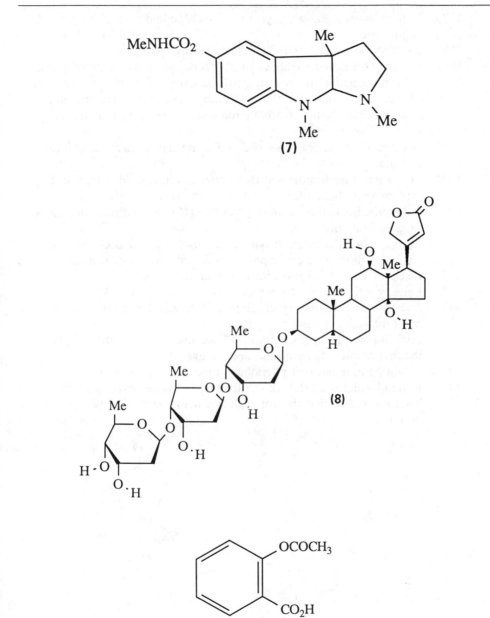

(7)

(8)

(9)

continued

Table 1.1.   *Continued*

1879	Murrel showed that glyceryl trinitrate (**10**) could relieve the pain of angina pectoris.
1881	Koch showed that $Hg(II)Cl_2$ killed anthrax spores.
1884	Knorr and Filehne introduced phenazone (**11**) as an antipyretic and thus stimulated an interest in synthetic drugs.
1891	Ehrlich coined the term "chemotherapy". He used methylene blue to treat malaria, the first synthetic material to be used to attack a specific disease.
1899	Hedonal (**12**) was prepared as a deliberate replacement for chloral hydrate.
1899–1901	Meyer and Overton devised the theory of oil/water distribution to explain anaesthetic effects.
1901	Tahamine isolated crystalline adrenalin (**13**), the first hormone to be isolated in a pure state.
1903	Veronal (**14**) a barbiturate synthesised by Conrad and Guthzeit in 1882 was shown to be a hypnotic by Fischer and von Mering.
1903	Eischom synthesised procaine (**15**) as a local anaesthetic.
1905	Langley published his theory of "receptive substances".
1906	Acetylcholine (**16**) was synthesised and its vasodepressor effect studied by Hunt and Traveau.
1909	Ehrlich patented arsphenamine (**17**) for use against syphilis. This was the first man-made chemotherapeutic agent.
1912	Hauptmann found that phenobarbitone (**18**) was antiepileptic.
1914	Kendall isolated crystals of the thyroid hormone thyroxine (**19**).
1919	Vogl recognised that the antisyphilitic drug merbaphen (**20**) was a diuretic.

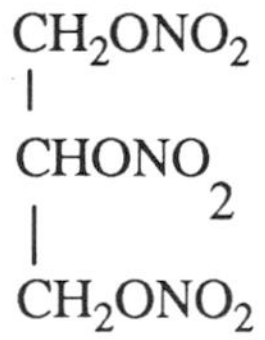

$$CH_2ONO_2$$
$$|$$
$$CHONO_2$$
$$|$$
$$CH_2ONO_2$$

(10)

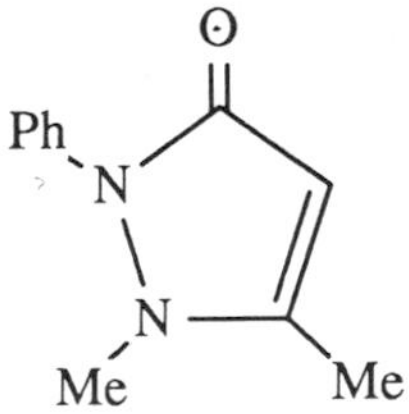

(11)

$$H_2N-\overset{O}{\overset{||}{C}}-O-CH_2CH_2i\text{-}Pr$$

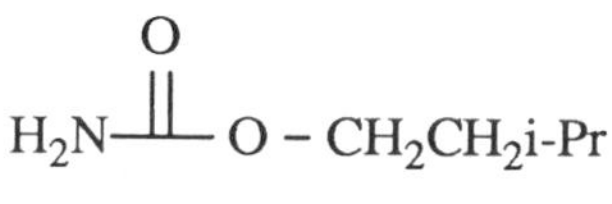

(12)

continued

Table 1.1.   *Continued*

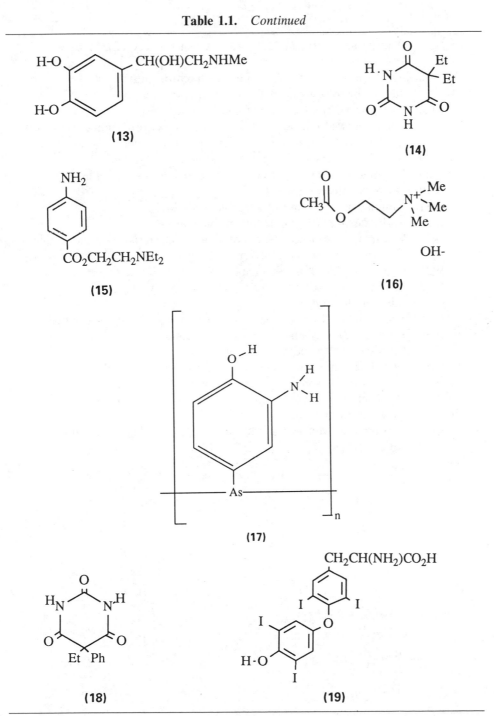

(13)

(14)

(15)

(16)

(17)

(18)

(19)

continued

Table 1.1.   *Continued*

1921	Banting and Best isolated insulin which was crystallised by Abel in 1926.
1924–32	Irradiation of foodstuffs to give antirachitic activity was shown to be due to the synthesis of vitamin D$_2$ (**21**) from ergosterol.
1926	Histamine (**22**) found in mammalian body.
1926	Loewi showed that acetylcholine was the neurohormone responsible for neurotransmission in the parasympathomimetic nervous system.
1929	Aurothio compounds suggested as therapy for arthritis.
1929	Fleming first observed the antibiotic activity of penicillin.
1929	Doisy isolated oestrone (**23**).
1931	King isolated vitamin C, ascorbic acid (**24**).
1931	Androsterone (**25**) isolated from bull's urine.
1932	Erlenmeyer espoused the concept of bio-isosterism, i.e. the similar biological activities of different chemical groups.
1932	Eddy introduced modern methods of analgesic testing.
1932	Domagk discovered the antistreptococcal activity of sulphamidochrysoidine (**26**).
1933	The structure of vitamin C was elucidated and synthesis achieved.
1933	Karer established the structure of vitamin A (**28**).
1934	Ruzicka synthesised progesterone (**27**).
1930–40	19 different hormones were isolated from the adrenal cortex.
1934	von Euler discovered prostaglandins.
1935	Darn reported that vitamin K (**29**) was essential for normal coagulation of blood.
1937	Putman and Merritt introduced the use of hydantoins (**30**) as anticonvulsants.

NaO$_2$CCH$_2$O

(20)

CH$_2$CH$_2$NH$_2$

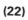

(22)

(21)

continued

Table 1.1. *Continued*

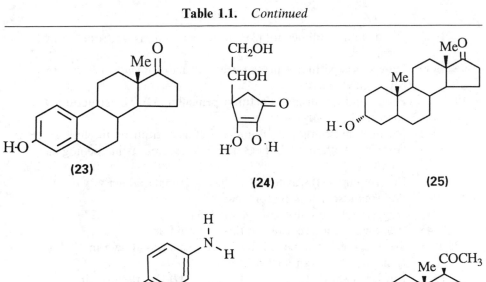

(23)

(24)

(25)

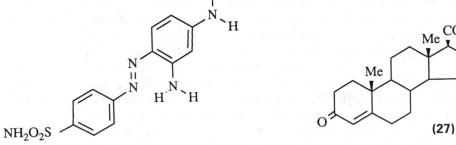

(26)

(27)

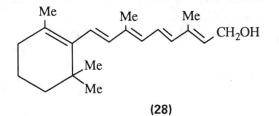

(28)

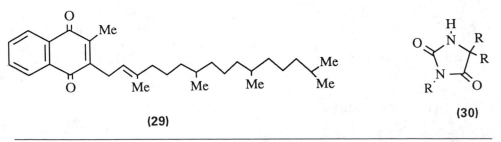

(29)

(30)

continued

Table 1.1.   *Continued*

1938	Dodds found stilboestrol (**31**) to be as potent as oestrone on i.v. dosing.
1939	Dubos showed that a protein-free extract of *Bacillus brevis* had bactericidal activity.
1939–41	Florey and Chain manufactured penicillin (**32**). The structure was confirmed in 1945.
1942	Nitrogen mustards were found to act as anticancer alkylating agents.
1943	Hoffman synthesised LSD (**33**) and discovered its hallucinogenic activity.
1943	Chloroquine (**34**) was found to have antimalarial activity.
1944	Waksman isolated streptomycin.
1945	Dugger isolated chlortetracycline (**35**).
1945	Woodward and Doering synthesised quinine.
1946–48	Synthesis of cortisone (**36**) by Sarett. This was shown in 1948 by Hensch to be an antiarthritic.
1946	von Euler showed that noradrenaline (**37**) was the principal chemotransmitter in the sympathomimetic nervous system.
1947	Antihistamines were shown to be anti-seasickness agents.
1947	Isoproterenol (**38**) was introduced as a bronchodilator by Lands.
1948	The existence of α and β adrenergic receptors was postulated.
1949	Lithium ions were shown to control manic-depression.
1952	Hitchings showed that 6-mercaptopurine (**39**) has antileukaemic activity.
1952	Reserpine (**1**) shown to be antihypertensive and tranquillising.
1952	Carpentier showed the antipsyhotic activity of chlorpromazine (**40**).

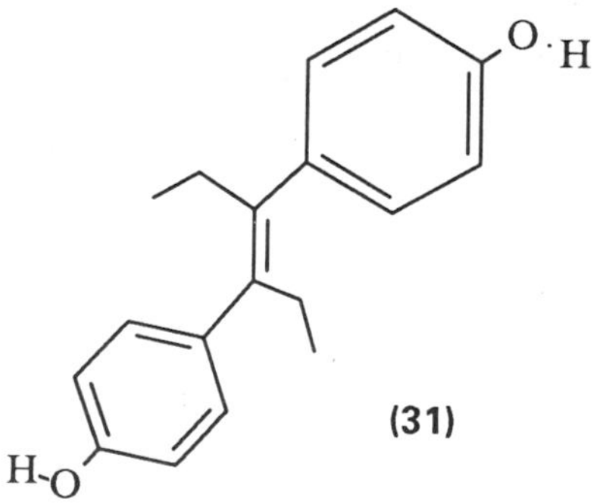

(**31**)

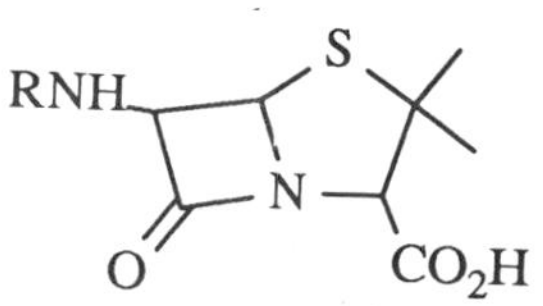

(**32**)

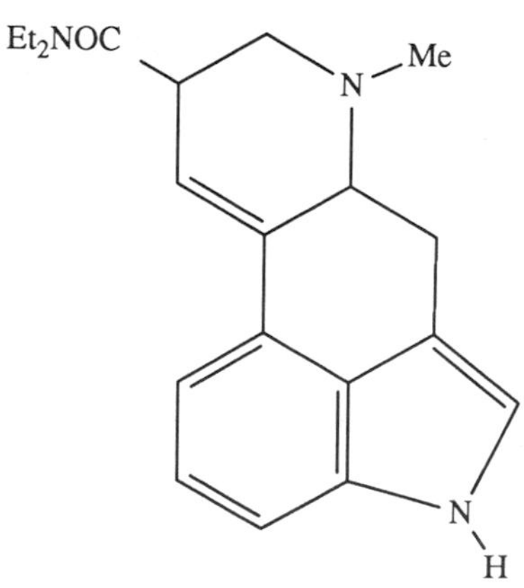

(**33**)

continued

Table 1.1.   *Continued*

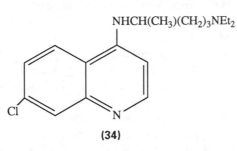

(34)

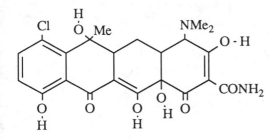

(35)

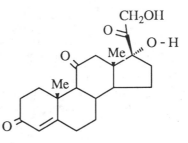

(36)

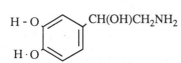

(37)

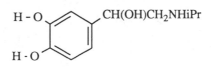

(38)

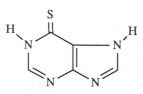

(39)

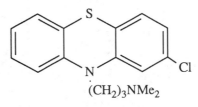

(40)

continued

Table 1.1.   *Continued*

1952	Isoniazid (**41**) was introduced as an antitubercular agent.
1953	Potassium phenoxymethyl penicillin (**42**) marketed as first orally active penicillin.
1953	The structure of DNA announced.
1955	α-Methyldopa (**43**) found to be antihypertensive.
1956	Cephalosporin structure identified; cephaloridine (**44**) the first orally active derivative was marketed in 1964.
1957	The growth-retarding effects of interferon on viruses discovered.
1957	Imipramine (**45**) found to be antidepressant.
1957	Chlorothiazide (**46**) introduced as a diuretic in congestive heart failure.
1958	The antipsychotic haloperidol (**47**) discovered.
1959	Beecham laboratories used aminopenicillanic acid (**48**) as a source of semi-synthetic penicillins.
1959	Enovid (**49**) was approved for use as the first oral contraceptive.
1959	*Journal of Medicinal Chemistry* founded by Beckett and Burger.
1960	Chlorodiazepoxide (**50**) marketed as an anxiolytic.
1961	Tranylcyclopromine (**51**) introduced as antidepressant.

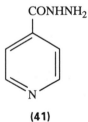

(41)

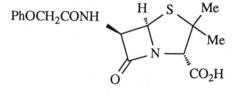

(42)

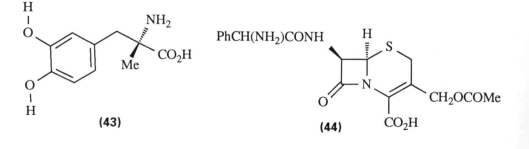

(43)   (44)

continued

Table 1.1.   *Continued*

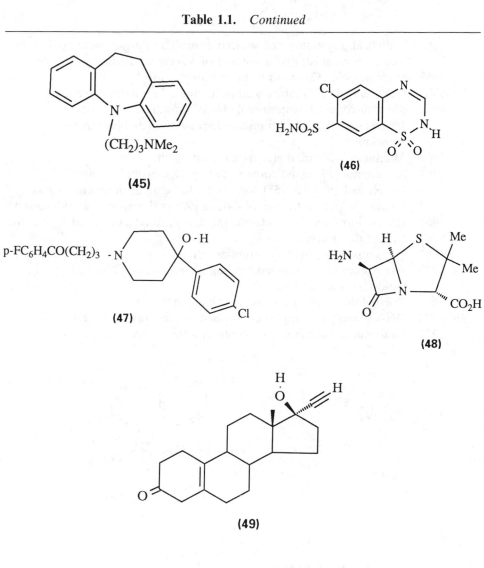

(45)

(46)

p-FC₆H₄CO(CH₂)₃

(47)

(48)

(49)

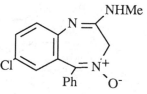

(50)

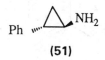

(51)

continued

Table 1.1.   *Continued*

1962   Statistical, regression and molecular orbital analyses were applied to
       medicinal chemistry by a number of workers, principally Hansch.
1963   Valproic acid (**52**) found to be anticonvulsant.
1963   Indomethacin (**53**) introduced as an antiinflammatory agent.
1964   Black introduced propranolol (**54**) as a *β*-adrenergic blocker.
1965   Janssen showed that tetramisole (**55**) was a broad spectrum
       anthelmintic.
1966   Allopurinol (**56**) marketed as antigout agent.
1967   Salbutamol (**57**) found to be a lung specific bronchodilator.
1967   1-Aminoadamantane (**58**) was shown to be an antiinfluenza agent.
1967   Cotzias pioneered the use of L-dopa (**59**) as therapy for Parkinsonism.
1967   Fisons introduced Intal (**60**) as the first prophylactic antiallergy agent.
1967   Gilbert discovered DNA ligase.
1968   Carbenoxolone (**61**) has antiinflammatory and antiulcer activity.
1971–73   The science of radioligand binding to receptors established by
       Goldstein, Pert and Snyder.
1971   Triethylphosphino gold used as an antiarthritic.
1972–73   DNA cloning techniques established by Boyer, Cohen and Berg.
1975   Endogenous morphine-like peptides were discovered.

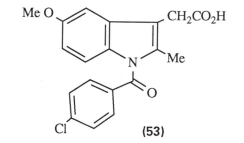

(52)

(53)

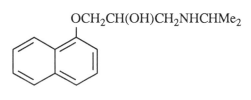

(54)

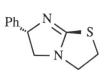

(55)

continued

Table 1.1. *Continued*

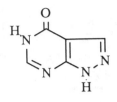

(56)

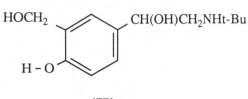

(57)

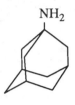

(58)

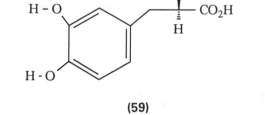

(59)

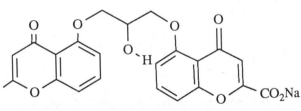

(60)

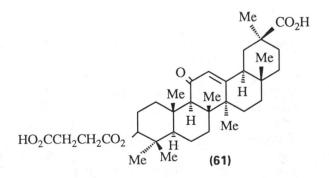

(61)

continued

Table 1.1.   *Continued*

1977   Cimetidine (**62**) was introduced by Smith, Kline and French as the
        first histamine H-2 antagonist.

1977   Acyclovir (**63**) introduced by Elion and Hitchings for the treatment of
        herpes infections.

1980   RU 486 (**64**) the first progesterone antagonist introduced by Roussel
        as an abortant.

1988   The first biotechnology products appear. These were tissue
        plasminogen factor, α-interferon, human insulin, human growth factor
        and erythropoetin.

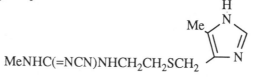

MeNHC(=NCN)NHCH₂CH₂SCH₂

(62)

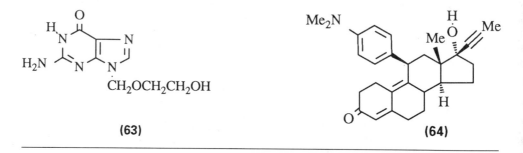

(63)   **(64)**

Perhaps the most beneficial innovation of the 19th century was the introduction of agents capable of rendering patients insensitive to pain during operations. Nitrous oxide was first used by Davy, ether was introduced by Long and chloroform by Simpson, so transforming what had previously been akin to crude butchery into surgery. Virtually overnight the attributes of a surgeon changed from the essential, but primitive ones of speed, brutal indifference to the suffering of the patient and insensitivity, to absurdly small survival rates, to the modern qualities of careful dissection and care for the patient. The new procedures were reinforced by the introduction of phenol as an antiseptic by Lister, which soon meant that many more people survived surgery. Today the risks and rigours of surgery are much lessened, an advance which has resulted in no small way from the efforts of the medicinal chemist in producing the array of pain-killers, anaesthetics, muscle relaxants and antiinfectives which are used as adjuncts to modern day techniques.

Perhaps not surprisingly the earliest natural substance to be investigated was opium. Serturner probably holds the record for the first isolation of a pharmacologically active substance from a natural product when he isolated, albeit in impure form, morphine (**4**, R = H) in 1805. Amongst the work stimulated by this breakthrough was the discovery of a quaternary salt which had curare-like activity establishing the precedent that it was possible to modify the biological activity of natural products by chemical means.

The table clearly illustrates that the great explosion in understanding and knowledge in chemistry and biology has contributed to a massive growth in the range of drugs available to treat diseases affecting both man and other animals. In fact the process has been one of symbiosis with the fundamental techniques of organic chemistry, structure determination and synthesis being driven by a desire to isolate pure materials of therapeutic significance from plant sources. The discovery that biological activity was not confined to natural products and that synthetic compounds could have activities different from, and often superior to, natural remedies then exposed the field to the full creative abilities of its chemists. As the fundamental anatomy, physiology and biochemistry of the body processes became available the targets for the medicinal chemist began to expand dramatically, a process aided by increasing understanding of drug action.

Over the last 200 years there have been many outstanding contributions to medicinal chemistry. At the end of the nineteenth century the most widespread of modern drugs, aspirin, was introduced, and Paul Ehrlich established the fundamental concept of chemotherapy, the selective destruction of invading organisms while leaving the host body unharmed. The 1930s and 1940s saw the introduction of antibiotics by Fleming, Florey, Chain, Dubos, Domagk and Waksman which enabled society to overcome the tremendous scourge of bacterial infections. In the 1950s and 1960s Hansch pointed the way to rational drug design, and the first medicines capable of providing a better quality of life to those afflicted with a range of mental disorders (and their families) appeared. Black demonstrated how to exploit differences in receptor subtypes to give highly selective drugs acting on the heart and, subsequently, the first chemical alternative to surgical treatment for ulcers. Over the same period Hitchings and Elion showed how to modulate disordered biochemical metabolic pathways to provide new antileukaemic, antitumour and antiviral agents. Finally, in the 1980s, molecular biology has enabled even greater insights into the biochemistry of the body, the provision of new specific drugs, and, with the expansion of computer technology, the path to truly rational *ab initio* drug design has opened for the medicinal chemist.

1.2.2 Selectivity

A continual aim of the work described above has been the search for chemicals capable of curing or alleviating a disease whilst causing minimum harm or disturbance to the entire organism: in other words the search for selectivity of action. This has been most cogently argued by Adrian Albert in a series of books dating from 1951 entitled *Selective Toxicity*. In these Albert has argued that, with the exception of replacement therapy, all drugs dosed to treat illness are in fact toxins, but the more the toxic action is restricted to the malfunctioning system itself the more selective is the action. He differentiates the subject into two distinct areas, notably chemotherapy and pharmacodynamics with three underlying mechanisms of selectivity: differences in distribution, comparative biochemistry and cytology.

The term "chemotherapy" was first introduced by Paul Ehrlich as "the use of drugs to injure an invading organism without injury to the host". In Ehrlich's time the definition referred essentially to invasion by bacteria, fungi, yeasts and viruses, but today the term has been expanded to include tumours whose rapid growth distinguishes them from normal cells. Thus an alternative definition has been given by Hitchings as "to the biochemical chemotherapist, it is not only a matter of faith, but an obvious fact that every cell type must have a characteristic biochemical pattern, and therefore be susceptible to attack at some locus or loci critical for its survival and replication".

While Ehrlich is rightly regarded as the founder of chemotherapy, it was in fact a Russian, Romanovsky, who in 1891 made the first recorded observation of a chemotherapeutic effect. He discovered by microscopic examination of the blood from patients suffering from malaria and undergoing treatment with quinine that the drug was working by damaging the malaria parasite itself more than the blood cells of the patient. Thus some feature of the parasite is more susceptible to the chemical action of quinine than are the blood cells of the patient.

Ehrlich, however, was the founder of the systematic approach to the discovery of chemotherapeutic agents and the inventor of the "chemotherapeutic index", the ratio of the minimal curative dose of a substance to its maximal tolerated dose, which enabled quantitative comparisons to be made between different compounds. His systematic structure–activity investigations of organoarsenicals led eventually to the introduction of arsphenamine (**17**), the first agent to be effective against syphilis. Subsequently, the selectivity of (**17**) was shown to be due to a combination of selective absorption by the parasite allied to a greater susceptibility of a number of its crucial enzymes, particularly phosphopyruvate kinase, over the mammalian counterparts.

A clearer example of selective distribution producing selectivity is provided by the tetracyclines which are preferentially absorbed by bacteria over mammalian cells. Once in the cells, they disrupt protein synthesis by blocking the binding of aminoacyl t-RNA to the A-site of bacterial ribosomes, thus a dose providing blood levels relatively nontoxic to the host is selectively toxic to the bacteria.

Differential biochemistry is a more widespread mechanism for selectivity. For example, the sulphonamides such as prontosil (**26**) act by being hydrolysed *in vivo*

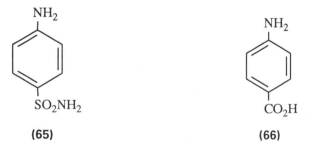

(65)   (66)

to sulphanilamide (**65**) which acts as a biostere, or structural mimetic of *p*-aminobenzoic acid (**66**), an essential factor for bacterial growth. However, (**65**) cannot be utilised by the bacterium, and cell growth ceases. A different biochemical selectivity

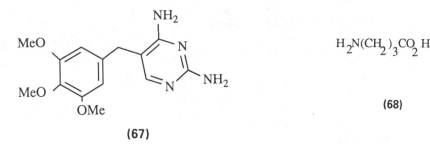

(67)   **(68)**

is illustrated by that of the antibiotic trimethoprim (**67**) which is approximately 60 000 times as active as an inhibitor of dihydrofolate reductase from *E. coli* as it is for the enzyme from human liver. The antiviral Acyclovir (**63**) represents a more complicated example of selective biochemistry. This is monophosphorylated by thymidine kinase, an enzyme which is induced by herpes viruses as it infects cells, rather than by the cellular kinases. Further phosphorylation of the monophosphate leads to the active 5′-triphosphate which is a potent inhibitor of herpes simplex virus-1 DNA polymerase owing to its competition with the natural substrate, deoxyguanosine triphosphate, and inhibition of the viral DNA polymerase is much stronger than that of the mammalian DNA polymerases α and β.

The final mechanism for selectivity, namely differences in cytology, is well illustrated by the antibiotic action of the penicillins. Bacteria differ from mammalian cells in that they alone have cell walls composed mainly of giant crosslinked peptidoglycans, and no such feature is found in mammalian cells. Penicillins and cephalosporins inhibit the biosynthesis of this polymer thus weakening the bacterium and making it susceptible to bursting under osmotic pressure.

Pharmacodynamics refers to the situation where the malfunctioning cells or tissues are part of the organism. Finding selectivity in these circumstances is more difficult because differences between the two species are likely to be less and the required response often needs to be a temporary one. Selectivity through differences in distribution is most easily seen with the brain which is protected by a poorly permeable "blood–brain barrier". This is a lipid-like barrier formed by the fusion of capillaries and epithelium to form a continuous cellular layer separating blood from interstitial space in the brain, and hydrophilic molecules cannot pass through this barrier unless specific transport mechanisms for them exist. However, Bodor has shown how this barrier can be penetrated but then used to retain a drug within the brain. Thus, for example, the inhibitory amino acid, γ-aminobutyric acid (**68**) which does not cross the blood–brain barrier to any appreciable extent can be converted to the much more liphophilic amido-ester (**69**). This substance readily crosses the blood–brain barrier where oxidative enzymes convert it to the hydrophilic pyridinium cation (**70**), and, whilst any of (**70**) generated outside the brain will be readily eliminated because of its water solubility, the pyridinium-generated cation within the brain cannot now traverse the barrier and is trapped. Subsequent hydrolysis releases (**68**) to act on inhibitory neurons, its action thus being largely restricted to the brain.

Other examples of pharmacodynamic selectivity can arise because not all neuro-transmitter receptors have exactly the same structure for a given physiological

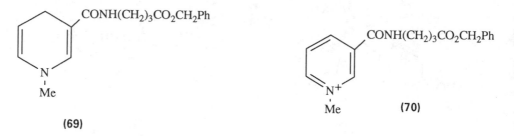

(69)

(70)

transmitter. Receptors will be discussed in more detail in a following chapter, so it is sufficient to state that the transmitter noradrenaline (37) acts through receptors which have been differentiated pharmacologically as α and β, with a further differentiation into subsets. Noradrenaline is the primary neurotransmitter in the sympathetic nervous system which has profound effects on, inter alia, the heart and lungs. The β-antagonist propranolol (54) has approximately 1000 times greater affinity for β compared to α-receptors and is widely used in treatment of cardiovascular disease. Likewise, the β_2- stimulant salbutamol (57) is an essentially selective stimulant of β receptors in the lung with very little effect on the heart.

A superb example of pharmacodynamic selectivity is the case of histamine. Histamine manifests a number of physiological responses and its antagonists have been used for many years for the treatment of hay fever and sea-sickness. Black, however, demonstrated that histamine also controls gastric acid secretion and its excessive excretion results in the formation of gastric ulcers, via its action on a subtype of receptor on which the classical antihistamines had no effect. This work led to the discovery of cimetidine (62) which acts as an antagonist of this histamine subtype receptor and is a potent antiulcer agent. Its widespread use has largely eradicated the need for surgical intervention which was previously the only effective treatment for such ulcers.

1.2.3   Enantioselectivity
The world is three-dimensional and asymmetric, and this includes the receptors and enzymes in all biological systems. Therefore the reaction of a chiral agent with a receptor is diastereomeric with each enantiomer possessing different binding abilities. Earlier drugs were largely obtained from natural sources and were usually isolated as a single enantiomer, and complications due to the presence of the alternative enantiomer were thus avoided. Synthetic chiral drugs have, until recently, usually been obtained as racemates with the implicit assumption that the presence of the "wrong" enantiomer is immaterial. In practice, this is unlikely to be true, with, the wrong isomer acting, at best, as inactive ballast although compromising 50% of the total product and, at worst, acting antagonistically on the receptor complicating the pharmacological profile. Moreover, the isomer can interfere with the pharmacokinetic, metabolism and distribution profile of the active principle, with these effects varying from species to species and further complicating the extrapolation of biological data from animal to man. Ariens in particular has highlighted this particular problem, and it is now accepted that chiral drugs should in most cases be developed as the

single appropriate enantiomer.

1.3   THE SCENE TODAY

1.3.1   Classification of drugs
The creativity and ingenuity of the medicinal chemist, biologist, pharmacist and physician have today produced a situation in which more than 5000 compounds have been characterised and investigated as potential therapeutic agents. Of this number, however, only some 1500 single and combination products are available in the British pharmacy.

Nevertheless, this is a large number of molecules, and efforts have been made to classify them in a systematic manner. In the early days of medicinal chemistry drugs were often classified and discussed by their chemical structures irrespective of their therapeutic effects. The inconvenience of this was underlined by the discovery of many agents with similar chemical structures but different biological activities. A more logical and useful method is to classify structure according to therapeutic effect with subsections for specific disease states dependent on underlying biochemical mechanisms when these are known. Table 1.2 presents such a classification which is used for *Annual Reports in Medicinal Chemistry*.

1.3.1.1   CNS or psychopharmaceutical agents
The central nervous system of man comprises the brain and spinal cord which control the thought processes, emotions, senses and motor functions. Antipsychotic agents alleviate the worst effects of severe mental disorders such as schizophrenia, whilst anticonvulsants control the involuntary convulsions of epilepsy. Analgesics are prescribed to relieve pain, antidepressants for severe depression, anxiolytics for anxiety and antiparkinson agents for the tremors and gait disorders of the major motor disorder Parkinson's disease. Sedative-hypnotics are used to promote sleep, stimulants to temporarily fight fatigue, and drugs for cognitive disorders are prescribed for the sufferers of Alzheimer's disease, a major affliction of the elderly which results in a severe and distressing loss of memory.

1.3.1.2   Pharmacodynamic agents
The term "pharmacodynamics" was introduced for the selective correction of a malfunctioning unit of the body. Such agents act on the dynamic processes of the body involving the heart, respiratory system and gastrointestinal tract. Antihypertensives, calcium modulators, antiischaemic, antithrombotic, antiarrhythmic, antianginal and vasolidating agents all act on some part of the heart and vasculatory system to reduce blood pressure, heart rate or force, or to improve blood flow. Pulmonary and antiallergic drugs affect the lungs and respiratory system, while antiglaucoma drugs affect the eye condition, glaucoma. Antiulcer and gastrointestinal drugs heal and prevent the recurrence of stomach ulcers and increase gastric motility.

Table 1.2. Classification of drugs based on their major biological effects

---

1. *CNS or psychopharmaceutical agents.*
   Antipsychotic agents
   Anticonvulsants
   Analgesics
   Antiparkinsonian agents
   Antidepressants
   Anxiolytics
   Sedative-hypnotics
   Drugs for cognitive disorders
   Stimulants

2. *Pharmacodynamic agents*
   Antihypertensive agents
   Calcium modulators
   Antiischaemic (antistroke) drugs
   Antiulcer-gastrointestinal agents
   Antithrombotics
   Pulmonary and antiallergic agents
   Antiarrythmics
   Antiglaucoma
   Vasodilators
   Antianginals

3. *Chemotherapeutic agents*
   Antimicrobials
   Antifungals
   Anticancers
   Antiparasitics
   Antivirals

4. *Metabolic diseases*
   Contraceptives
   Antiandrogens
   Antiinflammatories
   Dermatologicals
   Antiatherosclerotics
   Antirheumatics and autoimmune disease drugs
   Antiobesity agents

1.3.1.3 Chemotherapeutic agents

As described above, chemotherapeutic agents are selectively toxic to parasitic organisms invading the body. Antimicrobials act on bacterial infections, antifungals on fungal infections, antivirals on viruses, and antiparasitics on parasitic infections such as worms and protozoa (e.g. the malarial parasite). The classification of chemotherapy has been broadened to include attack on the disordered bodily tissues seen in invasive tumour growth (anticancer drugs).

1.3.1.4   Metabolic diseases and endocrine function

While this group is a miscellany of agents not conveniently classified in the previous groups it does include a great number of medically important drugs. Contraceptives interfere biologically with the conception process (traditionally in the female), antiandrogens are of importance in prostate cancer, whilst antiinflammatories, especially the nonsteroidal antiinflammatories (NSAID), are very widely used as palliatives for mild pain, joint disorders, and rheumatism. True disease-remitting antirheumatic agents modulating the underlying immune disfunction of the disease are still not available. Dermatologicals are usually applied topically to alleviate skin disorders, and antiobesity drugs are used to treat eating disorders.

In most, if not all of the above categories of drugs, different underlying biochemical mechanisms are responsible. A number of these processes will be discussed in future sections.

1.3.2   Industry/commercial aspects

Over the twenty years from 1966 to 1985 a total of 663 "new chemical entities" were evaluated in man as potential therapeutic agents and, of this number, 98% originated from the pharmaceutical industry with the remainder arising in universities and independent research institutes. Inevitably the vast majority of scientists active in drug discovery work in the industry and it is of interest to consider some of the factors which have shaped the evolution of the industry and which continue to affect it. The pharmaceutical industry is essentially restricted to Western Europe, the United States of America, and, more recently, Japan.

1.3.2.1   The evolution of the pharmaceutical industry

As stated previously the origins of the drug treatment of illnesses are lost in the mists of unrecorded time. Nevertheless, it can be assumed that the preparation of the remedy and the treatment of the patient were conducted by the same individual and it is likely that the preparation of the treatment was on demand from fresh herbs and other local sources. The establishment of large armies would have created the need for stocks of remedies, and such "pharmacies" are known from the Egyptian, Greek and Islamic civilisations. The practice of the storage of such preparations in ceramic vessels was adopted by Northern Europeans from Islamic North Africa and was the forerunner of modern therapy.

With increasing urbanisation and the development of independent trading states, the apothecary's shop which specialised in the preparation and sale of remedies came into being. At this point the combined practices of treatment of the patient and the preparation of the remedy began to diverge, much to their mutual benefit. Traders could concentrate on obtaining supplies of herbs and natural products from steadily increasing areas of the world and on producing better quality products with defined properties, whilst treatment was left to those with such interests. Nevertheless, the two areas have constantly overlapped and the practice of consulting pharmacists on medical matters continues to this day although the actual formulation of drugs by pharmacists has essentially ceased.

By the beginning of the 19th century a pattern of retail pharmacies supplied by traders and wholesalers had been established in Western Europe and the United States. Some firms which were later to become extremely well-known, such as Allen and Hanbury's, were established at this time. There now began also a process of change from simple sorting, cleaning and packaging of materials to one of isolating active principles such as quinine and morphine. The American industry was founded around 1820 in Philadelphia as a number of firms established means of preparing such basic materials as quinine, morphine and calomel, whilst the resultant profits enabled the industry to grow. A further boost was provided in the 1860s by the Civil War when the firms of Eli Lilly and E. R. Squibb were sufficiently mechanised to be able to satisfy large Government contracts for the supply of opium, quinine and ergot. However, in Britain and America "research" covered the separation of new materials and reformulation and not the synthesis of drugs. The birth of the synthetic drug industry took place in Germany in the years after 1880.

At this time a crisis in the dyestuff industry led to the search for new colours and also new products. This programme resulted first in the successful antipyretic drug pyramidon, tuberculin and salvarsan from Hoechst, aspirin from Bayer, and veronal from Schering. Thus by the onset of the First World War there was a well-established research based pharmaceutical industry in Germany. Similar changes were occurring in America but not in Britain, despite the founding of the Wellcome Physiological Research Laboratories in 1894, or in France where industry based research began only well into the 20th century.

Around the end of the 19th century the distinction arose between "professional" manufacturers making products to be dispensed by the medical profession and the "patent medicine" makers selling direct to the public. However, the profits to be made from the latter activity led the ethical manufacturers to seek ways of combining the two activities. The system of doctors prescribing medicines was established although pharmacists continued to diagnose and prescribe, much to the disquiet of the medical profession. The relationship between the industry, physicians and government which was also becoming an issue at the time will be dealt with later.

Before the First World War the Swiss chemical industry was extremely small, but during the war they were able to supply dyestuffs to the Allied powers and thus prospered. As the market slumped at the end of the war they invested the profits into pharmaceutical research to such good effect that three companies, Ciba-Geigy, Sandoz, and Hoffman-La-Roche soon became major world players.

The years between the wars saw great increases in scientific sophistication and the understanding of diseases, with the introduction of many new drugs. As a consequence research in the industry was recognised as an essential activity. British firms such as May and Baker, Glaxo, Boots, and BDH began to employ significant numbers of research workers and to establish solid reputations. Despite this, British companies were unable in wartime conditions to exploit the discovery of the potent activity of penicillins by Chain and Florey at Oxford in the early 1940s, and its mass production required the skills of American workers in Peoria, Illinois.

The great boom in the pharmaceutical industry after the Second World War was fuelled by the discovery of a range of life-saving antibiotics, notably the penicillins, streptomycin, aureomycin, and the tetracyclines. These were rapidly followed by psychopharmaceuticals, antivirals, and new agents for many aspects of heart disease. Allied to a number of takeovers and mergers these developments led to a multinational industry of immense resources and influence.

1.3.2.2   The industry today

Following the Second World War the industry entered a period of unprecedented growth due partly to the increasing standard of living in the developed countries and partly to the discovery of a succession of new agents which created a climate of expectation for "wonder drugs". The effectiveness of penicillin during the war showed the great therapeutic necessity for such agents, and the subsequent discovery of streptomycin by Waksman in the late 1940s showed that this was not to be a unique agent. This discovery also showed how other agents might be found and thus initiated an explosion of research activity. The commercial and therapeutic success of agents such as aureomycin and the tetracyclines finally established research from being a peripheral activity to a central one for a company's future success. In the 1960s Roche introduced the anxiolytic benzodiazepines, ICI the β-blockers for heart disease, and Smith Kline and French the antiulcer agent, Tagamet. In all these cases vast new markets were created with the result that in 1988 the worldwide sales of ethical pharmaceuticals was estimated to be £65 thousand million divided as shown in Table 1.3. Along with the increased markets, research costs have also risen and today most major pharmaceutical companies spend between 10 and 15% of their gross turnover on research, a figure equalled only by major defence contractors. Furthermore, in contrast with such companies the costs of pharmaceutical research are not borne by governments on a cost plus profit basis, but by the firms themselves out of current and future sales.

Table 1.3.   Value of world pharmaceutical sales in 1988 (£m)

Country	Estimated value	% world market
USA	17 900	28
Japan	15 100	23
West Germany	5 300	8
France	4 400	7
Italy	4 300	7
UK	2 300	3
Canada	1 500	2
Spain	1 500	2
Rest of world (excluding Eastern bloc)	12 700	20

This period has also been characterised by two major developments, namely increasing internationalisation as companies have sought to establish themselves in all major geographical markets for access to potential sales and the creative and technical talents of their populations, and an increasing wave of large company mergers and takeovers.

Takeovers were initially used as a way in which a company could move into a country and acquire an existing market share, for example Merck Sharp and Dohme's acquisition of Morson in England, while mergers and consolidations were the means by which Glaxo originally achieved a platform for future growth. The late 1980s however, have seen a burst of such activity fuelled by companies anxious to share research interests and economies of scale. Thus the following "marriages" have taken place: Kodak-Sterling, Ayerst-Wyeth, American Home Products-Robins, Smith Kline-Beecham, Novo-Nordisk, Merrell Dow-Marion, Bristol Meyers-Squibb, Fujisawa-Lyphomed, Merieux-Connaught Biosciences, Roche-Genetech, Rhône-Poulenc-Rorer, and, most recently, Du Pont and Merck. All this activity left the world's top companies ranked as in Table 1.4 in 1989. By the time this book is published, Glaxo will have probably risen to the first position in the pharmaceutical league table, and the combined Rhône-Poulenc-Rorer company will be ranked at least in the top ten.

Table 1.4.   Top ten pharmaceutical companies 1988–89

Company	Sales ($m)
Merck & Co (US)	4983.7
Glaxo (UK)	4577.8
Hoechst (WGer)	3958.0
Bayer (WGer)	3712.6
Ciba-Geigy (Switz)	3531.7
Takeda (J)	3471.4
American Home Products (USA)	3218.0
Sandoz (Switz)	3417.0
Eli Lilly (USA)	2279.8
Abbot (USA)	2599.0

1.3.2.2.1 *Products*
Table 1.5 lists the twenty top selling branded pharmaceutical products of 1989, providing an illuminating insight into the ailments and treatments of Western man. Thus while antiulcer preparations are first and fourth best sellers, no fewer than eight of the twenty products treat some aspect of cardiovascular disease. Additionally, there are three antiinflammatory agents, three antibiotics, two bronchorespiratory agents, one oral contraceptive, and an antiviral drug.

Within the United Kingdom, sales by the UK pharmaceutical industry reached £5607m in 1988 (£4411m to the National Health Service) and £1735m to export divided by therapeutic class as shown in Table 1.6.

1.3.2.2.2 *Research*
Pharmaceutical research needs resources, scientists and investment. The money, as indicated above, is enormous; for example, Merck alone will spend $885m in 1990

Table 1.5. The top 20 best selling medicines worldwide in 1989

Brand name	Company	Therapeutic class	Sales ($m)
Zantac	Glaxo	H_2 antagonist	2373
Capoten	Bristol-Meyers Squibb	ACE inhibitor	1267
Vasotec	Merck	ACE inhibitor	1195
Tagamet	SmithKlineBeecham	H_2-antagonist	1030
Tenormin	ICI	β-blocker	1020
Voltaren	Ciba-Geigy	NSAID	975
Adalat	Bayer/Takeda	Ca antagonist	850
Ceclor	Eli Lilly	cephalosporin	696
Cardizam	Marion	Ca antagonist	658
Naprosyn	Syntex	NSAID	645
Omnipaque	Sterling/Dailchi/ Schering/Hafslund Nycomed	contrast medium	620
Rocephin	Hoffmann-La Roche	cephalosporin	597
Feldene	Pfizer	NSAID	585
Mevacor	Merck	hypolipaemic	556
Ventolin	Glaxo	bronchodilator	555
Zovirax	Wellcome	antiviral	537
Augmentin	SmithKlineBeecham	antibiotic	497
Zatiden	Sandoz/Sankyo	antiasthmatic	484
OrthoNovum	Johnson&Johnson	oral contraceptive	450
Procardia	Pfizer	Ca antagonist	440

Table 1.6. Pharmaceutical sales by main therapeutic classes in UK (£m) 1988

Category	Value
Central nervous system	303
Cardiovascular system	409
Blood and blood-forming organs	22
Respiratory system	367
Alimentary tract system	459
Genitourinary (inc. sex hormones)	91
Hormones (exc. sex hormones)	38
Muscular and skeletal system	304
Dermatologicals	112
Sensory organs	67
General antiinfectives	395
Antiparasitics	12
Veterinary preparations	161
Other medical preparations	375

and the remainder of the American industry a further $8000m. It is usually estimated that the balance of these costs is approximately one third to research and two thirds to development (see next section). However, money is not sufficient without trained scientists, and this, in turn, requires a university system with sufficient throughput of high-quality graduates and postgraduates in sciences such as chemistry, biology, biochemistry and pharmacy. However, this is not enough, and there is also a need for a climate which encourages research. This is perhaps best illustrated by Table 1.7 which surveys the country of origin of new chemical entities which were placed in development (though not necessarily onto the market) between 1960 and 1983. A more up to date listing would probably include representation from Japan, whilst one for 1995 most certainly will. Over this period the United Kingdom had a greater than expected ranking on the basis of research spend.

While different countries have had different degrees of success in pharmaceutical research, so have different firms. This is illustrated in Table 1.8 which lists the number of drugs in development amongst the top twenty pharmaceutical companies in 1989. As will be examined in greater detail in the next section, it is to be expected that a

Table 1.7. The origin of new chemical entities (1960–1983)

Country	Number originated
USA	223
UK	87
West Germany	75
Switzerland	55
France	36
Belgium	29
Italy	22
Denmark	19
Sweden	19
Netherlands	15

very large number of these agents will not reach the public, but nevertheless these figures indicate that there will be a significant influx of new drugs towards the end of the century.

1.3.2.2.3   *The development of drugs*

The development of any drug is a lengthy, costly exercise which requires the combined activities of a large number of chemists, biochemists, biologists, pharmacists and clinicians. To consider the process in more detail, it is conveniently divided into a number of phases. The first phase is considered to cover the period from initiation of the project to the identification of a molecule possessing the appropriate combination of chemical and biological properties predicted to give it a therapeutic advantage. The decision to undertake research in a particular disease results from the consideration of a number of scientific, medical and economic factors such as the

Table 1.8.   The top 10 research and development
companies in 1989

Company	Number of R&D drugs
Bristol-Meyers	103
Merck	98
Ciba-Geigy	96
Rhône-Poulenc	94
Johnson & Johnson	92
Lilly	91
Elan	90
Roche	90
Hoechst	88
SmithKlineBeecham	81

number of people afflicted by the diseases, the effectiveness of current therapies, and current knowledge of the relevant disease processes. Since the costs of a drug development are enormous (£150m in 1992), the future sales of the potential medicine must clearly repay all research costs and provide appropriate sales profits.

It is in the discovery phase that medicinal chemists play their major role. A lead structure, that is a molecule with some suggestion of the researched pharmacological activity, must be identified and then extensively modified to obtain the optimum profile of biololgical activity relative to unwanted side effects. There are a number of possible sources for this lead structure or prototype molecule. Traditional or folk medicine provides a source from which many an active compound has been isolated and subsequently modified to provide an effective medicine. Intal (**60**) was discovered in this way albeit the final chemical structure was very far removed from the prototype molecule. Another approach depends upon the observation of a particular side effect in a drug in clinical use. In fact salicylic acid and its derived drug, aspirin, was observed to be antipyretic after it had been first introduced as an antiseptic suitable for internal use and observation of patients in the clinic showed that associated fevers were reduced. A more systematic starting point is the understanding of a dysfunction of the body biochemistry underlying a particular disease state and the use of this knowledge to design agents capable of modulating this. Notable examples of this approach include the design of the histamine H_2 antagonists used for the treatment of gastric ulcers, the antivirals described previously, and the cholesterol-reducing hydroxymethylglutaryl-CoA reductase inhibitors. This enzyme is critically involved in the biosynthesis of cholesterol, a vital constituent of mammalian membranes and steroid biosynthesis which, when present in unnaturally high concentrations in blood, is a major factor contributing to heart disease, a major cause of death in Western society. Inhibition of this enzyme blocks the biosynthetic processing of cholesterol and thus reduces circulating cholesterol blood levels. Serendipity, the art of making discoveries by chance, is still a valuable contributor to new leads discovery through high throughput screening. The word is from the writings of Horace Walpole who in a letter of 28 January 1754 stated, "The three princes of Serendip, Balakrama, Vijayo and Rajahsighu as they travelled were always making discoveries by accident and sagacity of things they were not in quest of…". (An alternative paraphrase is that there are many good medicinal chemists, but lucky ones are valued.) The design of modern drugs from the modification of lead structures will be disclosed in detail in Chapter 5.

At the end of the discovery phase a candidate drug will have been synthesised, but its activity will have been determined in animal models of the disease state and only very limited toxicity testing will have been completed. The next phase in development is to assemble the necessary toxicity data required by legislation to allow the compound to be investigated carefully and progressively in man and eventually the patient. During the development process the new drug must be studied in two animal species over long periods to provide evidence of any long-term toxicity risk and cancer-inducing potential. Today the highly expensive carcinogenicity tests are not undertaken without first doing preliminary mutagenicity testing in bacteria (the Ames test), which is a relatively quick and cheap test requiring milligrams of material which will save unnecessary expenditure of resources, and, most importantly, test animals (primarily rodents).

Until recently all such toxicity testing had to be completed before a new compound could be administered to humans. The legislative situation in the United Kingdom has recently changed, and a Clinical Trials Exemption Certificate will now be granted allowing a single dose to man after satisfactory 14 days repeat dose testing in animals, and extending the testing to 28 days allows up to 10 days repeat dosing in healthy male volunteers. The purpose of this preliminary testing is threefold, namely to observe any unwanted effects, to establish that the compound is actually absorbed in man, and to obtain an indication of its pharmacokinetic profile. Patients suffering from the targeted disease are not investigated in this phase (Phase 1). Provided that the results of these initial studies are satisfactory, it will now be possible to continue with the development of the drug to demonstrate efficacy in patients (Phase 2). Table 1.9 summarises the typical toxicity testing needed so that this phase of development may proceed. During this phase, the process chemist will be working to convert the original laboratory synthesis into one which will allow sufficient quantities of material to be manufactured safely, economically, and with due care for the environment for the long-term trials and testing. Great care in modifying the synthetic processes is needed since the regulatory authorities will demand evidence for consistent manufacture of the pure raw material in all subsequent batches.

At this stage the pharmacist will have converted the raw material and preliminary formulation used in initial trials into a properly formulated form suitable for the designated method of administration. The clinical trials will be carried out in patients suffering from the targeted disease, will take place in a number of medical centres, and are done "double blind", namely with neither the medical staff nor the patient knowing whether the drug substance or a placebo is being dosed, a statistician ensuring that the results of the study are clinically significant. On most occasions the trial drug will eventually be tested against a known effective reference drug for the disease under investigation.

Table 1.9.   Permitted length of exposure in man following animal toxicity

Intended duration of dosing in man	Duration of toxicity tests (d)
Single doses or repeat doses on 1 day	14
Repeat doses up to 7 days	28
Repeat doses up to 30 days	90
Repeat doses beyond 30 days	180[a]

[a]In this case, carcinogenicity data will probably also be required.

Only at the end of this phase when the new drug has been shown to be truly effective in the disease state and free from unacceptable side effects can an application be made for a product licence to market the drug in the country concerned. The clinical trials conducted so far cannot be sufficiently extensive to detect a low-incidence side effect. Thus the compound will be subject to long-term monitoring, or post-marketing surveillance, over the early years of its availability to the doctor until it is felt that a complete safety profile has been produced. Regrettably, there will always be cases where a drug will be found to be unacceptably toxic in a very small number of patients and will have to be withdrawn some years later.

The modern development process is extremely expensive (costing up to £150m in 1992) and the attrition rate for new chemical entities is extremely high. American studies indicate that of twenty compounds entering subacute toxicity only ten go into full toxicity testing and less than one eventually reaches the clinician. The twenty were chosen from a much larger group of synthesised compounds originally evaluated (frequently 5000–10000). Table 1.10 summarises the development process.

Table 1.10.   The drug development process

Phase	Principal activity	Scientific input	Time scales (years)
00	Concept testing QSAR Project selection	Medicine/biology Chemistry/mol.biol. Biopharmacy	Indeterminate
0	Preclinical evaluation	Toxicology/biology Biopharmacy/pharmacy Process chemistry	1
I	Clinical tolerance	Pharmacy/biopharmacy toxicology	0.5
II	Clinical efficacy	Biology/biopharmacy	1
III	Long term clinical tolerance/efficacy	Biology/biopharmacy Toxicology	3
	NDA application		

1.3.2.2.4 *Achievements*

An overview of the progress which has been made in drug therapy of the major diseases over the past 50 years is given in Table 1.11.

Excellent or good drug treatments of bacterial, topical fungal, and parasitic infections, hypertension, allergic and bronchial asthma, anaesthesia, epilepsy, peptic ulcers and hormone and vitamin deficiencies have been accomplished. Moderate control of systemic fungal and some viral infections, ischaemic heart disease, heart failure, skin diseases, organ transplantation, mental disorders, pain and Parkinson's disease has also been achieved. There remain, however, many diseases which can still only be poorly treated by modern drugs. Amongst this latter group are, notably, the viral infections (including AIDS), peripheral vascular disease (although the recently introduced HMG-CoA reductase inhibitors may vastly improve this situation), Alzheimer's disease and rheumatoid arthritis and other autoimmune diseases.

This is only the situation in the economically developed Western and Japanese world, however. For the rest of the world, the economic situation, ignorance and a lack of health care organisation result in a distressingly different picture. According to the World Health Organisation about 15 million children aged 5 or less die each year largely from preventable diseases. Vaccine preventable diseases, such as polio, tetanus, measles, diphtheria, pertussis and tuberculosis, still claim 3 million lives and incapacitate or cripple a similar number of survivors. Acute diarrhoeal diseases affect a further 4 million children although, thankfully, the supply and use of oral rehydration packs is now growing rapidly, which should help improve this appalling situation. A further 4 million children die each year from acute respiratory infections, mainly pneumonia, probably through a combination of poor nutrition, poor environment and inadequate or inaccessible health facilities.

Tuberculosis, a disease which has largely been eradicated in the developed world through a combination of improved hygiene, vaccination and drug treatment, still affects an estimated 1.7 thousand million people with 10 million new cases and 3 million deaths yearly. Intestinal worms affect 2.2 thousand million people; malaria some 270 million and schistosomiasis a further 200 million of our world population. The sexually transmitted AIDS epidemic looms larger with several million cases predicted by the end of the century.

Clearly, the health care and the contribution of the pharmaceutical industry has come a long way in a relatively short time (less than 50 years), but an enormous amount remains to be done before all the world population can enjoy fruitful and healthy lives with a good life expectancy.

1.3.2.2.5 *Patents*

The costs of researching, discovering and developing a new medicine are enormous (up to £150m). In contrast, the costs of synthesis, production and formulation are very much less *per se*. Thus the only way that the costs of research can be recovered is by allowing the inventing company a period of grace during which it can market its new discovery without competition, a degree of protection provided by the use of patents.

Patents were introduced when it was realised that all businesses had more to gain

Table 1.11.   Progress in medicines research over the past 50 years

Disease	Prognosis	Typical drugs
Infections		
Bacteria	Excellent	Sulphonamides, β-lactams and others
Fungi	Good (topical) Moderate (systemic)	Griseofulvin, Ketoconazole
Animal parasites	Good	Ivermectin, Antimalarials
Viruses	Excellent	Vaccines
	Moderate	Acyclovir (herpes)
	Poor/moderate	AZT (AIDS)
Cardiovascular		
Hypertension	Good	Methyldopa, propranolol, ACE inhibitors e.g captopril, Ca-channel blockers e.g. nifedipine,
Ischaemic heart disease	Moderate	β-blockers, Ca antagonists. Surgery
	Moderate/poor (Infarction)	Acute-streptokinase, tpa; mevinolin; cholestyramine,
Heart failure	Moderate	diuretics e.g. thiazide; ACE inhibitors
Peripheral vascular disease	Poor	Possibly HMG-CoA inhibitors
Cancers	Poor/moderate	Methotrexate, cisplatin, steroids, tamoxifen, interferons, sex hormones
Skin diseases	Moderate	Retinoids, anti-inflammatory steroids
Immune diseases		
Allergy and bronchial asthma	Good	H_1 antagonists, glucocorticoid steroids, β_2 stimulants, intal,
Rheumatoid arthritis	Poor/moderate	Glucocorticoid steroids, NSAIDS, immune suppressants
Organ transplantations	Moderate/good	Cyclosporin, immune suppressants, glucocorticoids.
Central nervous system		
Mental illness	Moderate	Chlorpromazine, neuroleptics, Imipramine, anti-depressants. benzodiazepines
Pain	Moderate	Pentazocine, buprenorphine

continued

Table 1.11. *Continued*

Disease	Prognosis	Typical drugs
Central nervous system		
Anaesthesia	Good	Halothane
Parkinson's disease	Moderate	Levodopa
Alimentary tract		
Peptic ulcers	Good	Cimetidine, H_2 antagonists,
Inflammatory bowel disease	Poor/moderate	Glucocorticoid steroids
Hormone and vitamin deficiencies	Good/excellent	Vitamins, steroids, peptide hormones, insulin

by encouraging the disclosure of developments than by the secrecy which until then had been the only means of preserving a new product or process for the inventor. The first act was passed in Venice in 1474 when the Council of the Venetian Republic decreed that "whosoever in this city shall make any kind whatsoever of new and ingenious devices will be able to ask the municipal authorities for protection against counterfeiting". Similar laws were passed in England, France and America. All these acts had as a common purpose the idea that useful inventions should be rewarded by a period of monopolistic trading. Today, virtually all countries in the world have some form of patent legislation although the precise nature of these laws, what they cover and for how long, does vary quite considerably (see Tables 1.12 and 1.13). This variation is the cause of much dispute and litigation and efforts are continually being made to achieve greater uniformity. One manifestation of this is the recent introduction of the European patent whereby a single filing at the European Patent Office produces national patent coverage in Austria, Belgium, Switzerland, Liechtenstein, Germany, France, Greece, Great Britain, Italy, Luxembourg, Netherlands, Sweden and Spain at the same time.

Most countries require that for a patent to be granted for a product or process, it must be novel, useful, and have an inventive step. The European Patent Convention in Article 52 expresses this as:- "European patents shall be granted for any inventions which are susceptible of industrial application which are new and which involve an inventive step".

The definition of industrial application is, of course, easy to satisfy, but the terms "new" and "inventive step" are more prone to debate. In most countries, with the notable exception of the United States, any form of prior disclosure will invalidate a patent since it is no longer "new" including theses, deposited in a University library or any presentation at an open meeting. However, the United States allows an inventor a period of one year between the disclosure of the invention and its patenting, although, of course, any independent disclosure by a third party would negate this application.

As far as "inventive step" is concerned, it is helpful once more to consider the

Table 1.12. Categories of patentable inventions (pharmaceuticals)

Country	Products	Processes	Use
European	Yes	Yes	Yes
Denmark	No	Yes	No
Hungary	No	Yes	No
Norway	No	Yes	No
Portugal	No	Yes	No
Finland	No	Yes	No
Turkey	No	Yes	No
USA	Yes	Yes	Yes
Canada	Yes	Yes	No
Mexico	No	Yes	No
Brazil	No	Yes	No
Argentina	No	Yes	No
Columbia	No	Yes	No
Venezuela	No	Yes	No
Japan	Yes	Yes	Yes
China	No	Yes	No
India	No	Yes	No
Pakistan	No	Yes	No
Australia	Yes	Yes	Yes
New Zealand	Yes	Yes	No
Algeria	Yes	Yes	No
South Africa	Yes	Yes	Yes

definition given in the European Patent Convention. Article 56 stipulates "An invention is considered as involving an inventive step if, having regard to the state of the art, it is not obvious to a person skilled in the art". Of course, this definition begs another question, notably, the definition of a "person skilled in the art", which appears in chemistry to have been settled as referring to a skilled technician in the particular field. American law, however, treats inventiveness in a different manner. It states that "a patent may not be obtained though the invention is not identically disclosed or described as set forth in section 102 of this title, if the differences between the subject matter sought to be patented and the prior art are such that the subject matter as a whole would have been obvious at the time the invention was made to a person having ordinary skill in the art to which said subject matter pertains". Thus in place of "inventive step" "nonobviousness" is currently used.

Over the years a number of criteria have been developed to give substance to these vague terms. For how long had there been a perceived need for the invention?, had there been prior attempts to solve the problem?, what are the unexpected results of the invention?, and is there anything in the prior art which could discourage an inventor from carrying out the research?

Table 1.13. Lifetimes of patents

Country	Years of validity from:		
	Filing	Publication	Grant
European	20		
Denmark	20		
Hungary	20		
Norway	20		
Portugal			15
Finland	20		
Turkey	15		
USA		17	
Canada	20		
Mexico		14	
Brazil	15		
Argentina	15		
Columbia			5[a]
Venezeula			10
Japan		15	
China	15		
India	14		
Pakistan	15		
Australia	16		
New Zealand	16		
Algeria	20		
South Africa	20		

[a]Renewable once

A product, a process or a use of the same can be patented but as can be seen from Table 1.12 not all countries allow all these to be patented. The actual process of patenting an invention begins with a patent agent compiling a claim based on chemical reports and, for pharmaceutical products, pharmacological data for the compounds which indicate the proposed biological activity in man. The patent must contain a description of the chemical process which is sufficiently detailed for "one skilled in the art" to be able to repeat, and, at some point, the true inventors of the claim must be identified. This must be done with great care since incorrectly naming the inventors could invalidate the patent and because in some countries significant financial rewards are attributed to the patentors of successful products. Neglecting an inventor with a legitimate claim in these circumstances will, at best, cause deep resentment, at worst legal action. The date of filing has also to be chosen with care because the lifetime of the patent is limited (Table 1.13). Obviously a company wishes to protect its inventions as soon as practicable but in Europe the lifetime of the patent begins with the date of filing and lasts only 20 years. However, as was described above, the development period for a new drug lasts at least 8 years and frequently

12 years, leaving the period of patent protection very much less than the 20 years. This clearly puts the pharmaceutical industry at a significant disadvantage compared to the electronics or engineering industries where development times are very short and where the patent protection may be much closer to the full 20 years. At the time of writing the European Commission is considering the extension of pharmaceutical patents to improve this situation.

In Europe the priority claim for a patent is the date of filing of the patent, while in the United States a properly witnessed notebook can establish priority. Once a patent has been filed in a country, or group of countries, there is a period of one year when further compounds or results can be added to the patent and the patent filed in different countries. Filing the patent of course does not mean that the claim is accepted, although different countries review claims differently. Belgium, for instance, files claims after checking that the application is in order and that there is a unity of invention (i.e. all the claims form part of a single unit) but not to see if the criteria of patentability have been respected. Other countries only grant the patent after thorough examination of all the claims, together with any prior literature and usually only after repeated questions to the claimant.

Only after the patent has been granted, and only in the country in which the patent was initially filed, may it be challenged. Such challenges can be decided by tribunals or the judiciary: different countries having different procedures. Finally, it must be pointed out that patent law is extremely complicated and this description is intended only as a general introduction.

1.3.2.2.6 *Biotechnology*

The major development in drug research in the 1980's has been the application of the techniques of molecular biology to the discovery of the mechanisms underlying many physiological processes. The great power of molecular biology lies in the fact that it is capable of producing workable amounts of proteins which normally only exist in trace quantities. Despite being present in such very small concentrations they do play vital roles in the normal, and abnormal, functioning of the body. Examples of these are the growth hormones, the cytokines which control much of the activity of the immune system, and the receptors for neurotransmitters. To isolate any of these proteins directly is virtually impossible because of their extremely low natural occurrence. However, it is feasible to isolate the specific DNA which controls the synthesis of any proteins. This genetic material can then be transferred into the genetic machinery of a yeast or bacterium such that the organism's natural replication mechanisms produces relatively large quantities of the target protein. Thus enough of a given material can be isolated to enable its structure to be determined, its functional activity to be identified, and interference with its natural role to be used as a potential target for novel therapeutic approaches to a particular disease. It seems likely that this extra dimension of understanding will be judged retrospectively to have been the most important contribution of molecular biology to medical science.

The technique has been extensively used to synthesise significant quantities of proteins which are themselves therapeutic agents. This particular use has resulted in considerable publicity in the public media with predictions of wonder cures and massive profits for the biotechnology companies concerned. On this basis a considerable number of biotechnology companies have been launched, using speculative venture capital funding particularly in the United States. What has been largely ignored is the long time and high cost of the development process required to establish the safety profile of any biological agent intended to be used in man (as for man-made molecules). Although some have proposed that, as such products are endogenous, mammalian proteins, they should not be subjected to the same toxicity evaluation that synthetic small molecules undergo; others have highlighted the extreme difficulty of establishing exact concurrence between any two high molecular weight proteins and support established safety guidelines. To date (1991) the biotechnology products already available to medicine include (with their indications):

tissue plasminogen factor (TPA) — thrombosis
α-interferon — anticancer
human insulin — antidiabetic
human growth hormone — growth disorders
erythropoietin — kidney dysfunction
hepatitis β vaccine — antiviral

In the USA the value of these products reached \$900m in 1989 and this is expected to grow to \$3b (b $= 10^9$) by 1993. The example of human growth hormone is particularly illustrative of the technology as this material, which is used to stimulate the growth of children suffering from dwarfism, was previously obtained from cadavers. However, this source had to be abandoned when certain stocks became infected by the virus which causes Creutzfeld-Jacob's disease. This is an incurable illness which causes premature senile dementia and early death and for which the virus is difficult to detect or destroy. The replacement of such potentially contaminated material by the biotechnology derived product which could not be similarly affected allowed treatment to be once more available to sufferers.

The future potential of biotechnology applications is enormous and its potential influence on future therapy very significant, either directly or indirectly.

1.3.2.3 *Industry – government interactions*
The direct involvement of governments in the affairs and business practices of the pharmaceutical industry began in the period 1894–1926. Before that period many countries had legislation which concerned the sale of poisons and the control of opium abuse, but in Britain and Germany there was considerable confusion about the illegality of selling a product substantially different from its description in a Pharmacopoeia. Similar weak legislation existed in America and it therefore appeared that there was little control over what was sold as a medicine. It will be recalled that by the end of the last century branded products from named manufacturers were being sold to be used "only under the direction of a physician". For a time it seemed that the only control needed was the sense of responsibility of the physician, the publishing of therapeutic results in learned journals, and the desire of the manufacturer to be seen to be above reproach. The realisation that this might be insufficient came with the introduction of the bacterial antitoxins, particularly diphtheria antitoxin in

Germany and France in the 1890's. These agents were potentially much more hazardous than others because they were injected into the bloodstream and they were used at the height of the illness. Understrength agents would be ineffective, adulterated ones dangerous, and most of the patients would be children. In Germany, many of these children were treated in children's hospitals which were under the control of the government. These circumstances led to the establishment of the Control Station for Diphtheria Antitoxin in 1895 which worked closely with the main suppliers, Hoechst, Schering and Merck to properly assess the strength and purity of the preparations. The value of the system was shown a year later when the medical journal *Lancet* tested a number of antitoxins from different manufacturers and found wide discrepancies between claimed and actual strengths, with those of Hoechst and Schering being superior.

American legislation followed tragedy: a situation which, unfortunately, has been repeated on subsequent occasions. In 1901 a tetanus infected horse was used to produce diphtheria antitoxins which subsequently killed 13 children, and a similar case involving smallpox antitoxin killed 9 in Campden, New Jersey. The subsequent outcry led to the 1902 act requiring the licensing of manufacturers and the labelling of products. This was followed by the 1906 Federal Food and Drug Act which made the specifications of the US Pharmacopoeia legally enforceable and imposed controls on the manufacturers of ethical pharmaceuticals.

In Britain a parliamentary select committee investigated the claims being made by both ethical and patent medicine manufacturers and recommended in 1914 that the promotion and sale of proprietary medicine should be closely regulated by the Ministry of Public Health. The chance to enforce this idea came with the widespread use of the toxic antisyphilitic salvarsan during the First World War. Licences were granted to Wellcome in the UK and Poulenc Frères in France to produce this agent provided that each batch was tested by the Medical Research Committee. The success of this scheme and the desire to fall in line with other countries led to pressure to extend the system to other agents.

This relatively small scale beginning has now evolved into an extremely complex series of regulations and legal requirements which cover virtually every facet of the Industry's operations. For instance, in the UK the use of animals in research is controlled by the 1986 Animals (Scientific Procedures) Act; the use of toxic, explosive, radioactive, and flammable substances and controlled drugs are all governed by separate acts. Clinical pharmacology must be approved by ethical committees and clinical research by the need to obtain licences from the Medicines Control Agency (MCA). All manufacturing plant has to be licensed by the Department of Health and is subject to investigation by the appropriate authorities from other countries to which the product is exported. Changes in manufacturing processes have to be approved by the Regulatory Authority and the labelling of packages must not only contain approved specified information but also coding which would allow recall of the product should there arise problems with a particular batch. No new product can be marketed without a licence from the MCA which lays down strict criteria of acceptability, and all old products are reviewed from time to time. This committee has the power to revoke the licence of a product which shows unacceptable properties or side effects on large scale human use. The price of the product is controlled by the principal customer, the Department of Health and Social Security via the Pharmaceutical Price Review Scheme which is a highly complex formula which credits manufacturers with research and manufacturing costs within the UK but aims to control profitability and marketing/sales costs to about 8–9% of UK sales. All distribution and warehousing facilities are subject to Home Office control, and if any of the products are regarded as dangerous under Schedules 3 and 4 of the Medicines Act of 1968 the degree of security and accountability will be especially stringent. It is fair to conclude that few other industries worldwide are so completely controlled by their governments. However, this degree of control is understandable in the light of the desire of democratic governments to improve the well-being of their citizens and the role that medical treatments play in achieving this. It is also fair to conclude that failures and past excesses by the industry have certainly helped to bring about this situation. Thus the thalidomide tragedy of the 1960s made inevitable increased legislation controlling the introduction of new drugs, particularly demanding increased toxicological testing in animals. In addition, public concern about excessive profits and the use of questionable marketing techniques increased pressure on an albeit productive industry. Finally, the situation has arisen in which governments carry some degree of the cost of medicines either directly through the National Health Service in the UK, or through state sponsored insurance schemes. Inevitably, health care costs have risen dramatically as people expect more and better treatment as they grow older and as they survive more life-threatening conditions. Governments seek to control all social costs, and medicines, which in fact constitute a relatively small part of the overall cost (c. 10–11% of health care in the UK, and which has remained static over the past 30 years), are a tempting target.

The pharmaceutical industry is in an unusual position with respect to its customers in that very little of its sales and product range are made directly to the consumer. Instead, it must sell to a third party, notably the doctor or hospital service, who then dispense the prescribed product to the customer, the patient. Advertising to the general public is largely forbidden, at least in the UK, and this removes much of the normal advertising outlets. Instead, use has to be made of the scientific and medical journals, sponsored symposia or direct approaches to the doctor. These are busy professionals, of whom about 59% inevitably never see a company representative or follow recent literature, and, despite a strict code of practice followed by members of the Association of the British Pharmaceutical Industry, some desperate methods have inevitably been tried to win their attention with extravagant advertising claims.

Thus the relationship between the industry and governments of all types is inevitably an uneasy one. On the one hand the industry is enormously successful both in improving the health of its fellow citizens and financially, and this very success breeds distrust and criticism. The pharmaceutical industry employs very large numbers of highly qualified professional people, uses few natural resources, and is generally a good export performer. Nevertheless, the pressures on the industry, particularly with regard to prices and profitability, continually increases, notwithstanding an average annual investment of some 15–20% of sales in research and development and a total spend of more than £1000m p.a. in the U.K. alone (1992).

1.3.2.4   The future

The industry has grown from modest pharmacy beginnings to the giant multinational organisations of today in a relatively short time. While many of these international companies are amongst the most profitable institutions in the world, there has been a succession of mergers and regroupings as individual companies have sought the economies of scale considered essential to maintain their competitive edge and the profitability required to sustain the enormous research investments necessary for success.

Most observers of the health scene agree that there will be increasing pressures on the industry and very great challenges to success resulting from the changing environment in which it operates. These challenges arise from a combination of scientific, sociological and political pressures, but they will result in the dilemma of research becoming even more expensive with high drug prices more difficult to maintain.

Increased scientific understanding of fundamental subjects such as biochemistry and physiology provides yet more targets for drug intervention but also increases the complexity of studies which have to be undertaken when thoroughly investigating the pharmacology of a new compound. Delays and discussions with regulatory authorities further extend the development process of new medicines and reduce the subsequent marketing time available, with essential patent protection, to recuperate all research costs.

Changes in public attitudes in many Western countries mean that a considerable proportion of citizens no longer regard research as "an essential", and alliances of patient groups, consumer organisations and politicians are much more willing to debate the merits of, and necessity for, new drugs. Clinical pharmacology is controlled by ethics committees with representatives who are more and more likely to question drug trials which are not seen as improving the quality of life. An interesting reverse situation has arisen in America where pressure groups acting on behalf of AIDS patients have put severe pressure on the Federal Drug Administration to curtail placebo controlled clinical trials on potential anti-AIDS drugs that showed promise of affecting the disease, to facilitate their development. The issue is not a simple one, being a conflict between the tried and tested method of proving the efficacy of new treatments in the past and the very real fears of a group of terminally ill patients for whom all delays in introducing therapy may be fatal.

The marketing methods of the industry have always been convenient targets for its major critics and this discussion is likely to increase. In response the industry will have to adopt a more pro-active stance recognising that it is no longer taken for granted as a positive benefit and that research for its own sake is no longer so readily supported. Animal experimentation is viewed with great disfavour by large groups of uninformed people and the industry has to promulgate its indisputable success in introducing new and effective medicines. Its marketing techniques will have to be refined and directed towards the great mass of healthy individuals who need to be convinced that one day they might need the products of the research. It has to show that new drugs are still needed in vast areas of medicine and that drugs are a cost effective way of improving the quality of life of large numbers of patients. Thus, for example, the cost of an antibiotic should be related to the savings resulting from shorter stays in very expensive intensive care units, and the costs of antiulcer H_2 antagonists to the costs of the surgical procedures previously used with their inherent risks.

To combat all these challenges the industry will have to become even more efficient and will have to discover innovative products more rapidly and develop them faster than ever before. Nonetheless the challenge of drug discovery and the introduction of new medicines for mankind remain the most rewarding of goals for the research scientists in the pharmaceutical industry.

1.4 MAJOR PROCESSES OF DRUG ACTION

The biological effects observed (both the desirable or therapeutic effects and the undesirable or side effects) after administration of a medicine are based on a sequence of chemical events (see Figure 1.1). These start when the medicine enters the body and culminate after the active principle reaches the target site and produces the biological response. These processes are complicated and it is by no means obvious to the layman why, for instance, the oral administration of an analgesic agent should alleviate the pain of gout in an extremity (the toe) when the site of action (the pain receptor) for the drug itself is in the brain. The relationship is perhaps even less evident when the process affected is a cerebral one such as memory or mental disturbance such as in schizophrenia.

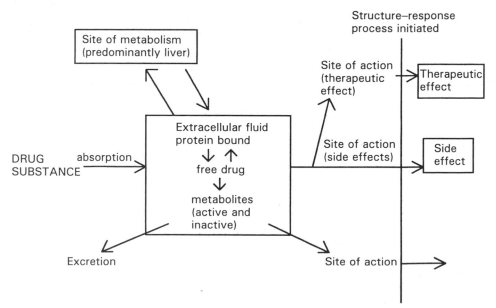

Fig. 1.1.   Major processes involved in drug action.

The approach to medicinal chemistry used in this text separates the complex processes taking part in drug action into three discrete phases, and the book as a whole is organised accordingly. An overview of the classifications used and the desired objectives for each phase are outlined in Table 1.14.

Table 1.14.   Principal phases in drug action

Classification	Pharmaceutical phase	Pharmacokinetic phase	Pharmacodynamic phase
Process taking place	Disintegration of dosage form Dissolution of active susbstance	Absorption Distribution Metabolism Excretion	Drug–receptor interaction in target tissue
Objective	Optimisation of *pharmaceutical availability* [Drug available for absorption]	Optimisation of *biological availability* [Drug available for action]	Optimisation of required *biological effect* [Induction of therapeutic effect]

1.4.1   The pharmaceutical phase

This phase covers the time from the administration of the drug substance as a pharmaceutical formulation, commonly a tablet or capsule taken by mouth, until the active component has been released into the body fluids. A typical tablet contains only 5–10% of active principle, 80% diluent, binder etc. and some 10% of agents designed to help the tablet to disintegrate as rapidly as possible under physiological conditions. It is obviously desirable, in cases where a high concentration of active principle is required, that the pharmaceutical preparation should break down rapidly, although there are circumstances where a long-term slow release of active principle is desirable and where the pharmacist must formulate a more appropriate preparation. The essential interest of this phase is the pharmaceutical availability of the active principle.

1.4.2   The pharmacokinetic phase

When the active principle has been released from its pharmaceutical formulation the process is described by the pharmacokinetic phase which covers the period during which the drug is transported through the living organism to its target tissue. The drug must be absorbed into the bloodstream, which means that within about four minutes the drug will have reached every organ in the body. To reach its target site the active principle will have to pass through numerous membranes which are of special complexity if its site of action is within the brain. Whilst in the blood stream, a drug substance (like all xenobiotica) can bind to blood proteins and also become subjected to metabolic attack in many organs, especially on passage through the liver. Although the drug will be distributed throughout the body only a small fraction of it is available for binding to the appropriate target structure. It must be stressed that the target tissue (its receptor) is not necessarily associated with the response tissue, but at the target tissue the drug molecule will trigger a stimulus either directly or indirectly which brings about the subsequent sequence of biochemical events leading to the observed pharmacological response. Once the initial stimulus has been triggered the physiological response is automatic and the process is consequently independent of the properties of the drug molecule. The site of action of the convulsant, strychnine, is in the central nervous system whereas its observed convulsive response occurs in the striated muscle. The major objective studied in this phase is the biological availability of the active principle released from its pharmaceutical formulation.

1.4.3   The pharmacodynamic phase
This is the phase of the greatest interest to the medicinal chemist; the drug substance interacts with its receptor site, usually a membrane protein, and initiates the ultimate biological response. The maximisation of this biological effect translated into a therapeutic effect and combined with a minimisation of deleterious or undesired effects of the molecule, is the main interest of medicinal chemistry.

After having initiated and suitably sustained the appropriate tissue response, the drug must be eliminated from the body where it would otherwise accumulate to produce toxic effects, relying on the metabolic processes which take place in the body. The overall time for the above process will vary enormously for individual drugs, for different categories of drugs, and from one patient to another. In general, the more water soluble the original drug substance is, the more rapidly it will be eliminated, whereas very lipophilic drugs may be absorbed and stored by the fatty tissues of the body and hence retained for a considerable time. The major objective of this phase and the major challenge for medicinal chemistry is the optimisation of the biological effect.

A drug which is absorbed into the intracellular fluids (principally blood) can exist in a number of derived forms, not all of which are necessarily therapeutically active. The processes of metabolism can give rise to active or inactive forms of the drug whereas excretion causes its loss from the body. From the extracellular fluid the drug circulates to its sites of action, primarily the cellular membranes of the major organs, where the appropriate secondary messenger systems and pharmacological effects are initiated, resulting in both the desired therapeutic effect and any side effects in treatment. All these processes will be discussed in greater detail in the following chapters.

2

The pharmaceutical phase

2.1 INTRODUCTION TO BIOPHARMACEUTICS

The pharmaceutical phase of drug development covers the science and technology of converting a drug into a form which can eventually be taken by, or administered to, the patient. The constraints on this process are that the formulation should be such that it can be manufactured, stored, and distributed without altering the biological properties of the drug. The formulation also has to be acceptable to the patient, and has to release the active principle into the body of the patient after ingestion.

In its early development, a candidate drug will have been evaluated in animal tests after administration by injection, either as a solution or in suspension. Thus a whole new series of problems arises in preserving the pharmacological characteristics of the compound in its new delivery system, and the name **biopharmaceutics** (the science of drug input) is used to describe the science of formulating a drug to achieve the optimum biological response. A typical problem encountered in biopharmaceutics is highlighted (Figure 2.1) to show the importance of such studies. The plasma levels of the antibiotic chloramphenicol for different polymorphs containing the same amount of active principle can be seen to be quite different. It is obvious from these that formulations containing B will be more effective, but what must also be highlighted, is that too high plasma levels may give side effects which could be just as injurious to a patient as the presence of too low, or ineffective, plasma levels.

Biopharmaceutics takes account of the relationships between:

(a) the chemical and physical properties of the drug
(b) the physicochemical and pharmaceutical properties of the dosage form
(c) the pharmacokinetic parameters of the active ingredient
(d) the biological, pharmacological and clinical effects of the drug.

The study therefore begins by considering the fate of the drug in man: a process known as its **disposition**, on what tissues or target organs it acts, and the chemical

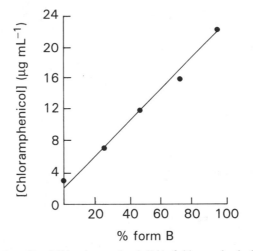

Fig. 2.1.   Correlation of 'peak' blood serum levels (2 h) of chloramphenicol versus percentage
concentration of polymorph.

transformations occurring in its distribution and elimination; that is, its **metabolism**. Once these are known an appropriate dosage form can be designed according to the five following basic principles:

(1) The dosage form should allow the drug to reach its site of action in the optimum time, to the greatest extent and with the minimum of inconvenience to the patient. Note that the optimum time is not necessarily a short time. Sometimes fast onset of activity is essential, but, as will be shown later, a more prolonged period of action is often very desirable.
(2) The processes by which the drug is eliminated from the body should be known before the most suitable route of administration can be determined.
(3) The drug must first dissolve in the fluids surrounding a membrane since it is virtually impossible for a solid to pass through biological membranes.
(4) Non-ionised forms of drugs will, in the absence of specific uptake processes, generally cross biological membranes more rapidly than ionised forms. The pH of the gastrointestinal tract can, therefore, significantly affect the rate of absorption of orally administered drugs and consequently the actual site of drug absorption.
(5) Any factor which affects stomach emptying will affect the rate of absorption of the drug, since in fact the intestine is the major site of absorption for orally administered drugs.

The relevance of these principles will become evident during this chapter.

2.2   PHYSICOCHEMICAL PRINCIPLES

2.2.1   Crystallinity and polymorphism in drug formulation

The existance of polymorphism, or the ability of a compound to exist in more than one crystalline state with different internal structures, will have significance for the development of a suitable dosage form for a new drug substance. Metastable polymorphs will tend to have an increased solubility and faster dissolution than a stable polymorph. This property may become important for a drug substance with an inherently poor initial dissolution rate profile, provided that the metastable form does not convert to the stable configuration during storage or in the gastrointestinal tract.

An example is provided by the antibiotic, ampicillin, where the anhydrous and trihydrous forms result in significantly different serum levels in human subjects after oral administration, the more soluble anhydrous polymorph producing higher and earlier blood levels (see Figure 2.2).

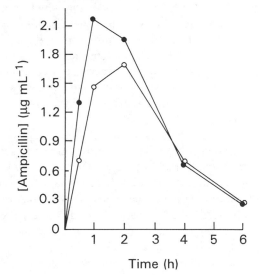

Fig. 2.2.   Mean serum concentrations of ampicillin in human subjects after oral administration of 250 mg doses of two solvate forms of the drug in suspension: ●, anhydrous; ○, trihydrous.

2.2.2   Particle size of the drug substance

The particle size of the drug substance is a major consideration in virtually all new formulations for oral and, notably, aerosol administration. The surface area per unit weight is increased by size reduction which aids both dissolution and the potential systemic bioavailability. Poorly soluble medicines are usually prepared in micro-crystalline or micronised form in order to optimise the absorption potential. During its lifetime as a medicine the therapeutic dose of spironolactone has been reduced twenty-fold, from 500 mg to 25 mg, by reformulation of the drug substance, notably by micronisation. Typically, reduced particle size is associated with more rapid dissolution, higher plasma concentrations, increased activity and reduced inter-individual variations for the drug substance. The effects of particle size in aerosol and dry powder inhalation devices on the penetration and retention of medicines in the bronchopulmonary system have also been studied. Particle size may also affect texture, taste and rheology of oral suspensions as well as their absorption.

The formulation scientist, however, has to balance the advantages of particle size reduction, which gives greater penetration in the airways or increased blood levels, against detrimental changes in flow characteristics and chemical properties, and frequently has to reach an optimum compromise.

2.3   FORMULATION SCIENCE

2.3.1   Dosage forms

The chemical substance which is a pharmacologically active ingredient synthesised by the medicinal chemist is not *per se* the medicine which is administered to the patient. There are a number of reasons why the raw material must be processed into a suitable dosage form to be of benefit. Formulation of the active principle into a medicine is based on prerequisites such as patient acceptance, ease of handling and transport, stability, and the need to administer accurate, reproducible doses of potent active principles. The medicine must be available to the patient in a variety of dosage forms with different characteristics that are easy to administer (see 2.4) and contain different prescribed doses.

Modern dosage forms consist of only some 10% of the active ingredient or drug, mixed with a variety of pharmacologically inert ingredients or excipients. These excipients perform a number of functions such as acting as bulking agents, colours, antioxidants, preservatives and binders. Simple tablet formulations typically contain three or four excipients although the number is usually higher. Although the excipients are intended to be biologically inert, they may modify the patient response to the drug substance by controlling the amount and rate at which it is made available from the site of administration. Whilst a rapid bioavailability of the drug substance from the dosage form is usually required, suitable sustained release forms can be formulated to release effective levels of a medicine over long periods when this is appropriate (section 2.5).

The manufacturing process or changes in the excipients contained in a medicine may have a profound effect on the bioavailability of a drug substance, and it is important to appreciate that it is never the drug substance, but a medicine which is administered to the patient. This may be illustrated by the very significant differences in characteristics of apparently equivalent dosage forms seen in the case of the plasma levels of two chemically equivalent chloramphenicol tablets, described previously (Figure 2.1).

The science of formulation is based on detailed studies of the physicochemical properties of the drug (section 2.1) and may rule out certain types of products. Thus, for example, drugs which have a limited stability in aqueous solution can, obviously, not be formulated in this fashion, but can be used in aqueous solution if they are reconstituted before use. The properties of the drug have to be married with the physicochemical properties of the recipients to produce a product with the optimal therapeutic efficacy.

2.3.2   Liquid formulations
Liquid formulations are frequently used in medicines and are administered by almost all routes from intravenous injections to topical lotions.

2.3.2.1   *Solutions*
Aqueous solutions are the most commonly used types of liquid formulations, but oils and other solvents can be employed where necessary. The major limitation of this type of formulation is the solubility of the drug in the chosen vehicle, but the solubility may be modified by judicious choice of excipients or vehicles. Drugs in solution are frequently not stable, especially in aqueous solution where hydrolysis may take place, but formulation factors may prevent this.

The organoleptic properties of a drug in solution are also important in oral products, and some form of taste masking is usually necessary. Nowadays noncarcinogenic materials are used, especially in paediatric products, to not only provide a sweet-tasting vehicle but also to increase viscosity of the preparation and slow taste recognition. Liquid preparations facilitate the growth of microorganisms and so most nonsterile products consequently contain a preservative.

2.3.2.2   *Suspensions*
Suspension formulations consist of a finely divided solid phase, dispersed in a continuous aqueous liquid, and are most frequently used for oral dosage forms. The main aim in the formulation of suspensions is to minimise caking of the solid ingredients—most easily accomplished by producing a flocculated system in the suspension. A floc is a loose cluster of particles held together in a random structure, which resuspend easily but clear rapidly. The ideal formulation is a partially deflocculated suspension that clears slowly but has long-term physical stability. Stability is usually improved by the addition of macromolecules or polymers or by altering the surface charge.

Specialised suspension formulations also exist in the form of inhalation aerosols which are widely used for asthma and allergic diseases. These systems are quite different from aqueous suspensions, and the drug is suspended in an organic solvent, usually a chloro or fluorocarbon propellant, together with suitable stabilisers such as long chain fatty acids or surfactants. Particle size distribution is critical and is limited to about 2–6 μm in order to achieve effective penetration of the alveoli and retention in the small airways.

2.3.2.3   *Emulsions*
Emulsions are similar to suspensions in that they contain a dispersed phase, usually a vegetable or mineral oil, suspended in a continuous phase which is usually aqueous. They were traditionally used for oral preparations of medicinal oils such as liquid paraffin, a use which has declined in recent years, but are now more frequently used

for other routes of administration. Mixtures of oil and water are inherently unstable, and surface active agents must be used to disperse the oil in the aqueous phase. The surfactant reduces interfacial tension facilitating droplet formation and also reduces the tendency of the droplets to coalescence by forming a protective layer on the surface of the droplet. Properly formulated emulsions will remain stable for prolonged periods.

A major application of this type of formulation is the use of fat emulsions for intravenous feeding, and emulsions are frequently employed as aerosol preparations contained in a pressurised canister containing a propellant gas when, on release, a foam is generated which is particularly useful for topical applications to body cavities, such as the rectum and vagina.

2.3.3   Semisolid formulations
Creams and ointments are typical semisolid formulations that are applied topically to the skin and mucous membranes. Although such formulations are convenient for local medication at the site of injury they may also be used to provide controlled systemic effects (see section 2.5). Excipients are chosen to facilitate penetration of the skin, and high concentrations of drug are used to maximise the concentration gradient across the skin barrier. It is important that these formulations cause no surface irritation and are cosmetically acceptable to the patient.

2.3.3.1   *Creams*
Creams are complex emulsion formulations comprising usually oil in water and referred to as vanishing creams since on application the water evaporates and the oil is absorbed into the skin. Such creams are not greasy on application, and the water evaporation further concentrates the drug on the skin surface. Unlike simple liquid emulsions these systems are extremely complex, nonhomogeneous mixtures of a dispersed phase, emulsifying agent and water organised in a variety of fashions (see Figure 2.3).

The emulsifying agents are usually waxes chosen for their ability to impart body and creaminess to the formulation, with the choice of wax, either anionic or cationic in nature, depending on the drug substance being used and the dispersion (oil) phase. Water-in-oil creams are also used, but in all cases the choice of excipients has a marked effect on drug availability from the formulation.

2.3.3.2   *Ointments*
Ointments are mixtures of fatty substances which are immiscible with water and are usually anhydrous, such as white soft paraffin (petrolatum), combined with emulsifying waxes to form emulsifying ointments which can form water-in-oil emulsions. These formulations feel greasy on application to the skin and form an occlusive layer which hydrates the skin, enhancing drug penetration. Hydrophilic ointments can also be prepared by using hydrophilic materials such as macrogels or polyethylene glycol as bases, thus resulting in a final product containing a lower water content.

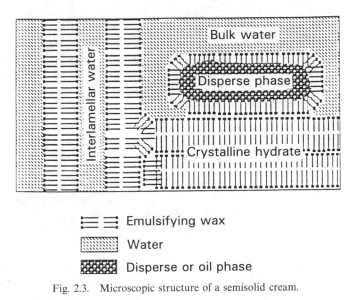

Emulsifying wax

Water

Disperse or oil phase

Fig. 2.3.   Microscopic structure of a semisolid cream.

2.3.3.3 Gels

Topical gel formulations arise from the gelation of organic or aqueous liquids by suitable excipients which form a continuous structure in the liquid providing solid-like properties. Gel formulations are valuable for the application of drug substances to the mucous membranes. The gelling agent has to be carefully chosen to avoid undesirable interactions with the drug substance which may limit its effective release or result in physical instability of the formulation.

2.3.4 Solid formulations

Solid dosage forms are the most widely used for the administration of medicines for a number of reasons, including patient acceptability and convenience, product stability and ease of manufacture. Although tablets and capsules are primarily used for oral administration of medicines to obtain the systemic effects of the drug substance, local effects are achieved by application of pessaries to other body cavities such as the vagina. The formulation and preparation of these dosage forms are dependent on the solid properties of the active ingredient such as particle size and shape, bulk density, hygroscopicity and powder flow characteristics, together with properties of the excipients used. Alteration of the formulation can be used to regulate the release of the active principle from the solid product and change the performance characteristics of the medicine. Tablets may also be coated to mask taste, improve stability and delay drug release (see section 2.5).

2.3.4.1 Tablets

Tablets are manufactured by the compaction of a powder mixture which contains a variety of binding agents serving different functions in the production of the finished product (Table 2.1).

Table 2.1. Tablet excipients

Excipient	Function	Examples
Diluent	Bulking agent used to adjust the tablet weight to desired level	Lactose, dicalcium phosphate, crystalline cellulose
Binder	Adhesive agent which holds together the powder during granulation and compaction	Starch, poly(vinylpyrrolidone), cellulose derivatives
Glidant	Added to improve the flow properties of bulk powder/granule masses	Colloidal silica, starch
Lubricant	Prevents tablet adhering to punches and dies, provides lubrication for punches moving in die	Magnesium stearate, stearic acid, sodium lauryl sulphate, talc
Disintegrant	Helps tablet break up when placed in an aqueous environment	Starch, sodium starch glycollate, crosslinked poly(vinylpyrrolidone)

A tablet of any desired size and shape is produced in a tablet press (Figure 2.4) which consists of two stainless steel punches and a die capable of generating pressures of the order of several tons. Millions of tablets are produced in a typical batch production at outputs up to 5000 per minute! The flow and compaction properties of the powder mass are consequently extremely important, and since most powders will not flow sufficiently fast for modern presses the powder is usually granulated in a form similar to that of instant coffee granules.

Wet or dry granulation processes may be used to prepare the powder mass for tablet manufacture, and the choice of formulation and method of manufacture depend on the dosage size of the medicine and the compaction properties of the drug substance. The relative proportions of the excipients and the compaction pressure in a tablet are important factors in determining the behaviour characteristics of the finished tablet. The essential considerations for a tablet formulation are its disintegration and delivery of the drug substance to the appropriate part of the gastrointestinal tract.

The finished tablet, which is usually round with flat or convex surfaces, may be coated with a material to further improve its properties for a number of reasons. Sugar coating has long been carried out to mask the frequently bitter taste of the tablet and improve its patient acceptability. Firm coating with polymers is nowadays used not only for protective purposes but to delay release of the active principle until its passage into the intestine from the stomach (enteric coating). This process is also used to prevent possible irritation of the stomach lining by certain drug substances.

The processes used in tablet formulation are rigorously controlled and the performance characteristics of the tablet are specified in national pharmacopoeias. The finished tablet is a highly sophisticated product optimising sometimes contradictory

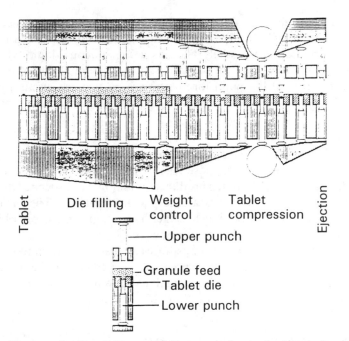

Fig. 2.4.   Diagram of a rotary table press. Tablet press cycle: punches 2–7, the lower punch falls to its lowest position and the space between the top of the punch and the die is filled with excess granules: the upper punches are inactive. Punch 8, the lower punch, is raised to a set height and excess granulate is expelled; the tablet weight is set by the quantity of granules remaining in the die; the upper punch is inactive. Punches 9–12, the lower punch drops to prevent loss of granules; the upper punch begins to fall and enter the top of the die. Punch 13, the granules are compressed between the two punches and the compression force is set by the spacing of the rollers. If the rollers are moved closer together, the compression pressure is greater. Punches 14–1, the upper punch is withdrawn and the lower punch rises to its full extent to eject the table, which is then removed and the cycle restarted.

requirements such as flow and compaction properties, ease of manufacture, cost implications, patient acceptability and, ultimately, the optimum performance of the medicine in the patient.

2.3.4.2 *Capsules*
A frequently used oral dosage form is the gelatin capsule which is used for a variety of medicines and other proprietary preparations, such as vitamins and tonics. The capsule consists of a hard or soft gelatin shell containing the active drug mixed with a variety of additives such as plasticisers, colorants and preservatives to improve performance characteristics of the gelatin. Hard gelatin capsules are obtainable preformed in a variety of sizes, colours and distinguishing appearance. As with tablet formulation the excipients are carefully selected to optimise flow and fill characteristics. Release of drug substance is dependent on the wetting properties of the formulation and subsequent dissolution of the active principle. Capsules may also be filled with coated granule or pellet mixtures to control the release of the drug substance in the stomach.

Soft gelatin capsules are obtained by the inclusion of high concentrations of plasticiser (glycerol) in the shell, and these capsules are not provided preformed. In this case the formulation is usually filled as a nonaqueous liquid which does not dissolve the capsule shell, and the capsule is pressed from sheets of gelatin around the fill between dies. This type of formulation is particularly useful for substances which are oily liquids or which are sensitive to tablet manufacture processes.

2.3.4.3 Moulded products

Medicines which are administered via other body cavities such as the rectum or vagina are usually obtained as suppositories or pessaries which are manufactured as solid moulded products. The molten product containing the suspended drug substance is shaped in a mould which serves as the packing material. The major excipient, referred to as the base or vehicle, may be either hydrophilic or hydrophobic depending on the physical properties of the active principle.

The bases used in pessaries and suppositories are usually chosen to melt just below body temperature to allow controlled spread of the medicine in the rectum or vagina and facilitate drug absorption. The formulated product must not be irritant, to prevent its premature ejection from the site of application.

2.4   ROUTES OF ADMINISTRATION OF MEDICINES

2.4.1   Introduction

Medicines may be administered to the patient in a variety of ways, but the desired therapeutic effect will be achieved only if the drug substance reaches the target cells in the body in a concentration sufficient for the appropriate effect and duration of action. Local application of a medicine to areas of the body is sometimes convenient, notably for ear and eye infections and for skin disorders, but medicines are usually delivered systemically, necessitating absorption of the drug substance from the site of administration into the general circulation of the body.

The age of the patient and their physical condition will have a significant effect on the route of administration chosen. Oral dosage forms are not easily administered repeatedly to very young children, and parenteral or rectal routes are convenient alternatives. Aged people are liable to underdose or overdose oral medicines if they are not supervised, and other routes need to be considered in certain cases. Compliance is also a major consideration for such patients as schizophrenics who may be unwilling to take antipsychotic drugs systemically each day. Slow release intramuscular injections which can be given once every two to four weeks may be a satisfactory alternative. Injectable medicines can be administered only by qualified staff and are frequently not as convenient as oral dosage forms for antibiotic treatments.

The stability of the primary drug substance itself under the physiological conditions to which it will be exposed, for example, the acidity of the stomach and its digestive enzymes, must be considered. The chosen route of administration will have a major effect on the duration of drug action, intravenous injection being the most rapid method of exerting the therapeutic effect, and consequently the most useful. The disease state and general physical condition of the patient will also be factors in the selection of the route of administration.

2.4.2 Oral

Oral dosage forms including tablets, capsules, powders, syrups and solutions are the most widely used dosage forms for medicines. Tablets and capsules together comprise well over 50% of all National Health prescriptions in the United Kingdom. The popularity of the oral route is due to a number of factors, notably convenience of self-administration and its suitability for most patient classes of all ages. The oral route is usually precluded only in major illness where the patient is incapacitated or the gastrointestinal tract is not functioning correctly in some way.

Although medicines are administered orally for local treatment of infections and ailments of the gastrointestinal tract, the large majority of medicines are administered by this route for their subsequent systemic effects in infection and disease. The majority of drugs for treatment of illness including cardiovascular diseases such as hypertension and central nervous system disorders such as chronic depression, which require daily treatment of the patient, are administered in oral formulations. In all such cases effective treatment depends on disintegration of the dosage form used in the GI tract and absorption of the active drug substance into the systemic circulation at effective blood levels. Oral administration is not the treatment of choice for those drug substances, such as peptide molecules, which are too unstable in the GI tract, or in those conditions where local application elsewhere in the body is preferable, for example by inhalation into the lungs in asthma therapy.

2.4.2.1   *Drugs acting locally within the GI tract*

Medicines administered orally for these effects include throat lozenges, gargles, cough syrups, antacids, laxatives, and anthelminthics and antibiotics for GI tract infections. Although local and acute infections of the throat and tonsils may be treated in this fashion, chronic infections should always be treated with systemic antibiotics. As well as the local soothing of the irritation leading to cough, the cough syrup must contain an antitussive agent which acts on the central nervous system, in order to inhibit the cough effectively.

Antacids, usually hydroxide or carbonate salts of aluminium, calcium and magnesium, are widely used for the symptomatic treatment of hyperacidity associated with minor stomach upsets frequently of dietary origin. They are also used as co-therapy in the treatment of gastric and duodenal ulcers and reflex oesophagitis where their action is simply to neutralise the excess acid secretion in the stomach.

Absorbents such as kaolin and charcoal are used for the nonspecific treatment of diarrhoea and stomach disorders, as are the bulk forming laxatives such as bran which swell enormously on hydration and passage through the GI tract.

Chemotherapeutic agents which are precluded from the systemic treatment of disease for reasons such as side effects or toxicity may be administered orally for local treatment of disorders within the gut if they are poorly absorbed or very rapidly metabolised, provided that therapeutic concentrations are achieved locally. For example, the anthelminthic mebendazole, which is virtually insoluble, is not absorbed to any significant extent after oral administration and is used for the effective treatment of tapeworm and threadworm infections.

2.4.2.2   *Drugs acting systemically*

Medicines prescribed for oral administration vary extensively and range from liquids to syrups, semisolids, capsules and tablets. The performance characteristics of oral products may be controlled from that of immediate local release in the stomach or intestine to that of a very slow controlled release through designated areas of the GI tract to provide once daily dosing.

Liquid dosage forms are presented in the form of solutions, emulsions and suspensions, a major advantage being that the dosage may be conveniently adjusted by dilution in individual cases. Ease of swallowing and palatability of such medicines are also reasons for their acceptability in paediatric and geriatric cases. Bioavailability of the drug substance is also likely to be maximised in liquid formulations.

Solid dosage forms are prescribed in the form of powders, granules, tablets and capsules. Powders and granules are usually prescribed in unit dose sachets as rapidly dispensable or effervescent formulations which are administered in water. As has already been stated, the most frequently prescribed dosage form is the tablet. Many oral forms have modified release characteristics such as those produced by interim coating, an inert protective coating introduced to protect the drug substance from exposure to the acidic stomach contents or to minimise the gastric irritation of certain drugs. Tablets are sometimes manufactured in a multiple layer format, each component of which will provide different release characteristics for the contained drug substance.

The effect of food on GI transit and absorption of the drug substance is a consideration of great importance especially for slow-release products. Gastric retention times can vary from a few minutes to several hours depending on the state of fasting and the diet. It is for these reasons that prescriptions usually specify the dosage regimen relative to food intake for the patient. Administration of a medicine which is designed for maximum absorption from the intestine after a large meal could result in its retention in the stomach for an extended period with a delayed or no subsequent therapeutic effect.

2.4.3   Parenteral administration

The term parenteral currently refers to the administration of medicines via injection, although the original Greek derivation referred to any route beside (*para*) via the gut (*enteron*). Parenteral dosage forms include sterile solutions, suspensions and solids for reconstruction, as well as intravenous infusion fluids. The main advantage of parenteral administration is the rapid onset of action achieved which is valuable in the case of unconscious, uncooperative or uncontrollable patients. These routes of administration also avoid preliminary metabolism in the GI tract or liver (first-pass effect), but injectable preparations must always be sterilised to be free of bacterial contamination, since some of the natural defence barriers of the body are circumvented.

2.4.3.1 Intravenous

A wide variety of administration routes may be used for parenteral formulations, of which the intravenous injection is most commonly used in medical care. Since this route requires the direct injection into a vein with concomitant risk, the drug substance must be completely in solution with no particulate matter present. Injections should be isotonic, whenever possible, with biological fluids and at the same pH to avoid local pain and tissue necrosis. The intravenous route avoids all the natural barriers of the body to absorption, and therapeutic blood levels are reached almost instantaneously. Duration of action is consequently very short and thus infusions are used where prolonged effects are required in the case of emergency. Precipitation of the drug substance from solution on dilution in the blood can result in pulmonary embolism.

2.4.3.2 Other parenteral routes

Intramuscular injection is a very convenient route which is more practicable for routine administration and inherently safer for the patient. The solution, or more usually in this case the suspension, is injected into relaxed muscle such as the shoulder or thigh which allows the drug substance to be absorbed over a prolonged period, using appropriate vehicles in which the drug substance has poor solubility. Pain and local irritation are frequently encountered via this route and may be obviated by the concomitant use of a local anaesthetic.

Subcutaneous injections are administered into the loose connective and adipose tissue immediately beneath the skin. This route is particularly useful in the case of medicines which are not effective after oral administration and permits self-medication by the patient on a regular basis as, for example, in the case of insulin for diabetics. Absorption is slower and less controlled than via other parenteral routes as it is determined by the subcutaneous blood flow. This may also be deliberately delayed by co-administration with vasoconstrictor substances, or enhanced by massage of the area surrounding the site of injection to increase local blood flow.

Local routes of injection are also used for specific purposes and conditions. Intrathecal injections are used for delivery to the ears with lower systemic side effects elsewhere. Intra-arterial injections are used to deliver toxic drugs such as the cardiac glycosides specifically to the target organ. Arthritic conditions are sometimes treated by intra-articular injection of the drug substance into the synovial sacs of the inflamed joints. Eye conditions such as infections and inflammation are sometimes treated by intraocular injection when topical and systemic therapy has failed.

Drugs administered by the parenteral routes enter the general circulation via the lymphatic or venous transport systems and pass through the lungs before entering the arterial circulation. The lungs act both as a storage and metabolic site for parenteral formulations and can significantly modulate the therapeutic effects of some drug substances.

Parenteral administration suffers from a number of disadvantages and problems. Patients, in general, are averse to injections, and qualified medical staff are usually needed for even their routine administration. Once administered it is difficult to counteract the effects of the drug substance in the case of overdose and care must always be taken to avoid the injection of air or particulate matter into the body.

2.4.4   Rectal administration

Medicines are administered rectally in the form of suppositories, enemas and ointments, and the vast majority of drugs prescribed in this fashion in the UK are for local actions notably in the treatment of haemorrhoids and constipation. Antihaemorrhoid preparations include local anaesthetics, analgesics, emollients and astringents whilst treatments for constipation cause relaxation of the rectum. In continental Europe, however, with different prescribing habits, drugs are extensively administered rectally for systemic use. Medicines frequently administered by this route include theophylline for asthmatic conditions, prochlorperazine for nausea and analgesics for early morning stiffness in arthritis.

Blood supply to the rectum arrives via the superior rectal artery and is removed via the haemorrhoidal veins. Whilst the superior vein leads into the portal system and hence the liver, the inferior and middle veins lead into the inferior vena cava. The absorption of a drug substance into these lower veins will avoid preliminary exposure to the liver and first-pass metabolism, and it is estimated that 50–70% of a rectally administered medicine will directly enter the systemic circulation without passing through the liver. The lymphatic system also contributes to this process in the rectum. The rectal route of administration is, moreover, advantageous for certain medicines which are unstable in the GI tract, such as peptides, or as an alternative to parenteral routes when the oral route is precluded for other reasons.

The mucosal membrane of the rectum is well supplied with blood and lymph vessels and so drug absorbtion is usually high, and can be significantly increased by absorption enhancers such as chelating agents (EDTA), nonsteroidal anti-inflammatory agents (NSAID) and surfactants. The base used in the suppository will have significance in drug absorption, as will the particle size of the drug substance. In spite of its potential advantages rectal administration remains an underused alternative to other forms of administration for medicines.

2.4.5   Vaginal and uterine administration

Medicines formulated for vaginal insertion include pessaries, tablets, creams, jellies, sprays, tampons and foams. Blood is supplied via the vaginal and uterine arteries and voided via the vena cava, consequently, as with rectal administration, first-pass metabolism in the liver is avoided by this route. Lymphatic circulation also drains from the vagina.

The principal indications for vaginal drug administration are local infections, such as vaginal thrush, and contraception including spermicidal creams used in conjunction with diaphragms. In certain situations the route is used for systemic actions such as with contraceptive steroids formulated into impregnated vaginal rings for long-term administration, the advantage being the maintenance of hormone levels at an effective concentration and easy removal of the dosage form if required.

The limitations of vaginal administration are similar to those of rectal dosage forms. It should be noted that absorption from the vagina varies enormously during the menstrual cycle and with age.

2.4.6 Nasal

Medicines may be administered via the nasal route either for their local effects, notably in rhinitis and other allergic conditions, as decongestants, or for systemic drug delivery. Drugs administered in this fashion are not subjected to first-pass effects in the liver or by the digestive tract enzymes and the route is gaining prominence for the administration of peptides such as buserelin, used for the treatment of prostrate cancer, and calcitonin which is used in osteoporosis. The respiratory region of the nasal cavity has a large surface area of cilia and microvilli from which absorption predominantly takes place. The vascular bed permits direct passage into the systemic circulation with peak levels of drug substance frequently being achieved within 15 minutes. For some drugs, such as propranolol and progesterone, the bioavailability after nasal administration compares with that of the intravenous route and is considerably better than that after oral treatment. Although peptide bioavailability is often only a fraction of that after intravenous injection, the ease of nasal administration often compensates for this disadvantage. Poor peptide absorption from the nasal cavity is now considered to be the result of enzymatic hydrolysis in the mucosa and not of the inherent polarity of the peptide.

2.4.7 Buccal and sublingual administration

The oral cavity itself is used for the absorption of medicines under certain conditions via two different dosage forms. Dosage forms may be positioned in the buccal region, between the cheek and the gum, or under the tongue (sublingual). The sublingual route provides a very rapid onset of action, necessary, for example, in the treatment of anginal attacks with glyceryl trinitrate. Sublingual tablets are small, and disintegrate and dissolve rapidly to allow rapid systemic absorption. The buccal route, however, is used for complete absorption where rapid onset is not essential. The tablet is formulated to disintegrate and dissolve slowly in the buccal cavity, releasing the drug substance over a prolonged period (30–60 minutes) thus giving an extended absorption.

Drugs administered via these routes are absorbed into the sublingual and buccal veins, hence via the jugular vein and superior vena cava into the systemic circulation. Unlike conventional oral administration the drug substance consequently avoids the first-pass effects from exposure to the GI tract and liver. Saliva secreted by the sublingual, submandibular and parotid glands dissolves the drug substance, a necessary prerequisite for its absorption. The drug substance has to be quite potent since the dose administered is necessarily low (10–15 mg), and its taste must be masked since this would result in salivation with subsequent loss of drug from the oral cavity.

A variety of drugs have been administered by these routes including the narcotic analgesics, propranolol, nifedipine and hormones. Drugs administered by the buccal and sublingual routes frequently have improved bioavailability compared with that from the oral route, and morphine has a better bioavailability by the buccal route than via the intramuscular. The major limitations for the administration of drug substances by these routes are the prerequisite for low dose levels, the masking of taste and the risk of irritation to the mucosa especially with prolonged treatment.

2.4.8   Transdermal administration

Medicines are traditionally administered topically for their local action on the skin and are usually formulated as ointments and creams. They are also applied in the form of drug powders, aerosol sprays and solutions, the objective of all formulations being to maximise local contact of the drug substance whilst minimising its absorption through the skin.

The transdermal route is now used for direct drug delivery to the systemic circulation and is another route which avoids the GI tract and liver. A single transdermal application provides a multi-day therapy improving patient compliance, extends the activity of drugs with a short half-life, and provides for rapid cessation of treatment if necessary. Such use, however, is limited to highly potent drugs. Physiological factors which are important in transdermal absorption include the state of the skin, damaged skin being much more permeable than intact skin, and the degree of hydration of the stratum corneum which also increases skin permeability. The anatomical location of the skin is also important as are its age and condition. The underlying cells of the stratum corneum are also capable of metabolizing drugs and affecting their subsequent bioavailability.

The most important physicochemical properties of a drug affecting its transdermal permeability are its partition coefficient and molecular weight. To reach the systemic circulation the drug substance must cross both the lipophilic stratum corneum and the hydrophilic viable epidermis. Although there is no direct correlation between percutaneous absorption and molecular weight of the drug substance, macromolecules penetrate the skin very slowly, if at all. Peptides and proteins are not effectively absorbed through the skin. Increasing drug concentration in the dosage form generally increases absorption via the skin until the vehicle is saturated. The pH of the formulation will also affect its penetration, ideally the drug being in the unionised form. Penetration enhancers such as dimethyl sulphoxide (DMSO) and urea dramatically increase transdermal drug absorption.

2.4.9   Pulmonary

Although inhalation of medicines is one of the oldest methods of effective treatment and has been used by asthmatics for their self-medication with natural products for centuries, it is the development of modern inhalation aerosols which has dramatically affected the treatment of asthma. The major advantage of inhalation drug delivery is that the drug substance can be targeted directly to its sites of action in the lower respiratory tract with a propensity for significantly reduced systemic side effects. Oral corticosteroid treatment for asthma was severely limited by their effects, particularly in children, and the advent of inhalation formulations has resulted in tremendous progress with steroid therapy. The large surface area of the alveoli, together with the excellent local blood supply, ensure rapid absorption into the bronchial mucosa and smooth muscle, with subsequent rapid onset of action of an administered drug. Drugs administered by inhalation avoid the GI tract and the liver, although the lungs themselves are also an efficient site of metabolism. The majority of drugs delivered via pulmonary administration are used for their local effects, notably in asthma, and include the bronchodilators, steroids and other prophylactic treatments for respiratory diseases. Mucolytics and antibiotics are also administered via this route to patients with severe respiratory infections.

The particle size of the drug substance is critical for optimum delivery in inhalation devices. If the particles are larger than $10\,\mu m$ they impact on the walls of the respiratory tract and never reach the alveolar sacs. If they are smaller than $1\,\mu m$ then they are likely to be exhaled from the lungs before impact. Only 10–20% of the administered drug substance will reach the alveolar sacs owing to these particle size constraints.

A number of dosage forms are used for pulmonary administration, but the most common form is a spray from a pressurised aerosol dispenser. The device contains the drug in suspension in an inert propellant usually a low-boiling fluorochlorohydrocarbon although new halogen-free propellants are being developed. On activation the propellant gas rapidly vaporises, leaving a dispersion of the drug in the inhaled air distributed throughout the airways.

Drugs may also be administered as micronised powders from breath-activated devices. The drug substance formulated with an inert carrier such as lactose is presented in hard gelatin capsules which are pierced in the device and inhaled with air drawn through it by mouth. The carrier is deposited in the upper airways and the drug substance of correct particle size $(1–10\,\mu m)$ penetrates deep into the respiratory tract.

Nebulisers are also used to administer drug substances conveniently in hospitals. The nebuliser converts an aqueous solution into a very fine mist of particles suitable for inhalation and is particularly useful for patients who have difficulty in using aerosol inhalers.

A number of disadvantages limit the use of inhalation devices, a notable inconvenience being incorrect use of the device itself. A high degree of coordination between breathing and activation of the device is also needed for optimum drug delivery and patients tend to either under- or over-dose the drug substance. Concerns have been expressed over the toxicity of aerosol propellants and also their global effects on the ozone layer, although their contribution to this is very small. Inhalation of the formulations used in these devices can also cause bronchoconstriction in certain cases, and some patients are reluctant to use their devices in public. Pulmonary administration is a very safe and effective way of administering medicines, however, particularly in asthma.

2.4.10 Summary
The advantage and disadvantages of the various routes of administration are summarised in Table 2.2.

Table 2.2.   Advantages, disadvantages and limitations of different routes
of administration

Route	Advantages	Disdvantages/limitations
Oral	Easy to administer Convenient Economical Safe (overdosage can be treated generally) Self-administration Painless Controlled release possible	Can cause nausea/vomiting Drugs may be unstable in GI tract Erratic absorption for poorly soluble drugs Food can affect absorption Patient must be cooperative and conscious Drugs subject to first-pass liver metabolism Slow onset of action Insufficient blood levels may be obtained

Parenteral	Useful for poorly absorbed drugs
	For unstable (GI) drugs
	Rapid onset of action
	Total and predictable levels
	Patient can be uncooperative or
	  unconscious
	Exact dosage given
	Large doses possible
	Prolonged release injection possible
	Compliance is total
	No first-pass effect
	Inject into specific area of body
	Peptide delivery made feasible
		Requires trained staff
		Self-administration unusual
		No going back once given
		Disliked by patients
		Painful
		Expensive
		Shorter shelf-life products
		Injection of bacteria, particles, pyrogens or
		  air can occur

Rectal	Little or no first-pass effect
	Useful when oral route dosage form cannot
	  be swallowed, *e.g.* infants
	Severe GI irritation is reduced
	Local actions possible
	Good alternative to oral/parenteral routes
	Avoids GI breakdown
	Can be used if patient is unconscious
	Peptide delivery may be possible
		Unpopular in UK and USA
		Slow, poor and erratic absorption
		Rectal irritation
		Inconvenient for patient
		General paucity of relative bioavailability
		  data

Vaginal	Avoids first pass metabolism
	Useful for delivery of hormones
	Local treatment possible
	Birth control devices
	Used for abortions instead of surgery
	Peptide delivery may be feasible
		Inconvenient for patients
		Erratic and unpredictable absorption,
		  particularly affected by
		  menstrual/hormonal changes
		Irritation
		Lack of bioavailability data

Nasal	Avoids first-pass metabolism Little or no breadown in nose Convenient Avoids GI breakdown Suitable for peptide delivery	Irritation Absorption affected by state of nasal mucosa
Buccal/ sublingual	Avoids first-pass metabolism Convenient Avoids GI degradation Quick onset of action Instant cessation of treatment possible Peptide delivery may be feasible	Duration of action determined by holding dosage form in place intact Palatability of drug Limited to low dosage drugs Cannot swallow, eat, drink while taking

continued

Table 2.2.   *continued*

Route	Advantages	Disdvantages/limitations
Transdermal	Avoids first-pass metabolism Avoids GI breakdown and absorption problems Prolonged action leading to good compliance Rapid cessation of treatment possible Local actions	Skin irritation Only suitable for potent drugs Tolerance may develop Erratic absorption affected by site chosen
Pulmonary	Actions localised so reduced side effects and doses Convenient Rapid onset of action No GI breakdown First-pass metabolism avoided	Only small proportion reaches site of action High degree of patient coordination required Propellant toxicity Irritation to bronchi Overdosage
Ocular	Local action only Prolonged action with inserts possible	Inefficient delivery to eye Hard to administer

2.5   CONTROLLED RELEASE DOSAGE FORMS

2.5.1   Introduction
The primary aim of dosage forms administered by the above routes of administration is to produce therapeutically effective blood levels of a medicine over periods up to several hours after which time it has been essentially eliminated from the body by the metabolic processes described in Chapter 3. An ideal sleep-inducing agent, for example, would merely trigger the natural sleep-promoting and control processes of the body whilst the drug itself would be rapidly deactivated metabolically, long before awakening from a normal period of sleep. In chronic disorders, however, extended treatment with a medicine is frequently necessary, as for example, in schizophrenia. By the very nature of the illness the patient is frequently unable to regularly self-administer the drug on a daily basis, and considerable effort has been expended to develop controlled release dosage forms capable of providing effective therapeutic levels of the drug substance over very long periods. Controlled delivery systems have been developed for the gastrointestinal tract and for transdermal drug delivery.

2.5.2   GI Tract delivery systems

2.5.2.1   *Rationale*
Delivery systems have been developed to alter *in vivo* release profiles of drug substances for a number of reasons:

(1) To provide a location-specific action within the GI tract.
(2) To avoid an undesirable local action in the GI tract.
(3) To provide programmed delivery of the drug substance.
(4) To increase absorption or bioavailability.
(5) To increase the effective half-life of a drug substance after administration.

2.5.2.2 *Matrix devices*

Matrix devices consist of the drug substance blended with a matrix which retards release of the drug. Examples of materials used to manufacture matrix devices are shown in Table 2.3.

Table 2.3. Examples of materials used to fabricate matrix devices

Insoluble	Erodible	Erodible
Ethyl cellulose	Shellac	Sodium carboxymethylcellulose
Cellulose acetate	Fatty acid esters	Hydroxypropylmethylcelluloses
PVC	carnauba wax	Hydroxypropylcellulose
Silicone	beeswax and other	Polymethyl methacrylates
Polyethylene	triglycerides	Polyhydroxybutyrate/valerate
	Stearyl alcohol	Polyethylene glycols
	Cellulose acetate	Polyvinylpyrrolidone
	phthalate and other	
	enteric coatings	

Nonerodible matrix dosage forms may fail to provide adequate control in the case of drugs where the therapeutic window is narrow and plasma levels must be maintained within strict limits for optimum therapy. Adequate release of drug substance within gastric emptying times is also difficult to control, but with a bioerodible matrix, however, the rate of drug release is dictated by the rate of erosion of the matrix rather than diffusion out of the matrix.

A variety of drugs, including ephedrine and certain antihistamines, have been formulated as matrix products for controlled release via the oral route . A typical application is the case of a sustained aspirin release preparation (Zapridin) where the rationale is to provide prolonged relief of arthritic pain whilst avoiding concomitant high plasma levels in the GI tract resulting in subsequent mucosal damage and ulceration.

2.5.2.3 *Gastric retention devices*

The concept of these devices is to provide dosage forms with a prolonged retention time in the stomach in order to provide gradual drug release into the lumen. This type of dosage form is particularly effective for drug substances for which absorption is reasonably high from the GI tract, but is applicable only to substances with a high degree of stability in acid media. Retention is controlled via the size and density of the dosage form or via adhesion to the gastric mucosa.

Early examples of such devices incorporated a drug reservoir attached to a balloon containing a suitable substance to inflate the balloon in the stomach by vaporisation, consequently retaining the device. Other approaches developed used swellable polymers which are expanded chemically in the stomach by crosslinking. By such means the frequency of dosing of drug substances may be reduced to once a day in favourable cases.

Hydrocolloid dosage devices have also been prepared which hydrate and swell on ingestion, generating a floating raft on the gastric contents, containing the active substance thus aiding its retention in the stomach. Solid foams such as polystyrene have also been used as supports to generate suitable low density dosage forms.

2.5.2.4   Bioadhesives
The basis for the original use of bioadhesives in oral dosage forms was the development of denture fixtures, the rationale being to prolong the presence of the drug substance in the upper GI tract. Further developments led to the use of cellulose derivatives designed to adhere to the buccal mucosa, thus providing several hours of drug delivery. As previously discussed, buccal delivery is a convenient method of avoiding first-pass metabolism in the stomach and liver. The use of bioadhesives which covalently bind to the GI tract mucosa is being investigated.

2.5.3   Transdermal delivery systems

2.5.3.1   Introduction
Transdermal drug delivery is, in principle, a scientifically attractive and noninvasive method of delivering medicines into the systemic circulation. Despite intensive research over a considerable period, however, very few drugs are currently administered by this method. The concept of topical application of drug substance has been known and practised for many centuries, and a wide variety of topical creams and ointments exist in pharmacy, albeit primarily for their local effects. Drug delivery by this route is both variable and poorly controlled because of significant variations in skin permeability over the various regions of the body. Such formulations have, however, clearly established the feasibility of using the transdermal route as an effective method of obtaining suitable systemic bioavailability.

2.5.3.2   Skin structure and function
In an optimum device the drug release rate should be less than the steady state flow of drug substance across the skin, ensuring that the device, and not the skin permeability, controls the rate of drug delivery (usually over a period of one to seven days). This will prevent excessively high dosage release and the consequent danger to those patients with an abnormally high skin permeability.

One of the primary functions of human skin is to provide a barrier to the ingress of xenobiotics to the body. The skin is the largest organ of the human body covering, on the average adult, an area of some two square metres. The anatomy of the human skin is illustrated in Figure 2.5. The skin in its simplest sense may be represented as a bilaminate membrane, and to reach the dermal vasculature (for rapid systemic circulation) the drug substance must penetrate both a lipophilic environment (stratum corneum) and an aqueous environment (viable epidermis and upper dermis). The processes entailed are outlined in Figure 2.6.

2.5.3.3   Advantages and disadvantages of transdermal drug delivery
The principal advantages are:

(1) Reliable and sustained plasma drug concentrations (oral multiple dosing frequently

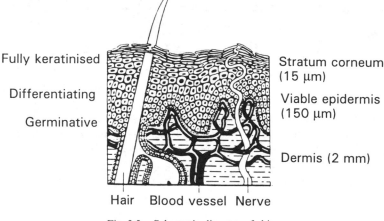

Fig. 2.5.   Schematic diagram of skin.

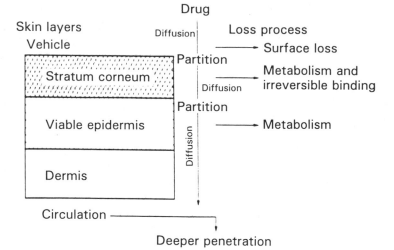

Fig. 2.6.   Sequential steps in percutaneous absorption.

results in peaks and troughs of plasma concentration).

(2) Avoidance of complicating factors such as gastric motility, pH, transit times and food intake associated with inter and intra-patient variations.

(3) Elimination of hepatic first-pass and GI metabolism.

(4) Reliability of drug absorption in diverse patient populations.

(5) Simple application, removal and control of dosing frequency together with a reduction in dosing frequency and increased patient compliance.

(6) Enhanced safety and convenience over other appropriate routes of administration such as intravenous infusion or intramuscular injection.

The principal disadvantages which are associated with the excellent protective functions of the skin barrier are:

(1) Percutaneous absorption, being a slow process, the method is of value only for very potent drug substances (active at a daily dose of 5 mg or less).
(2) The constant systemic levels achieved may be counterproductive if tolerance to the drug develops.
(3) Local application may cause irritation or allergic reactions.
(4) Biodegradation of the drug may occur owing to the microorganisms present on the skin surface, or enzymes present in the epidermis.

2.5.3.4 *Examples of drug applications*

Clonidine is a potent antihypertensive agent used alone, or in combination with diuretics for the treatment of mild to moderate hypertension. Although effective, it has to be taken two or three times a day to maintain therapeutic levels, the resulting fluctuations in plasma concentration of the drug being considered to be responsible for many of the side effects such as drowsiness associated with oral therapy. The transdermal system (Catapres, Boehringer Ingelheim) which provides steady state plasma levels for up to seven days represents a significant potential for improved patient compliance.

Estradiol is used for the treatment of symptoms associated with the menopause in middle-age women, and the value of oral therapy has been demonstrated for many years. A substantial fraction of an oral dose is very rapidly lost by first-pass metabolism in the liver, however, necessitating the administration of very high doses of the drug with the associated side effects such as hypertension and hyperlipidemia. The transdermal delivery device (Estraderm, Ciba-Geigy) achieves the necessary steady state plasma levels of the hormone for periods of up to four days, and the patch formulation is well-tolerated.

Nitroglycerin is a very potent smooth muscle relaxant which is used for the treatment of angina pectoris and congestive heart failure. The substance suffers from extensive first-pass metabolism and hence has a very short half-life after oral administration, thus limiting its use for prophylactic treatment. Several transdermal devices are now available for nitroglycerin administration which provide controlled release of the active substance over extended periods, and present many of the expected advantages. In some patients a limitation of these transdermal patch formulations is the rapid development of tolerance to the drug, which may arise as soon as twelve hours after commencing treatment. Many other drug applications are being developed for a number of drugs, and despite the limitations already encountered the route appears to offer great potential for future drug administration.

3

Pharmacokinetic phase

3.1 INTRODUCTION

The processes entailed in transport of a drug substance from its point of entry into the living organism (notably the human body) to the sites of action where it initiates its pharmacological effects followed by its clearance are described as the pharmacokinetic phase. During this phase the drug substance interacts with the many tissues which need to be transgressed and the numerous membrane barriers which need to be traversed. Necessary prerequisites for understanding this phase of concern in medicinal chemistry are an understanding of the roles of the fundamental building blocks of the living organism, the cells, and of the structure of the diverse membranes which form a physical barrier to the processes taking place in this phase. These aspects will be discussed in detail in Chapter 4. The physicochemical properties of a drug desirable for its passage through the various membranes to its sites of action can be deduced from the structural features of the cell and its mechanisms for assimilating materials. This knowledge can then be used to quantitatively relate the biological activity of a series of molecules to their chemical structures and the derived relationships can then be used in a predictive sense to optimise the ideal therapeutic profile of a chemical substance—the ultimate challenge for the medicinal chemist.

There are four discrete processes in the pharmacokinetic phase during the biological disposition of *xenobiotica*, notably their absorption, distribution, metabolism, and excretion (ADME), and the processes of metabolism and excretion are collectively defined as clearance.

3.2 ABSORPTION PROCESSES

3.2.1 Introduction

Absorption covers all processes which a drug substance may undergo after its administration before reaching the systemic circulation. Loss of drug due to metabolism by the microflora of the gut, by the enzymes of the gut wall, or from its initial passage through the liver are all processes which will affect the absorption. The absolute bioavailability of a drug is defined as the percentage of the drug substance contained in a defined drug formulation that enters the systemic circulation intact after initial administration of the product via the selected route.

3.2.2 Gastrointestinal absorption

The most frequently used route of drug administration is the oral route, whereby most of the dose is absorbed from the small intestine into the portal vein through the liver and hence into the systemic circulation. Significant quantities of drug substances thus administered are absorbed directly through the stomach wall into the intestines. Drug absorption from the gastrointestinal (GI) tract is a complicated process which is influenced by many factors. The physiology of the GI tract is of primary importance as are the chemical properties of the gut contents. The physico-chemical properties of the drug itself, its degree of ionisation, solubility in the gastric medium and lipophilicity all influence its rate of absorption. Other important factors in solubilisation of the drug substance include its crystal structure, polymorphic form and particle size. The actual pharmaceutical formulation of the drug also significantly modifies drug absorption facilitating or impairing this process. Physiological factors such as food intake, stress or the physical state can also affect absorption as can the co-administration of other drug substances.

The acidic medium of the stomach and the alkaline medium of the intestine also chemically modify drug molecules, as may the microflora of the intestine and the enzymes present in the intestinal walls, before their absorption into the systemic circulation. A major consideration in oral administration of drug substances is the fact that most of the drug has to pass through the liver, which is the major metabolising organ of the body before entering the general circulation. Easily metabolised drugs may be extensively deactivated as a result by a process known as the "first-pass effect". The oral route is, however, the preferred route of administration wherever possible for most drugs.

3.2.2.1 *Physiology of the GI tract*

The gastrointestinal tract passes from the mouth to the anus and consists of four physiologically discrete layers (Figure 3.1). To be absorbed the drug substance must diffuse through the inner mucous coat into the submucous coat capillaries. The physiological function of the stomach is to store food until it has been sufficiently broken down to allow it to proceed further down the GI tract. Digestive juices including hydrochloric acid and pepsinogens are secreted from cells in the body and fundus of the stomach (Figure 3.2), either in response to central stimuli triggered by sight or smell of food, or directly by gastrin released by the presence of food in the stomach. The gastric mucosa are pitted by glands which contain the chief cells, which secrete pepsinogens, and the parietal cells which secrete hydrochloric acid which activates the pepsinogens to the pepsin enzymes. The pH of the lumen of the stomach under fasting conditions is within the range pH1 to pH3, but this rises to pH3 to pH5 after food intake. The acidity of the stomach may consequently cause significant decomposition of acid labile drug substances before absorption, notably in the case of the macrolide antibiotics such as erythromycin. The lining of the stomach is covered with a thin layer of mucous which is slightly alkaline on the mucosal side and acidic on the lumen side, resulting in a steep pH barrier to absorption which is referred to as the mucosal pH barrier.

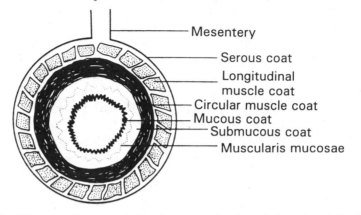

Fig. 3.1.   Diagrammatic representation of a cross-section through the gastrointestinal tract.

Absorption processes

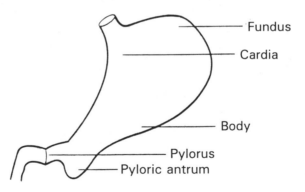

Fig. 3.2.   Gross anatomy of the human stomach.

The small intestine is divided into three regions, the duodenum, jejunum, and ileum. The duodenum is described as the section from the pyloric sphincter to the ligament of Treitz, some 20 cm in length. Within this section the bile and pancreatic juices empty into the small intestine at the ampulla of Vater. Most of the small intestine, some 260 cm in length, is divided into the jejunum and ileum in the proportion 2:3. The mucosal surface of the small intestine is superbly designed to facilitate absorption of small organic molecules (Figure 3.3). The finger-like projections, villi, of the mucosal surface are richly supplied with capillary blood vessels, nerves and lymph vessels, which provide an enormous area for contact with, and subsequent absorption of, drug formulations designed for oral absorption. The pH of the small intestine is more variable than that of the stomach, rising from pH5 to pH6 in the duodenum to about pH7 in the jejunum, values being one pH unit lower after food intake.

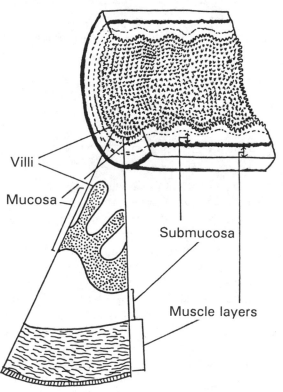

Fig. 3.3.   Mucosal surface of the small intestine.

The ileum terminates in the ileo-caecal valve at the entrance to the colon which itself terminates at the rectum (Figure 3.4). After food intake the valve opens regularly to allow migration of the intestinal contents into the colon. The mucosal surface of the colon contains no villi, and thus has a much smaller relative surface area for absorption, although some absorption does still take place from this region.

3.2.2.2   Factors affecting absorption

Gastrointestinal transit time is of major importance to the pharmacist when considering drug absorption since the extent of absorption of poorly or slowly absorbed substances will be very dependent on time spent in the small intestine with its very large surface area.

After feeding, peristaltic contractions in the stomach progress the gastric contents towards the rectum. Large particles of relatively indigestible material remain in the stomach whilst smaller particles pass through the pylorus into the small intestine. Once emptied from the stomach both large and small particles, as well as liquids, are transported at roughly the same rate through the small intestine.

Intestinal transport, either in the fed or fasting state, usually takes between 3 hours

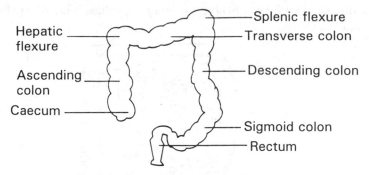

Fig. 3.4.   Gross anatomy of the human colon.

and 5 hours. Colonic transport which is significant for certain poorly absorbed drug substances and specific slow release formulations takes between 30 and 39 hours.

It is currently accepted that only the unionised form of a drug substance crosses the lipophilic gastrointestinal membrane and that, consequently, acidic drugs should be absorbed from the stomach more easily than basic drugs. Basic drugs should be more extensively absorbed from the duodenum with its greater pH, with correspondingly reduced absorption under these conditions for acids. However, the extraordinarily large surface area of the duodenum does mean that significant quaternary ammonium salts and sulphonic acids which are completely ionised are poorly absorbed under all conditions. Polar substances may also penetrate cells under certain conditions, possibly via porous channels present in the very large surface of the small intestine. The solubility of drug substances in the GI fluids is also a consideration in their absorption since acidic substances will tend to dissolve more slowly in the acid contents of the stomach than basic compounds, and, in addition, certain acidic substances of low solubility may even precipitate in the stomach milieu.

Another important factor to be considered in drug absorption is the relative solubility in lipids and water as measured by the octanol-water partition coefficient (log P, see Chapter 5). The importance of this is obvious when it is considered that biological membranes are essentially lipid and fluids largely aqueous. However, the existance of waterfilled pores of diameter of 6 Å in the jejunum and 3 Å in the ileum between the epithelial cells of the mucosal layer contradicts an impression of a continuous organic layer and allows the passage of unexpected species. In fact it is found that approximately 90% of drugs or their salts which have log P values between -2 and $+4$ are described as being well absorbed. It is only with extreme values, i.e. < -1 and $> +3$ combined with poor solubility that problems arise. Otherwise, despite possible exceptions absorption appears to be relatively insensitive to log P. At high values of log P (>3) the absorption rate reaches a plateau value, whilst at low values (< -1) the rate is also slow and also may not increase with increasing log P.

Owing to the much larger surface of the small intestine the rate of absorption of all drug substances is much greater from this region than the stomach and gastric emptying times consequently have a pronounced effect on drug absorption.

The presence of food or liquid in the stomach has an important effect on gastric emptying times and hence absorption. Gastric emptying time is also dependent on pH, volume and constitution of the stomach contents. Drugs dissolved in large volumes are more quickly emptied from the stomach than when dissolved in small volumes. Solid meals tend to empty more slowly than liquids and can take long periods when containing high concentrations of fat or fibre. Drug absorption can consequently be dramatically affected by ingestion with or after food. For slow release products gastric emptying is a factor of considerable importance.

Microorganisms are always present in the large intestine of mammals, which presents an ideal medium for the growth of many such organisms. The distribution and types of microorganism present vary within the gastrointestinal tract. In man, the main organisms are anabolic bacteria found mainly in the colon, although small colonies of organisms are present in saliva. The stomach and jejunum are usually sterile although Lactobacilli and Streptococci are found. The bacteria of the large intestine are capable of modifying many administered drug substances, reducing their absorption, but these byproducts are usually different from cellular metabolic products. Metabolic products are usually a result of oxidation or conjugation, whereas microbial byproducts usually result from reduction or hydrolysis. Of course drugs which are extensively absorbed from the duodenum and jejunum will not be exposed to the microflora of the large intestine.

The gut wall itself is capable of metabolising certain drugs during absorption. The mucosal cells lining the gut wall contain enzymes similar to those found in hepatic tissue which are capable of degrading drugs but to a much lower extent. These enzymes seem to be concentrated in the duodenum and jejunum although enzymatic activity occurs throughout the gut. Certain food constituents may induce intestinal enzyme activity in man and animals, as does smoking.

Food, drink, and co-administration of the drugs may affect absorption not only by affecting gastric emptying times as previously discussed but also by other factors. Certain drugs, e.g. tetracycline, may complex with food substances, notably milk products owing to the presence of metal ions especially calcium and magnesium, but also protein molecules, and thus their absorption will be reduced. The absorption of poorly soluble drug substances is often improved by co-administration of a fatty meal. Cholestyramine, an anionic resin polymer, used to bind and reduce cholesterol levels in the GI tract, also binds other substances such as warfarin and thiazide diuretics, also reducing their absorption.

The physical properties of the formulation prepared may also have a dramatic effect on the absorption of a selected drug substance with major factors being the particle size and crystal structure of the product. In general, reducing the particle size of a drug increases the rate and extent of its absorption. Interaction of the drug substance with inactive components of the formulation (Chapter 2) may dramatically impair absorption as may sugar coating of tablets. Poor absorption characteristics may be improved by the use of lipid adjuvants which form oil / water emulsions to achieve higher concentrations of lipophilic drugs than would otherwise be possible. In general, unsaturated fatty acids enhance absorption more than saturated fatty acids.

3.2.3 Rectal absorption

The physiology of the rectum makes it much less suitable for drug absorption than the small intestine although, perhaps surprisingly, some drugs are very well absorbed by this route. The anatomy of the rectum is illustrated in Figure 3.5. The ampulla recta is some 15–20 cm in length and the membrane surface is comparable to that in the remainder of the large intestine but without the corresponding villi and microvilli. The available absorbing surface of the rectum is about 0.05 m² compared with the 70 m² of the small intestine. The rectum is usually empty and undergoes little on-going movement. The blood supply to the lower rectum drains into the inferior rectal and middle rectal veins, which then empty into the inferior venal cavity thus by-passing the liver. The superior rectal vein, on the other hand, drains into the portal system passing through the liver before entering the general circulation. However, anastomoses occurring between the rectal veins results in reversal of the previously described processes. An important advantage of the rectal route is, consequently, the potential to avoid first-pass metabolism in the liver or gut before systemic circulation.

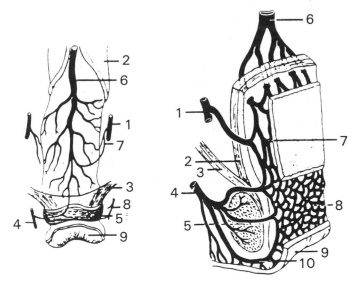

Fig. 3.5. The venous drainage of the human rectum: 1. middle rectal vein; 2. tunica muscularis; stratum longitudinale; 3. levator ani; 4. inferior rectal vein; 5. external sphincter; 6. superior rectal vein; 7. and 8. submucous venous plexus; 9. skin; 10. maringal vein and subcutaneous plexus.

The amount of liquid contained in the rectum is small (5 ml) and not sufficient to dissolve sparingly soluble drugs. Most drug substances are administered in suitable formulations, solubility in aqueous solutions being more important than for other routes of administration owing to the limited amount of fluid available, with release of drug from dosage forms being directly related to aqueous solubility.

The most widely used rectal dosage form is the suppository which consists of a suspension of the drug in cocoa butter or a derived semisynthetic hydrogenated product or fatty acid derivative of glycerine. The essential property of all suppositories is to remain solid at room temperature but to melt quickly at body temperature (37°C).

The rectal route is a widely accepted and often preferred route of administration in many European and South American countries but is not extensively used in the UK, the USA, or Japan. Rectal dosage forms are frequently more easy to administer to small children than oral dosage forms, and the rectal route is the preferred route if the patient is vomiting or the drug substance is extensively deactivated after oral administration.

3.2.4   Transdermal absorption

The skin presents a major barrier to the absorption of drugs by the transdermal route and is illustrated in vertical section in Figure 3.6. The skin can be classified in four distinct layers from the outside surface, namely the stratum corneum, the epidermis, the dermis or corneum, and the subcutis.

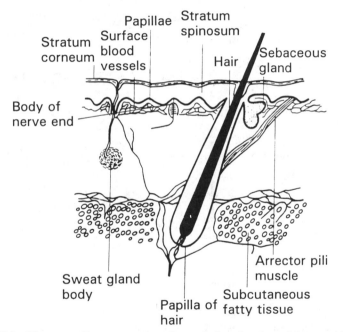

Fig. 3.6.   Diagrammatic representation of a vertical section through human skin.

The stratum corneum consists of dead cells which have become keratinised and varies between 6 and 15 μm in thickness (14 to 27 cells) except for the palm of the hand and the sole of the foot which are much thicker. The surface cells which are arranged in columns are constantly shed, the cell membrane consisting primarily of lipids with the cells containing α-keratin filaments embedded in a protein matrix. The stratum corneum is covered by a thin waxy film of aqueous and lipid components, and the extracellular spaces are filled with lipidic material excreted from cells in the epidermis, the lipids composed of high melting point mono and di-glycerides, fatty acids and phospholipids which provide the firmness of the intercellular structure. The resulting structure is, consequently, the most difficult layer for drug substances to penetrate and is frequently the limiting factor in transdermal absorption.

The epidermis, which is between 0.3 and 1 mm thick, consists of layers of clearly differentiated cells (Figure 3.7). The stratum lucidum is a thin amorphous layer which contains no cell nuclei or boundaries. The stratum granulosum is another thin layer of cells which are flattened and characterized by granules in the cells. Underneath is the stratum spinosum which is a lining layer of polyhedral cells which become flattened adjacent to the stratum granulosum and have a shiny or prickly appearance caused by adhesion between cells. The stratum basale is the lowest layer and consists of a single layer of columnar cells forming a boundary with the corium. This layer is heavily indented by the numerous folds of the corium and those two layers are continually dividing to produce new cells, which subsequently migrate to the surface layers. Transit time for a cell until it is shed from the skin surface is about 28 days, a layer of cells being lost from the stratum corium every day.

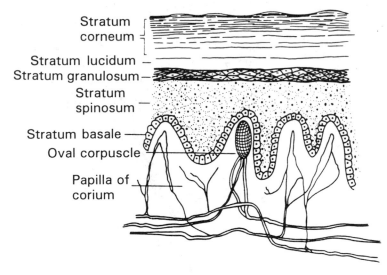

Fig. 3.7.   Diagrammatic representation of the epidermis.

The upper dermis is arranged into numerous folds which are extensively served by a network of blood vessels and nerves, known as the papillae of corium, which allows rapid exchange of materials between the epidermis and vascular network. The dermis which consists of collagen and elastin fibres embedded in a mucopolysaccharide matrix contains the sweat glands and fine hair follicles. The subcutis consisting of loose fibres together with stored fat cells contain the origins of the follicles of the thick hairs. To achieve significant systemic concentrations after transdermal administration a drug molecule must penetrate the stratum corneum and the epidermis to reach the blood vessels of the papillae of corium.

The vehicle used to formulate the drug substance can have a significant effect on the rate of permeation of the drug substance. Water is most frequently used either as a formulation or to rehydrate the skin. The stratum corneum normally contains about 45% water and on contact with water can dissolve up to five times its dry weight. Dry stratum corneum, on the other hand, is some ten times less permeable and hydration increases its permeability some two- to three-fold.

Hydration of the skin for absorption is extremely important and many topical formulations simply increase hydration of the stratum corneum by reducing water loss with an impermeable layer of a paraffin or wax base or with a high water content in the formulations, which are usually aqueous based creams. The use of a surface active agent frequently enhances penetration of drug substances. Dimethyl sulphoxide has been extensively investigated as a penctration enhancer but its use has been limited by its irritant and basic properties. A number of amides are capable of enhancing penetration of the skin barrier and have minimal side effects.

3.2.5 Intranasal absorption

Intranasal administration of drug substances has been used for many centuries, notably for the administration of stimulants such as nicotine (snuff) and hallucinogens such as cocaine. More recently the route has been applied to the administration of drugs such as steroids and peptides which are inactivated or have severe side effects after oral administration. The preparation of suitable formulations necessitates an understanding of the physiology of the nose if they are not to prevent its normal functioning. By virtue of its functions the nose ensures intimate contact of air with its mucosal surface and results in fluid secretion which is transported to the nasopharynx where it is swallowed. Thus bioavailability by the intranasal route is frequently very low and only 1–2% of that via intravenous injection. For certain drug substances, notably peptide hormones, this is frequently much greater than can be accomplished by oral administration. Many other drugs such as steroids which are inactivated in the GI tract, β-blockers which are susceptible to high first-pass effects, and drugs such as metaclopromide used to control nausea and vomiting are effectively administered via the intranasal route.

Formulations have of necessity to be non-irritant to the nasal mucosa and must not reduce the ciliary clearance. Drugs are usually delivered via metered dose nebulisers, inert chlorofluorohydrocarbon suspensions, or dry powder inhalation devices.

3.2.6 Buccal absorption

Drugs which are unstable at the pH of the GI tract, or are deactivated by the enzymes or microflora present, may be administered by the buccal route. The membranes of the mouth have been extensively investigated for drug absorption and the terms buccal and sublingual absorption are both frequently used, although for most purposes they should be considered synonymous. The major advantage of this route is due to the fact that such administration will result in systemic absorption without prior passage through the liver with consequently no first-pass effects. The dose administered must be limited to around 10 mg, however, since larger doses risk being swallowed and hence delivered conventionally.

As for other routes of administration, absorption depends on the fraction of unionised material (pKa) available at the buccal membranes and is also dependent on the partition coefficient of the drug (optimally log $P \sim 3$). In typical formulations the drug substance is present as a solid dose form, and substances with a high partition coefficient usually have low aqueous solubility which is often improved by judicious choice of salts. A careful balance between these properties is necessary, however, because buccal absorption is more dependent on lipid solubility than is absorption across the mucosa of the GI tract.

Several categories of drugs are administered by the buccal or sublingual routes notably the potent narcotic analgesics such as morphine and buprenorphine, where the bioavailability is frequently poor by the oral route, and certain cardiac drugs such as nitro-glycerine and isosorbide dinitrate where rapid onset of their effects is needed. Drugs administered by the sublingual route frequently demonstrate a desirable sustained effect due to storage in the buccal membranes.

3.2.7 Vaginal absorption

The vaginal route has traditionally been used for the logical administration of many agents to treat specific local infections and conditions occurring in the female, notable examples being antibiotics, antifungal agents, steroids and prostaglandins. The vagina is anatomically and physiologically very similar to the rectum, containing a dense network of blood vessels, and the vaginal cell surface is composed of micro-ridges eminently suited to drug absorption. As for rectal absorption, drugs should possess reasonable aqueous solubility having to traverse the aqueous media including vaginal secretions and also the lipsodal/aqueous membrane barrier. In general, solubility will be more important than the pH of the formulation although an unionised drug is more rapidly absorbed than the ionised species. Intravaginal administration may also avoid first-pass effects to some extent, most notably for the steroids.

Although antibiotics are frequently administered to the vagina for local infections, their systemic bioavailability is usually low by this route with the exception of metronidazole. Peptide hormones have also been effectively administered by the vaginal route.

3.2.8 Lung absorption

The lungs provide a very convenient and efficient route of administration for certain classes of drug substances. The lungs are extremely well provided with blood supply owing to their essential physiological role. The whole of the cardiac output passes through the alveolar capillary unit with its extensive capillary endothelium, and both alveolar epithelial and endothelial layers are very thin in order to facilitate gas exchange.

Hydrophilic drugs are absorbed by a nonsaturable diffusion process at a rate which decreases with increasing molecular weight. These compounds traverse the membrane through the aqueous pathway or through aqueous pores. Lipophilic molecules which cross the alveolar epithelium more rapidly than hydrophilic compounds also do so by a nonsaturable diffusion process dependent on increasing partition coefficient. Although many drugs are very well absorbed systemically via the lungs (frequently almost as rapidly as from an i.v. injection) this route is usually restricted to medicines used for the treatment of respiratory tract diseases. This route is the presentation of choice for antiasthmatic drugs, notably the bronchodilators such as salbutamol and the steroids such as betamethasone. The drug substance may be formulated either in an aerosol preparation containing an inert fluorochlorohydrocarbon under pressure or in a dry powder device, when it is delivered with an inert powder carrier. Drugs are much more potent when administered via the lungs, resulting in lower dosage and consequent reduced risk of systemic side effects—an effect which is particularly notable for the steroids. For optimum delivery into the small airways the administered drug substance must have a particle size of around 6 μm; too small and the particle material is exhaled, too large and the material does not reach the lower airways. More than 80% of the dosage in such formulations is not delivered to the lungs but trapped in the mouth and throat and subsequently swallowed.

Certain drugs, notably sodium cromoglycate which is an effective antiasthmatic, are totally ineffective after oral administration owing either to poor bioavailabilty or extensive metabolism, and can be administered only via the lungs.

3.3 DISTRIBUTION

3.3.1 General principles

In contrast to the absorption processes just described, the distribution and clearance phases are independent of the characteristics of drug presentation such as the dose of active substance used, its formulation and route of administration. The consideration of the distribution of a molecule becomes important as its investigation moves from the early evaluation of activity in *in vitro* models into the more complex *in vivo* biological systems such as isolated receptor preparations or perfused organ systems. An ultimate understanding of drug distribution is, however, dependent on its evaluation in the intact living organism since distribution controls access of xenobiotica to the diverse tissue sites of the body (nonspecific affinity) as well as to the precise physiological targets (specific affinity) required for effecting the requisite pharmacological effects.

The distribution of any administered substance is a complex dynamic process during which the chemical compound enters the body tissues from the systemic circulation. The process occurs immediately after intravascular administration and follows absorption after oral administration. The dynamics of distribution are regulated by the rate at which the substance enters the general circulation and are, consequently, affected by the conditions of administration and other factors such as blood flow and the permeability of membranes and the various biological barriers, together with the selective affinity of the drug for specific tissues. The residence time of the substance in any tissue depends on the efficiency of the systemic elimination processes (clearance) which, together with the degree of tissue affinity, determine its rate of return to the systemic circulation, thus resulting in a change of concentration gradient at the tissue. The interaction of these factors therefore regulates the entry of an active substance into its effector biophase (receptor) and determines the resultant pharmacological response. It is true that the design of compounds to optimise *in vivo* their intrinsic activity at the receptor is one of the major challenges facing the medicinal chemist.

3.3.1.1   *Affinity*

The distribution of a molecule is largely affected by its affinity for the various tissues of the organism and particularly by its relative solubility in the various constituents of the biophase which present a succession of aqueous (plasma, intra, and extracellular fluids) and lipid (membranal) components. This affinity is governed by the intrinsic properties of the molecule which are both physicochemical and structural in nature. The physicochemical affinity of a drug molecule thus depends on the balance between its hydrophilic and lipophilic properties and may be measured by its partition coefficient (P). The rate of transfer through a lipid membrane is linearly related to the value of log P until a certain maximum rate is reached; only compounds with an intermediate value are likely to cross both lipid and aqueous barriers and, conse-quently, be extensively distributed throughout the body to reach the specific site of action. These considerations form the basis for the nonlinear (parabolic) models of quantitative structure derived by Hansch and others (Chapter 5) which demonstrate that an optimal partition coefficient exists for biological activity in a series of homologous compounds with a range of partition coefficients.

The affinity which is determined by the molecular structure of a xenobiotic defines its interaction with endogenous protein or lipid macromolecules and, to some extent, account for variations in structural specificity in a series of homologues. In the extreme, the presence of an asymmetric site in a molecule is sufficient to cause stereo-specificity of both drug disposition and biological response for the two enantiomers. Two types of binding between xenobiotics and the endogenous macromoleules can be differentiated:-

(1) Specific binding with an effector molecule which induces a biological response. This response may be a pharmacological effect (or side effect); activation of an enzyme responsible for the biotransformation (metabolism) of the xenobiotic; or activation of membrane proteins responsible for its trans-membrane movement. This type of binding is usually of high affinity, very structure dependent, and is sensitive to any asymmetry in the compounds

(2) Nonspecific binding does not usually result in specific biological responses but may significantly affect the pharmokinetics and notably the distribution of a xenobiotic. Nonspecific tissue and plasma protein binding are of particular importance where both ionic and lipophilic forces are present and affect the available plasma fraction present at a given membrane for further distribution. The overall affinity of a compound for a given tissue can be measured by determination of its tissue to blood partition coefficient.

3.3.1.2   *Physiological factors affecting distribution*

Physiological factors can profoundly affect the distribution of drug substances. and the processes in blood/tissue disposition are summarised in Figure 3.8.

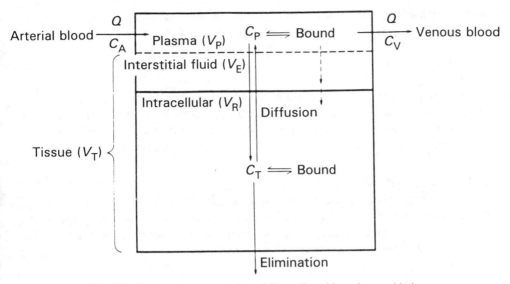

Fig. 3.8.   Schematic representation of tissue disposition of a xenobiotic.

The key factors are:

(1) The intensity of blood flow, which determines blood/tissue concentration gradients.
(2) Blood to tissue diffusion across the various membrane barriers, notably the capillary endothelium and cellular membranes.
(3) Blood and tissue binding

The distribution of xenobiotica may be perfusion-rate or diffusion-rate limited depending on the absence or presence of blood to tissue diffusion limitation. Assuming that perfusion limitation occurs, the amount of substance in tissue A_T is given by equation (1):

$$\frac{dA_T}{dt} = QC_A - QC_V - \text{elimination rate} \tag{1}$$

where C_A and C_V denote the respective arterial and venous concentrations.

For a tissue not taking part in drug elimination, assuming a constant arterial concentration (e.g. during constant rate infusion) the tissue concentration time curve is given by:

$$C_T = K_P C_A [1 - \exp(-k_T t)] \tag{2}$$

where K_P denotes the tissue to blood partition, and k_T is a first order-rate content. K_P is dependent on both the physicochemical and structural affinities of the xenobiotic and k_T is proportional to blood flow and inversely proportional to the affinity:

$$k_T = \frac{Q}{K_P V_T} \tag{3}$$

At a constant rate of presentation the amount of drug substance taken up by a tissue therefore increases until a steady state is achieved. The steady-state tissue concentration $(C_{T,SS})$ is directly related to the affinity of the drug for the tissue:

$$C_{T,SS} = K_P \, C_A \qquad\qquad (4)$$

Thus, at steady state the distribution of the substance in a given tissue depends only on the affinity of the substance for the tissue. In continual blood flow it plays a major role in early distribution, notably for compounds which diffuse readily through lipid membranes (i.e. those which have a high lipid to water partition coefficient).

3.3.1.3   The distribution compartment
Tissues and organs with similar distribution characteristics can be grouped in a single distribution compartment. This is defined as a space in which the drug distributes with the same dynamics to achieve a homogeneous steady-state concentration. The space is characterised by an apparent volume (V) which relates the amount of drug (A) in the compartment to the concentration

$$C = \frac{A}{V} \text{(at any time } t) \qquad\qquad (5)$$

The distribution volume will initially vary unless an equilibrium is achieved instantaneously. After an intravenous bolus injection an initial distribution phase is generally observed corresponding to the penetration of highly perfused tissues, and the apparent volume of this initial distribution space usually comprises the plasma volume and the total body water volume (the central compartment). Equilibration in this compartment is generally rapid because of blood flow. Simultaneous penetration into deeper compartments occurs where affinity governs the achievement of the steady state. The total volume of distribution, or steady state distribution volume, is the sum of the volumes of each compartment at steady state.

3.3.2   Critical factors affecting distribution
Distribution of a drug substance from the systemic circulation into the diverse organs and tissues of the body necessitates its diffusion through the tissue matrices and cell walls. Physiological factors and the physicochemical properties of the drug substance both affect the rate and extent of its distribution. Nonspecific distribution processes such as the route of administration, absorption, and of drug clearance will also affect blood to tissue concentration gradient and hence distribution.

3.3.2.1   Blood flow
The blood flow is a primary factor affecting drug distribution, influencing both its qualitative and quantitative uptake in all tissues. A schematic distribution of the body vascularisation in relation to administration and elimination is shown in Figure 3.9.

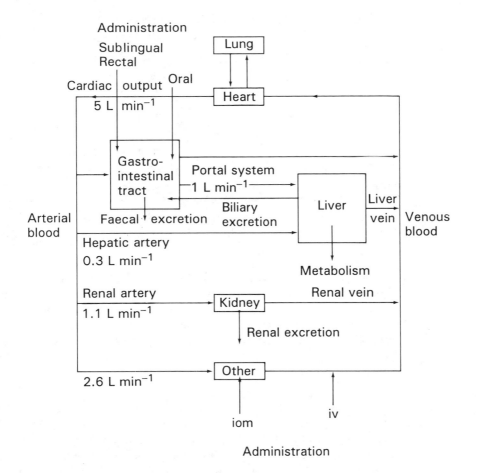

Fig. 3.9.   Schematic distribution of body vascularisation in relation to administration and elimination routes.

The rate-limiting step of drug distribution is either the blood flow rate which determines delivery of the drug to tissues, or transmembrane transfer processes which take place are both at capillary and cellular levels. Marked differences in blood flow occur between the various organs which can result in qualitative differences in initial distribution of the drug substance throughout the body as indicated in Figure 3.10. The lungs receive the total cardiac output, from which arterial output is distributed to the other organs as illustrated.

The liver and kidney are the primary organs engaged in drug elimination and receive 52% of the cardiac output, indicating their importance in determining the disposition of xenobiotica. Muscle and brain tissue are also highly perfused organs although brain uptake is diffusion rate rather than perfusion rate limited.

Variations in blood to tissue partition coefficient can profoundly affect the development of the pharmacological response, whilst long equilibration times with

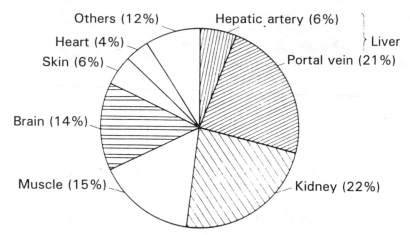

Fig. 3.10.   Schematic distribution of blood flow in man (percentage of cardiac output).

tissues can also affect drug removal from the body and hence its plasma half-life. Blood flow also varies significantly between species, resulting in significant inter-species distribution of a given drug substance and the consequent differences in pharmacokinetic profiles. In some disease states, most notably circulatory failure, the physiopathological status of the animal may profoundly affect blood flow as a result of decreased cardiac output thus resulting in increased exposure of the brain and heart to an administered drug.

3.3.2.2   Protein binding

The binding of drugs to macromolecules in the body is a major contributor to the distribution of a drug. The affinity of a drug substance for acceptor proteins depends on its physicochemical properties and the conformation of the acceptor protein, and may be specific or nonspecific in nature. Serum protein binding represents a very important example of nonspecific binding affinity which markedly affects drug distribution. Only unbound drug substance can penetrate the interstitial fluid, the lymph, and subsequently the cells by passive diffusion. Material bound to the blood proteins represents a circulating reservoir of potentially available drug substance which can affect distribution with time.

   The main protein present in blood and tissues is albumin which accounts for most of the nonspecific binding for the majority of drug substances. Albumin also carries endogenous materials such as bilirubin and fatty acids. The amount of albumin present in a tissue depends on the extracellular fluid present with some 60% of exchangeable albumin usually being found outside the circulation. Protein–xenobiotic complexes result from two types of binding:

(1) reversible binding due to ionic, hydrogen, hydrophobic or Van der Waals' bonding;
(2) covalent irreversible binding, frequently a cause of specific drug toxicity such as cytotoxicity, genotoxicity or oculotoxicity.

Depending on the binding capacity of circulating plasma proteins and the tissue proteins a drug substance may be confined to the vascular space, distributed in the tissues, or present in both the vascular space and selective tissues. Drugs which do not enter intra cellular space have low volumes of distribution. High values for distribution volume which exceed that of total body water (42 L) have no physiological significance other than providing a rough estimate of extrovascular distribution in the body. Only a weak correlation exists between plasma and tissue binding although the same physicochemical factors are present. Within a homologous series a relationship exists between plasma protein binding and distribution volume. Interindividual variations in drug distribution for a given drug substance are frequently observed, depending on the physiopathological status of the individual, notably changes in protein concentration, lean body mass and body fat distribution.

3.3.2.3   *Membrane transfer*

Of fundamental importance in tissue distribution is the ability of a drug molecule to cross biological membranes. The three major processes of membrane transport are passive diffusion, carrier-mediated diffusion, and pinocytosis, all of which are dependent on the physiochemical properties of the drug and the biochemical properties of the membrane concerned.

Biological membranes are essentially lipid–protein structures (see Chapter 4) so that the lipophilic/hydrophilic properties of the molecule will determine its affinity for the membrane and its consequent passage by passive diffusion. The driving force for such a diffusion process is dependent on the drug concentration gradient on both sides of the membrane. This process is unsaturable and no structure specificity is required for this transfer process. Only the unionised lipid soluble fraction of the molecule is transferable through the membrane. A difference in pH between the two compartments separated by the membrane will affect the distribution of incompletely ionised substances like weak acids and bases. Small hydrosoluble molecules, on the other hand, may diffuse through membranes via aqueous channels. Diffusion is then controlled by the molecular charge and volume of the solute relative to the pore sizes in the membrane, typically 5–10 Å, although this may be considerably larger (50–100 Å) in capillary membranes.

Large lipid insoluble or ionised molecules, on the other hand, may be transported by carrier-mediated systems present in certain membranes. The solute molecule binds to a surface component of the membrane and the resultant solute–carrier complex diffuses through the membrane. When the solute is released the carrier returns to the external surface. The process may be passive, where the driving force is still the concentration gradient of the solute (facilitated diffusion), or active where the transport process is associated with energy production. In this situation the solute may move against a concentration gradient (active transport). In these situations structural specificity may be high and the processes are subject to competitive inhibition by analogues or other molecules (including endogenous compounds) which competitively bind to the carrier. Drug interactions are frequently a result of such competitive processes. Since these transfer processes are dependent on energy derived from cell metabolic processess they may be also inhibited by substances which interfere with this metabolism. Both transport processes are saturable and may lead to nonlinearity in both pharmacokinetic behaviour and elimination processes.

Transmembrane transport may also occur by pinocytosis. This results from invaginations of the membrane which lead to intracytoplasmic vesicles, entrapping fluid and molecules into the cells. Enzymatic degradation of the vesicles subsequently releases the drug substance into the cytoplasm of the cell. Pinocytosis is a slow, nonselective process of uncertain biological significance, possible playing a role in the cellular uptake of peptides, proteins and other macromolecules. The process requires energy and may be noncompetitively inhibited by metabolic poisons.

3.3.3   Distributions of specific interest

3.3.3.1   *Central nervous system*
The distribution of drug substances into the CNS is of fundamental importance since many drugs manifest either directly or indirectly pronounced CNS effects. The pharmacological receptors for psychotropic drugs are situated within the CNS as are the target cells for many other agents such as antineoplastic and antibiotics. Peripherally acting drugs such as the antihistamines and β-blockers manifest their side effects via penetration of the CNS. To enter the CNS drug substances must penetrate two specific anatomical barriers namely the blood–brain barrier (BBB) and the blood–cerebrospinal fluid barrier (CSF).

The blood–brain barrier results from the structure of the complex cerebral capillary network and its protective features. The capillary endothelium consists of a cell layer with a continuous tight intercellular junction containing no pores together with characteristic astrocyte cells which are elements of the supporting tissue. These are found at the base of the endothelial membrane and form a solid envelope around the capillaries and also secrete trophic factors essential for the maintenance of the blood-brain barrier biology. To be distributed within the brain all compounds must cross this multilayered barrier either by passive diffusion or active transport. The primary role of the BBB is to maintain the brain in a stable liquid environment, modification of which could cause neurological disturbance. The barrier is effective not only against xenobiotics but also endogenous metabolism products such as the neurotransmitters whose cerebral concentration must be strictly regulated lest major changes severely affect the functioning of the CNS.

Polar nutrients such as hexoses, amino acids and water-soluble vitamins are transported by active transport mechanisms, and, in some cases, these membrane carriers also act as receptors.

The blood–CSF barrier is essentially composed of the epithelium of the chloroid plexus which is responsible for the active secretion of CSF. The capillaries in the chloroid plexus contain pores but the plexus epithelial cells are joined by continuous tight junctions as found in the BBB. Substances normally enter the CSF via the chloroid plexus, the epithelium of which is very similar in structure and function to renal epithelium. Transport through this barrier may also be via active transport systems. Although similar mechanisms operate for diffusion into both the CNS and

CSF the degree of relative uptake can be quite different. Thus for instance, some antibiotics, notably cephalotin and trimethoprim, achieve much lower levels in the CNS than the CSF, whilst for the β-blockers the reverse is true. The blood–brain barrier may be modified under a number of physiological and pathological conditions, such as metabolic acidosis or alkalosis, hypertension, old age, psychotic states and inflammatory conditions. Certain drugs, notably the psychotropics, may also affect membrane permeability. Certain areas of the CNS are not protected by the BBB, notably the hypothalamus which controls prolactin secretion and the trigger area which controls emesis. Intranasal administration of certain drugs may also result in penetration of the CNS via the submucosal areas of the nose and the subarachnoid space of the olfactive lobe.

The physicochemical properties of a drug substance which apply to transport across other membrane barriers also apply to transport across the BBB. Diffusion is facilitated for drug substances with a low ionisation at physiological pH and a high lipid solubility. A linear relationship is usually observed between lipophilicity and biological response for a series of homologous drugs for a range of log P values, beyond which there is a limited penetration of the BBB and hence limited biological activity. The lipophilicity range for most series of drugs with CNS activity is typically from a log P value of 1.2 to 2.4 with a value of log P around 2 being considered optimum. Molecular weight, which may limit passive diffusion (penetration decreases with increasing molecular weight) and active transport (notably of ionised substances), may also significantly affect penetration of the BBB and hence the biological activity of a xenobiotic.

3.3.3.2 *The bacterial membrane*

Regardless of the site of infection in the body and the resulting tissue distribution necessary for effective treatment, antibiotics face another barrier on the route to their target, namely the bacterial cell wall. This additional barrier, which protects the invading microorganism, is notable both for its rigidity and permeability. Bacteria may be classified into two groups, Gram-positive and Gram-negative, the structures of which are represented schematically in Figure 3.11.

Gram-negative bacteria possess an additional outer membrane consisting of a biolipidic layer containing lipopolysaccharides and phospholipids with waterfilled pores. The peptidoglycan layer, however, is thinner than in Gram-positive bacteria. Some bacteria also have an additional external envelope or capsule which is rich in proteins and polysaccharides, with the membrane being characteristic for a given bacterial strain, but it may be modified in mutants. The inner cytoplasmic membrane contains the enzyme systems which assist in the active transport of nutrients and the synthesis of membrane constituents.

Mutant bacterial strains become resistant to antibiotics because of their ability to increase synthesis of degradative enzymes and to generate protein receptor sites which irreversibly bind the antibiotic family.

Bacterial wall penetration is affected by the same processes as passage through other membrane barriers—diffusion (primarily passive) taking place in the external membrane whilst the internal membranes are transgressed by active processes.

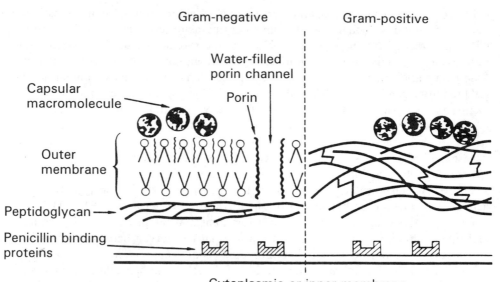

Fig. 3.11.   Schematic representation of the structure of bacterial membrane.

Antibacterial agents cross the additional external membrane of Gram-negative bacteria either by nonspecific passive diffusion through membrane channels or diffusion across the biolipic layer. The mechanisms of transfer for certain antibacterials through bacteria membranes are summarised in Figure 3.12.

Mechanism	Location	Antibacterials
Passive diffusion	Outer membrane	Aminosides
		Chloramphenicol
		Cycloserine
		β-Lactams
		Quinolones
		Tetracyclines
	Cytoplasmic or inner membrane	Chloramphenicol
Facilitated diffusion	Outer membrane	Fosfomycin
		Peptides
Active transport	Cytoplasmic or inner membrane	Aminosides
		Cycloserine
		Peptides
		Tetracyclines

Fig. 3.12.   Mechanisms of transfer of antibacterials through bacterial membrane.

Many structure activity relationships have been carried out for antibiotics, but few studies deal with the relationship between transmembranal passage of the bacterial cell and the physicochemical properties of the antibacterial family. It is necessary that the hydrophobic properties be distinguished from the electrical charge on the drugs. It should be noted that hydration shells around charged groups cause hydrophilicity of the drug thus facilitating penetration through porin channels. This is particularly seen for zwitterionic β-lactams and these channels favour cationic passage over anionic. In zwitterionic compounds hydrophobicity is of little consequence for membrane penetration; in contrast the penetration of anionic cephalosporins is closely related to their hydrophobicity as measured by the partition coefficient. Size becomes a factor only for anionic compounds of high molecular weight, although considerable differences are observed for different bacterial strains of the same family. The relationship between the physicochemical properties of antibacterial agents and the efficiency of diffusion is complex. This is because of the complexity of the bacterial cell wall, the existence of specific carriers, and the presence of porin channels.

3.4 CLEARANCE

3.4.1 General principles

3.4.1.1 Physiological and kinetic aspects

The concept of clearance of a drug substance includes all elimination processes which act to remove it from the physiological areas and which are facilitated if affinity is weak. Clearance of xenobiotics is achieved either by irreversible elimination or by biotransformation into derivatives with lower affinity characteristics, thus increasing their elimination rate. Clearance, consequently, is an all-important consideration which limits duration of the active substance in the organism, consequently modifying its duration in the biophase. An understanding of its nature is therefore necessary in designing the desired therapeutic regimen.

The clearance concept was first introduced to describe the renal excretion of endogenous compounds such as creatinine and urea, and was defined as the ratio of renal excretion rate to the arterial concentration of the compound. The concept which was introduced as a measure of kidney function has been extended to other eliminating organs such as the liver and lungs, and elimination pathways for endogenous and exogenous compounds (xenobiotics) and the physiological processes concerned are like those for distribution as illustrated in Figure 3.8.

The organ elimination rate of xenobiotics is expressed as:

$$\frac{\mathrm{d}A_\mathrm{E}}{\mathrm{d}t} = Q\,(C_\mathrm{A} - C_\mathrm{V}) \tag{6}$$

where the amount, A_E eliminated per unit time is calculated from equation (1), under steady-state conditions where $\mathrm{d}A_\mathrm{T}/\mathrm{d}t = 0$

The steady-state arteriovenous gradient normalised to the arterial concentration defines the extraction ratio E (equation (7)) which characterizes the intrinsic capability of the organ to extract a xenobiotic:

$$E = \frac{C_\mathrm{A} - C_\mathrm{V}}{C_\mathrm{A}} \tag{7}$$

The organ clearance Cl, is the product of blood flow and the organ extraction ratio and can vary from zero ($E = 0$, noneliminating organ) to the upper limit of organ blood flow ($E = 1$):

$$Cl = \frac{\text{Elimination rate}}{C_A} = QE \qquad (8)$$

Clearance is expressed in volume per unit time and may be defined as the volume of reference fluid (blood, plasma) cleared of a xenobiotic (total, unbound) per unit time. Clearance from an organ is thus the proportionality constant between the elimination rate and the arterial concentration. It is measured by the slope of the elimination rate–arterial concentration relationship (Figure 3.13) and obeys first-order kinetics. In such situations organ clearance is independent of the arterial concentration and, consequently, the administered dose. As drug concentration increases, diffusion from the arterial blood may become saturated (capacity limited) and the elimination rate is no longer proportional to the arterial concentration, approaching a maximum value, V_{max} (Figure 3.14).

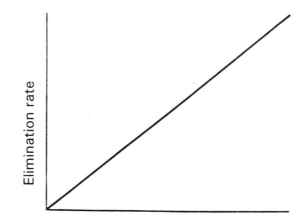

Fig. 3.13.   Kinetic aspects of organ elimination; first-order elimination.

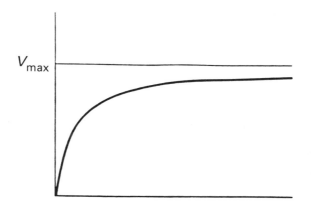

Fig. 3.14.   Capacity-limited elimination.

Such an elimination rate–arterial concentration obeys Michaelis–Menten kinetics (Chapter 4):

$$\text{Elimination rate} = \frac{V_{\max} C_A}{K_m + C_A} \tag{9}$$

where K_m, the Michaelis–Menten constant, denotes the concentration at which the elimination rate equals half the maximum. The clearance is no longer constant but inversely proportional to the drug concentration, and, consequently, the administered dose:

$$Cl = \frac{V_{\max}}{K_m + C_A} \tag{10}$$

When C_A has a much lower value than K_m the kinetics become first order since clearance is approximately the ratio of $V_{\max}$ to K_m, and the elimination rate becomes proportional to concentration. Within a given range of doses and concentrations all elimination pathways will thus follow first-order kinetics resulting in constant organ clearance. When C_A has a much higher value than K_m the elimination rate becomes essentially constant, approaching $V_{\max}$ (zero-order kinetics).

3.4.1.2 *Pharmacokinetic considerations*

The complete clearance of a xenobiotic from the body is the addition of each separate clearance which is characteristic of the separate elimination pathways. The two basic elimination processes are excretion, essentially renal and biliary in which the xenobiotic is eliminated unchanged and metabolism, mainly via the liver, where the xenobiotic is chemically transformed before elimination. The processes of drug metabolism will be discussed later in this chapter.

If all elimination pathways have first-order kinetics, the overall elimination of a xenobiotic will exhibit linear pharmacokinetics, and plasma levels will be proportional to the administered dose (Figure 3.15). The total body clearance, in this case, will be independent of the dose, route of administration, and the dosage regimen.

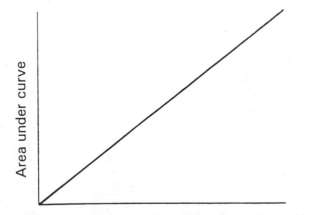

Fig. 3.15.   Plasma level versus dose relationships in linear pharmacokinetics.

When overall elimination is dependent on an elimination pathway with concentration and dose-dependent clearance, then total body clearance will also depend on concentration and dose-dependent clearance, and the plasma levels will no longer be proportional to dose (Figure 3.16). For such nonlinear pharmacokinetics, however, there will be a range of doses for which the kinetics approximate to linear, and most drugs exhibit linear pharmacokinetics in the normal therapeutic dose ranges. Particular attention has to be paid to those drugs with dose-dependent kinetics at therapeutic levels (notably the antiepileptics) since the clinically safe dose may easily be exceeded with resultant side effects.

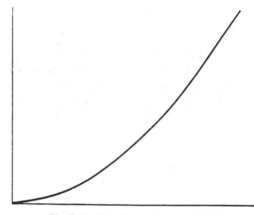

Fig. 3.16.   Nonlinear pharmacokinetics.

3.4.2   Critical factors affecting hepatic clearance

3.4.2.1   *Physiological aspects*
The liver is the primary organ concerned in clearance of a drug substance both because of its enormous blood supply and its capacity to chemically transform or metabolise xenobiotics. Hepatic clearance is consequently complex, depending on two independent processes, namely metabolism by the hepatic enzymes and biliary excretion, both of the parent substance and any subsequent metabolites, via the bile into the GI tract.

Since the blood supply to the liver is both via the hepatic artery and the portal system (Figure 3.9) orally administered drugs pass through the liver before their systemic circulation and are subjected to the hepatic elimination processes before becoming systemically available to all other tissues. Significant chemical transformation of the drug substance may take place (first-pass effect) which may have a profound influence on the bioavailability and pharmacological effects (activation or deactivation) of the drug substance. Xenobiotics may also be degraded or metabolised in the gastrointestinal lumen or in the GI membranes before passage through the liver, but this is a minor contributor to the first-pass effect. Extensive first-pass metabolism will result in low absolute bioavailability and a different ratio of metabolites to parent substance compared with the intravenous route (direct access to the systemic circulation) resulting in differences in biological responses. Extensive first-pass metabolism may also result in unpredictable pharmacokinetics with consequent implications for the drug effect and the clinical efficacy.

Hepatic clearance may vary from species to species and within the same species. Many physiological factors (such as age, sex, physical stress) as well as pathological factors (liver dysfunction, disease) affecting blood flow and enzymatic activity can also influence the first-pass effect. For compounds which undergo extensive first-pass metabolism other routes of administration may be used (see section 3.2).

3.4.2.2   *Metabolic and biliary clearance*
Most drug substances are biotransformed before clearance, relatively few being excreted unchanged via the kidney. The major processes of drug metabolism will be discussed in detail later. The primary role of metabolism is to decrease the lipophilicity of the parent compound molecule in order to facilitate its clearance as more polar metabolites via biliary and renal excretion. Whilst such metabolism generally results in loss of biological activity for most drugs, on some occasions increased or altered pharmacological effects and toxicity are observed. The enzymatic processes of metabolism are capacity-limited processes and, consequently, are a primary cause of nonlinear pharmacokinetics.

Metabolism of drug substances is a major concern for the medicinal chemist since many QSAR are derived by using *in vitro* correlations of biological activity and become invalid *in vivo* in cases where extensive metabolism takes place. Hydrophilic compounds which are relatively polar are generally little metabolised and are mainly eliminated directly by the renal and biliary routes. As the lipophilicity of compounds increases, clearance of drugs changes from renal to metabolic both for orally and intravenously administered drugs.

Bile flow, resulting from secretory activity of the hepatocyte, is generally slow (1 mL/min in man), but biliary clearance may be high as secreted compounds concentrate in the bile and achieve very high bile to plasma concentrations. Transfer of drug substances across the biliary epithelium into the bile occurs by active secretory processes with different transport mechanisms for anionic, cationic, and neutral compounds. Materials excreted in the bile are stored in the gall bladder and subsequently released into the intestine from which they are eliminated in the faeces or reabsorbed through the intestinal membrane completing an enterohepatic cycle (Figure 3.9).

The presence of polar groups in a drug substance facilitates biliary excretion, lipophilic molecules tending to be reabsorbed across the hepatic canaliculi. Higher molecular weight (>500) favours biliary excretion; xenobiotics and their metabolites with lower molecular weight are preferentially excreted in the urine. The relative amounts of urinary and biliary excretion will vary between animal species for each xenobiotica.

3.4.3   Critical factors affecting renal clearance

3.4.3.1   *Physiological factors*
The kidney, with the liver, constitutes the major route of excretion for the majority

of drug substances and their metabolites. Renal clearance is the result of the three physiological processes, glomerular filtration, tubular secretion, and reabsorption, which together produce urine. The functional unit which controls these processes is the nephron (Figure 3.17) which consists of a glomerulus linked to a tubule. Urine is formed in the glomeruli by passive filtration of blood through a membrane barrier consisting of epithelium with very wide pores, only blood cells and high molecular weight proteins (molecular weight exceeding 68 000) escaping filtration.

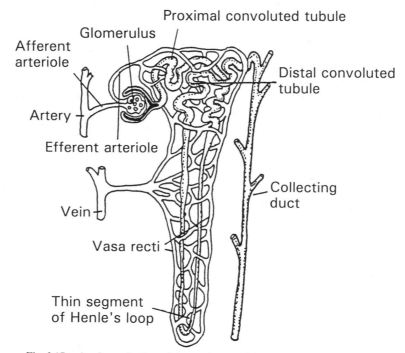

Fig. 3.17.   A schematic view of the nephron and its associated blood supply.

The glomerular filter also acts as a negatively charged barrier preventing filtration of anionic compounds. Any free fraction of a drug substance that is not bound to proteins, erythrocytes or other blood components is excreted by glomerular filtration. Tubular secretion occurs primarily in the proximal convoluted tubule, but only ionised fractions are secreted. The active transport processes are saturable and, consequently, drug binding to plasma proteins is not a limiting factor. Anionic and cationic forms are not excreted in the same segments of the provisional tubules.

Reabsorption also takes place along all sections of the tubules, and, although active transport processes exist for certain physiologically important substances, the reabsorption of most drugs is a passive process depending upon the pH of the urine and urinary flow. Urinary pH can vary from pH 4.5 to pH 8.5 significantly affecting the degree of ionisation of an excreted drug and hence passive absorption of the non-ionised fraction. Acid urine results in reduced excretion of weak acids and promotes that of weak bases. Drug absorption is also inversely related to urinary flow and depends upon the relative permeability of the drug across the tubular membrane.

3.4.3.2 Physicochemical factors

Overall elimination of an unchanged drug or its metabolites by the kidney depends both on the molecular weight, which affects the renal biliary balance, and the lipophilicity of the compounds, renal excretion being favoured by decreased lipophilicity (expressed by log P). The degree of ionisation of the drug and its metabolites is also a factor governing tubular reabsorption rates. Plasma protein binding also affects renal excretion of all drugs which are predominantly excreted by glomerular filtration and has been invoked to explain significant differences in renal excretion observed for certain drug stereoisomers.

3.5 SITES OF DRUG METABOLISM

3.5.1 Liver

The liver is the major site of metabolism for xenobiotics in the body and drug substances, subsequent to their systemic availability, may be subjected to a rapid initial metabolism before exercising their desired therapeutic effects. The liver is amongst the largest organs in the human body weighing around 1.5 kg in man and, unlike other tissues, has a dual blood supply. The liver receives its blood supply via the hepatic artery (25%) and portal vein (75%), and, since the major portion of the gastrointestinal blood supply drains into the portal system, all orally administered drugs pass through the liver before reaching the systemic circulation (the first-pass effect). Thus the liver with its considerable metabolising activity has a very considerable influence on the status of an administered drug and on the concentrations of subsequent metabolites available for exerting pharmacological effects on all other tissues.

The extent to which xenobiotics are metabolised by the liver or other tissues is dependent not only on the intrinsic metabolic activity of the organ but on a number of physiological and physicochemical factors. Blood flow, protein binding, and lipid solubility of a drug substance all exert a significant effect on drug metabolism. When the intrinsic clearance is high relative to blood flow, indicative of high binding of the drug in the liver, the first-pass effect for a drug becomes of major significance. Lipophilic drugs inevitably bind more readily to numerous intracellular membranes and the uptake of a drug is related to its ease of passage through the hepatocellular membrane. Highly lipophilic drugs may be stored in these membranes from which they may be released for their metabolism, biliary elimination, or subsequent systemic circulation.

The enzyme systems primarily responsible for the metabolism of drug substances (which may result in the formation of inactive or active metabolites of the xenobiotic) are stored in the endoplasmic reticulum, the normal physiological role of which is for protein and fatty acid synthesis. A large number of essential glycoproteins, fatty acids, prostaglandins, cholesterol and the bile acids are synthesised and transformed in the liver. A number of other enzyme systems occur elsewhere in the hepatocyte and also contribute to drug metabolism, resulting in the importance of the liver as the primary drug metabolising site in the body. The enzymes found in drug metabolism in all tissues are conveniently classified into two types, notably those which carry out oxidative and reductive transformations (phase I reactions) and those which derivatise or conjugate (phase II reactions). Phase I reactions are nonspecific for drug structure and may carry out numerous metabolic transformations, whilst phase II reactions are specific for certain chemical groupings within the drug structure with the object of enhancing water solubility (decreasing lipophilicity) of the parent substance. The metabolic reactions carried out in all tissues are described in detail later.

3.5.2   Gastrointestinal tract

For convenience most modern medicines are administered orally and pass into the body via the gastrointestinal tract. Traditionally the gastrointestinal tract was considered to take part only in the absorption process, and any presystemic metabolism via this route was considered relatively unimportant. The gastrointestinal tract, together with its resident microflora, however, has a metabolic capacity approaching that of the liver. The mucosa of the small intestine contain a wide range of phase I and phase II enzyme systems, some of which are highly adaptive to the presence of xenobiotics and can be stimulated by their presence to the levels found in the liver. In the absence of the xenobiotics, however, the enzyme activity may disappear completely. Alcohol metabolism in the gastrointestinal tract by the enzyme alcohol dehydrogenase is comparable to that in the liver. Ester hydrolysis and conjugation reactions are the most important transformations carried out by the gut wall. Glutathione conjugation is an important protective mechanism against toxicity induced by xenobiotics, and this enzyme plays an important role in the intestine.

The gastrointestinal tract is not normally sterile (unless treated by antibiotics), and the microflora of the gut present a diverse and highly adaptive metabolic challenge for a wide range of administered drugs. The absence of microflora produces morphological changes in the intestine resulting in the stomach upsets occasionally seen after oral antibiotic therapy. Owing to the acidic environment of the stomach the microflora are usually confined to the lower gut and consist of facultative anaerobes such as staphylococci and lactobacilli with strict anaerobes such as Bacteroides and Bifidobacteria, the most abundant. Although the microflora population of the adult is usually stable in the healthy state it may be influenced by diet or drug therapy. Presystemic metabolism by the microflora is likely to be minimal for well absorbed drugs but can be extensive for poorly absorbed substances which remain for extensive periods in the gastrointestinal tract. The major part of metabolism occurs in the hind gut and is relatively important, consequently, for those drugs administered as suppositories (per rectum) as opposed to orally.

Microfloral metabolism is significantly different from the phase I and II reactions which take place in the tissues since the relevant processes are hydrolytic, reductive and cleavage reactions. The consequence is, therefore, the generation of metabolites which are more lipophilic, have increased pharmacological (and toxicological) activity, and are more slowly eliminated. The major hydrolytic reaction accomplished by the gut microflora is glucoronide hydrolysis, which means that many substances which have been excreted in the bile as inactive glucoronides will be regenerated and reabsorbed, with their consequent pharmacological properties, via the enterohepatic circulation.

Reductive reactions by microflora are prevalent, with the most important entailing nitro and azo group reductions, but also notably aldehydes, alcohols, sulphoxides and double bonds. Diverse reactions carried out by the microflora include dehydroxylation, decarboxylation, dealkylation, dehalogenation, deamination and aromatisation.

3.5.3 Kidney

The kidney possesses the majority of enzyme systems found in the liver, and these are located in the cortex of the smooth endoplasmic reticulum of the proximal tubules. It is the proximal tubules which are exposed to the greatest quantities of glomerular filtration on the luminal side and the highest blood concentrations of the drug on the contraluminal side. The drug metabolising enzymatic activity of the kidney is considerably lower than that of the liver, however. Glucoronide conjugation in the kidney, for instance, is estimated to be only 3–4% of that of the liver. Impairment of renal function not only affects clearance of drugs eliminated via this organ, but also reduces levels of cytochrome P-450 which also affects drug metabolism.

3.5.4 Lung

The lungs are important for the metabolism of xenobiotics as they have the versatility of the liver, although of a much reduced capacity. Inhaled substances are extensively metabolised in a first-pass effect by the lungs. The lungs have an important role in the metabolism of endogenous compounds which reach the lungs via the pulmonary circulation. Biogenic amines such as noradrenaline and S-hydroxytryptamine are selectively metabolised, resulting in their pharmacological deactivation. Angiotensin I, on the other hand, is activated by cleavage to the octapeptide angiotensin II by the angiotensin converting enzyme (ACE).

The lung carries out a number of oxidative reactions (cytochrome P-450) as well as reductive and hydrolytic reactions, the hydrolysis of epoxides being a major defence mechanism for the body. Conjugation with glutathione, glucuronic acid, sulphate and N-acetylation also occur in the lung. The anaesthetics which are administered by inhalation are, surprisingly, not metabolised by the lungs and manifest their toxicity in the liver and kidney.

3.5.5 Other tissues

Practically all tissues of the body contain drug metabolising enzymes although of little significance in terms of general metabolism of xenobiotics. The skin, the largest organ of the body, contains a large number of oxidases, reductases and esterases primarily located in the epidermis, although its primary role is as a lipophilic barrier to hydrophilic compounds.

The blood-brain barrier likewise provides a protective barrier but also contains enzymes producing phase I and phase II reactions. The sulphation of biogenic amines in the blood–brain barrier is of metabolic importance. The metabolism of endogenous amines in the brain is of importance for their physiological effects.

The blood is an extremely important source of esterase activity for carboxylic acids and, for certain drugs such as procaine and malathion, hydrolysis is faster than in the liver. Aspirin, cocaine, heroin and other morphine esters are extensively hydrolysed in the blood. N-acetylation of certain drugs such as sulphanilamide and sulphamethazine also occurs in the blood.

3.6   BIOTRANSFORMATION

3.6.1   Introduction

It must be appreciated that the pure drug substance which is adminstered in a pharmaceutical formulation is normally extensively transformed by the metabolic systems of the body; such transformations resulting in the generation of active or inactive metabolites and, of great significance for toxicity, the generation of highly reactive unstable intermediates. It is, in principle, feasible to design new drug substances to optimise pharmacological effects or, reduce or eliminate toxicity and side effects of the original molecules, taking advantage of its biotransformation subsequent to its systemic availability.

3.6.2   Prodrugs

A prodrug is a compound which has to undergo an initial *in vivo* biotransformation to elicit its pharmacological response. The prodrug itself is pharmacologically inactive and is used to improve both the pharmacodynamic properties of the parent substance such as side effects and toxicity, as well as biopharmaceutical properties including drug stability, absorption and duration of action. There are many obstacles that prevent or limit drug action, and the prodrug is designed to minimise the undesirable property and yet to be cleared both rapidly and efficiently *in vivo* by enzymatic or chemical reactions. The protective moiety has by definition to be rapidly and innocuously eliminated otherwise the prodrug itself will have significant pharmacodynamic and pharmokinetic implications for clinical toxicity.

Enzymatic conversion of a prodrug depends on the presence of an appropriate enzyme in the body to cleave the protective moiety from the drug, and it depends on sufficient concentrations of the enzyme to generate the active principle consistently. Some enzymes used in the cleavage of prodrugs (usually hydrolases) are listed in Table 3.1.

Few processes exist for chemical cleavage of prodrugs by nonenzymatic processes, these being essentially limited to pH-dependent hydrolysis in the stomach (pH 1–4), the intestine (pH 5–8) and the blood (pH 7.4). The pH differences of these organs have been exploited, however, to obtain prodrugs with increased gastric stability (and a reduced gastric irritation) which are subsequently cleaved to the active substance in the intestine or blood.

A large number of applications of the prodrug principle in optimising drug performance characteristics exist and are the subject of numerous works and reviews.[1] Taste is a frequently encountered problem with drug substances as many molecules possess an extremely unpleasant taste when dissolved in the saliva. Decreasing aqueous solubility, notably in ester derivatives, obviates this problem; chloramphen-

Table 3.1.   Some of the enzymes used in the hydrolysis of prodrugs

Prodrug linkage	Hydrolysing enzyme
Ester	
Short-medium chain	Cholinesterase
Aliphatic	Ester hydrolase
	Lipase
	Cholesterol esterase
	Acetylcholinesterase
	Aldehyde oxidase
	Carboxypeptidase
Long-chain aliphatic carbonate	Pancreatic lipase
	Pancreatin
	Lipase
	Carboxypeptidase
	Cholinesterase
Phosphate, organic	Acid phosphatase
	Alkaline phosphatase
Sulphate, organic	Steroid sulphatase
Amide	Amidase
Amino acid	Proteolytic enzymes
	Chymotrypsins A and B
	Trypsin
	Carboxypeptidase A and B
Azo	Azo reductase
Carbamate	Carbamidase
Phosphamide	Phosphoramidases
β-Glucuronide	β-Glucuronidase
N-Acetylglucosaminide	α-N-Acetylglucosaminidase
β-Glucoside	β-Glucosidase

$$O_2N - \langle\!\!\!\!\bigcirc\!\!\!\!\rangle - CH(OH)CHCH_2R$$
$$\quad\quad\quad\quad\quad\quad\quad | $$
$$\quad\quad\quad\quad\quad\quad NHCOCHCl_2$$

(1a) R = $O_2C(CH_2)_{14}Me$
(1b) R = OH

icol palmitate (**1a**) is tasteless whilst the parent antibiotic (**1b**) is extremely bitter.

Pain at the site of injection is a frequent occurrence with the intramuscular injection of certain antibiotics and can be caused by precipitation of the drug substance resulting in haemmorrhage, oedema, inflammation and tissue necrosis. The phosphate ester of clindamycin (**2b**) has significantly greater aqueous solubility than the parent substance (**2a**), resulting in no local effects at the site of injection, the prodrug being hydrolysed to the active antibiotic in the body.

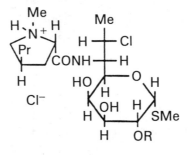

(**2a**) R = H
(**2b**) R = HPO$_3^-$

A frequent side effect experienced on drug administration is gastrointestinal irritation which can result, in extreme cases, in severe ulceration. Aspirin (**3**) which causes some degree of gastric disturbance, is a prodrug of salicylic acid which is the antiinflammatory agent but produces severe irritation of the GI tract.

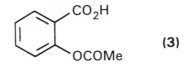

(**3**)

Many drugs which are efficiently absorbed from the gastrointestinal tract undergo presystemic first-pass metabolism and chemical deactivation before their systemic bioavailability, greatly limiting their utility. The corticosteroids are extensively metabolised and rapidly deactivated after their oral administration, but their effects can be much improved, using acetonide, ester and ether prodrugs such as triamcinolone (**4**). Lipophilic prodrug derivatives of steroids (**5**,R = ester) such as testosterone (**5**,R = H) have also been used, releasing the parent substance slowly from an intramuscular depot to significantly extend its hormonal effects. Similar depot release formulations have been used with antipsychotic agents such as fluphenazine (**6**,R = H) to better control schizophrenic patients over long periods.

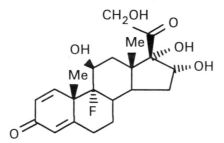

triamcinolone   (**4**)

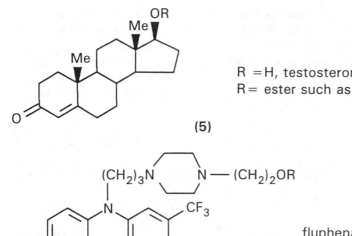

R = H, testosterone
R = ester such as $COCH_2CH_2$⟨cyclopentyl⟩

(5)

$(CH_2)_3N$⟨piperazine⟩N — $(CH_2)_2OR$

CF_3

fluphenazine, R = H

(6)

3.6.3 Hard and soft drugs

A primary objective of drug design is to optimise the desired biological activity within a novel series of molecules to obtain a potential new medicine. The maximum biological activity of the chemical series is not the only parameter of consideration, however, and the preferred drug substance may well be the candidate with a reduced side effect or toxicity profile. Considerations of the biopharmaceutical profile of the series may become of primary importance since it is possible to influence the metabolic profile in a series of analogues and hence the pharmacokinetic properties of the drug substance by modifying its chemical structure and hence its biotransformation without significant impact on its interaction with the pharmacological receptor or enzyme.

A drug substance which is resistant to biotransformation and is excreted unchanged is referred to as a "hard" drug, such a drug substance persisting in the body for long periods without being converted into potentially toxic metabolites. Drug response is elicited at lower doses with less patient variability and the potential for fewer drug–drug interactions. Enhanced metabolic stability is achieved by the identification and chemical protection of labile groups in the molecule or by their replacement with more stable substituents. The half-life of tolbutamide (**7**,R = Me) can be significantly increased by replacement of the oxidisable methyl group by chlorine as in chlorpropamide (**7**,R = C_l), although many other biotransformations will also contribute to its prolonged biological activity.

R —⟨benzene⟩— $SO_2NHCONH(CH_2)_3Me$

(7)

tolbutamide,   R = Me
chlorpropamide, R = Cl

Soft drugs, on the other hand, are rapidly deactivated by extensive biotransformation into inactive metabolites, ideally by hydrolysis or phase II reactions and not oxidative transformations which can potentially generate toxic intermediates.

Chemically labile substituents such as esters are incorporated into noncritical areas of the molecule, such as alkyl side-chains, which, on hydrolysis, generate products with no intrinsic biological activity. An extensive review of the principles and applications of soft drug design has been published.[2] Atracurium (**8**) is a neuromuscular blocking agent which is extensively metabolised by plasma esterases and nonenzymatic Hofmann elimination *in vivo* generating low-molecular-weight products with no receptor activity.

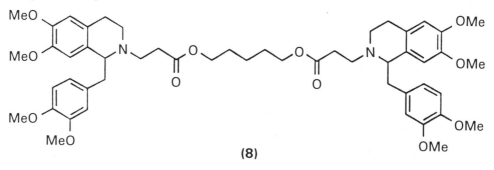

(8)

3.6.4   Bioactivation

Many xenobiotics undergo metabolism in the body to generate very unstable intermediates which are capable of reacting with and modifying the macromolecular proteins, nucleic acids and lipids of the organism in addition to the low molecular weight cellular components to cause toxic damage. The hypothesis was proposed in 1966 to explain the high toxicity of certain chemical carcinogens,[3] but also accounts for many other types of tissue damage which occur, such as cellular necrosis, mutagenesis and blood dyscrasias. The reactive metabolites generated by bioactivation cause their toxicity by covalent binding, generation of superoxides or similar species, peroxidative decomposition of cellular lipids, and enzyme cofactor depletion. Covalent (irreversible) binding to nucleophilic tissue constituents are essentially alkylation reactions which disrupt essential physiological processes such as energy production and protein synthesis or affect membrane permeability. As a consequence of their major role in metabolism many of these processes will occur in the liver, accounting for the hepatotoxicity of certain classes of chemicals such as the halogenated hydrocarbons. The generation of free radical oxygenated intermediates can result in the degradation of essential lipids and the depletion of cellular cofactors as a consequence of their interaction with essential recycling reactions.

3.6.4.1   *Reactive metabolites*

Toxic chemicals are biotransformed by lethal synthesis, oxidative and reductive activation, by conjugation and activation of tissue oxygen. These processes generate electrophiles, free radicals and neutral species such as carbenes and nitrenes which produce the resultant tissue injury. Cytochrome P-450 is the most important enzyme system generating electrophilic species from, for example, epoxides, hydroxylamines, nitroso and sulphur derivatives, although other enzymes such as prostaglandin synthetase and nitro reductase also generate electrophilic metabolites.

Free radicals are most commonly generated via NADPH cytochrome P-450 reductase or related flavin reductases, the reactive intermediates causing either direct toxicity or toxicity subsequent to the generation of superoxide from further metabolic reactions. Many endogenous amines such as adrenaline and DOPA as well as xenobiotics are reduced to intermediates which are capable of generating superoxide or hydrogen peroxide from oxygen by electron transfer reactions. Superoxide is converted chemically to more active and toxic forms of activated oxygen including singlet oxygen and the hydroxy radical. Besides the direct toxic effects of oxygen radicals which lead to membrane damage, the destruction of intra- and extracellular proteins and DNA mutation may result in indirect toxic effects like mutagenesis and carcinogenesis. Free radicals participate in recycling reactions and substained circulating levels of free radicals within cells deplete reducing cofactors, thus causing hypoxia. Since free radicals can initiate chain reactions and subsequent propagation reactions leading to membrane damage, the toxic implications are far greater than those of electrophiles. Examples of chemical families which undergo bioactivation are shown in Table 3.2.

3.6.4.2   Sites of action
The stability of a reactive metabolite dictates the sites of action where it may manifest its potentially toxic effects. Very reactive intermediates of a very short half-life will react with the enzyme molecules responsible for their production and are suicide inhibitors for the activating enzyme. The less reactive the metabolite is, the further it may travel before interacting with some functionality such that the toxicity may be expressed in other organs of the body. Stable intermediates frequently manifest toxicity in the excretory organs such as the kidney, bladder and small intestine when sufficient concentrations are present. Detoxification of active metabolites arises by competitive metabolic transformations and by cellular defence mechanisms invoking glutathione and related transferases, peroxidases and reductases. Glutathione, the major cellular nucleophile, has a number of important functions concerned with cellular integrity, notably protection of SH groups against deactivation by heavy metals, reactivation of deactivated SH enzymes, conjugation with toxic chemicals and metabolites, and detoxification of endogenous peroxides and reactive oxygen species.

The detoxification of reactive oxygen species is an essential feature of aerobic life and the living organism has evolved many defence mechanisms to counteract the destructive reactions of oxygen metabolites. These mechanisms use nonenzymatic radical scavengers such as the vitamins A, C and E together with a number of enzymatic systems. The antioxidant enzymes include the superoxide dismutases, glutathione peroxidase and other haemoprotein peroxidases, all invoking catalysis by metals such as copper, manganese, tin and selenium. These enzyme systems are ubiquitous in nature, indicating the importance of their role in preventing damage by oxygen metabolites in the living organism.

Many potentially toxic chemicals take part in a number of metabolic activation steps before generating their toxic metabolites. Thus metabolites generated in one tissue may be transported to another organ before being converted into a toxic

Table 3.2.   Activation of chemicals to toxic metabolites

Activation reaction	Examples	Biological effect
Haloalkanes $\xrightarrow{P\text{-}450}$ acyl halides, radicals	Chloroform, carbon tetrachloride, halothane	Toxicity
Substituted alkanes $\xrightarrow{P\text{-}450}$ epoxides (?)	Ethyl carbamate, aflatoxin B_2	Carcionogenicity
Alkanes $\xrightarrow{P\text{-}450}$ epoxides	Styrene, acrylonitrile	Toxicity, carcinogenicity
Furans $\xrightarrow{P\text{-}450}$ diketones	4-Ipomeanol	Toxicity
Polycylic aromatic hydrocarbons $\xrightarrow{P\text{-}450}$ epoxides, diol epoxides	Benzo[a]pyrene, 7,12-dimethylbenzanthracene, naphthalene	Carcinogenicity
Halobenzenes $\xrightarrow{P\text{-}450}$ epoxide radicals (?), quinones (?)	Bromobenzene, pentachlorophenol	Toxicity
Polyhalogenated biphenyls $\xrightarrow{P\text{-}450}$ epoxides (?)	Polychlorinated biphenyls, polybrominated biphenyls	Toxicity
Acetanilides $\xrightarrow{P\text{-}450,\ peroxidases}$ quinoneimines, semiquinone radicals (?)	Acetaminophen	Toxicity
Aromatic amines $\xrightarrow{P\text{-}450,\ flavin\ monooxygenase\ peroxidases}$ hydroxylamines and esters	2-Naphthylamine, benzidines	Carcinogenicity
Aminofluorenes $\xrightarrow{P\text{-}450,\ flavin\ monooxygenase\ peroxidases}$ hydroxylamines and esters, radicals, nitroso compounds	2-Aminofluorene	Carcinogenicity
Hydrazines $\xrightarrow{P\text{-}450,\ flavin\ monooxygenase}$ CH_3, CH_4^+, diazomethane (?)	Procarbazine, dimethylhydrazine	Toxicity, carcinogenicity
Thiocarbonyls $\xrightarrow{flavin\ monooxygenase}$ sulphenes, sulphines	Thioacetamide	Toxicity

intermediate which may even manifest its target organ toxicity elsewhere. Hexachloro-butadiene, for example, is conjugated with glutathione in the liver and transferred to the kidney where it is activated to a nephrotoxic metabolite by the action of a C-S lyase.

3.7   METABOLIC PATHWAYS

3.7.1   Introduction

Metabolic reactions are conveniently divided into phase I and phase II reactions. Phase I and functionalisation reactions result in the oxidation, reduction or hydrolysis of the parent molecule to give appropriate metabolic products which are substrates for subsequent phase II or conjugation reactions, a typical sequence being the conversion of benzene to phenylglueuronic acid via phenol.

Both phases may occur independently of each other, however, as well as successive phase I reactions followed by a variety of phase II conjugations. The ultimate metabolic profile is often complex, showing a large number of metabolites, including the parent molecule. The general pathways of drug metabolism are summarised in the following sections. Metabolic reactions are of fundamental importance in defining the pharmacological activities and disposition of drug substances in the living organism and, in general, will result in progressively reduced biological effects and facilitated elimination. Phase I reactions result in functional modifications of the parent molecule which may, as described earlier, result in bioactivation (see section 3.6.4) whereas Phase II reactions, on the other hand, radically alter the structure and physicochemical properties of the molecule. The physicochemical modifications resulting from metabolism result in increased polarity, water solubility and increased molecular weight, facilitating elimination via the kidneys and liver in the urine and faeces. Metabolic studies are thus a major consideration in modern medicinal chemistry, playing an important role in optimising the desired therapeutic profile of a new series of biologically active compounds.

3.7.2   Phase I or functionalisation reactions

3.7.2.1   Oxidations

A large number of oxidative reactions are carried out by the living organism, and all the elements present in xenobiotics, notably the ubiquitous carbon, but also nitrogen and sulphur, are oxidised and also undergo a variety of other transformations including dealkylation, dehalogenation and deamination reactions.

The great majority of these oxidations are carried out by the haemoprotein cytochrome P-450 which is embedded within the phospholipid environment of the microsomes derived from the endoplasmic reticulum of living cells. A large number of P-450 isozymes derived primarily from the liver and adrenal mitochondria have now been characterised. The cytochrome P-450s are mixed function oxidases activating molecular oxygen to insert one atom into a variety of lipophilic substrates with the other being reduced to water. The reaction sequence includes reduction of the haem iron atom by the flavoprotein NADPH-cytochrome P-450 reductase, with subsequent activation of molecular oxygen in an ion Fe (II)–oxygen complex. On release of the oxidised molecule the iron of the cytochrome is reoxidised to Fe(III).

A number of flavoprotein and molybdenum containing oxidases free from cytochrome P-450 have also been characterised. Monoamine oxidase, a flavoprotein widely distributed in mammalian tissues and notably the brain where it is responsible for the breakdown of neurotransmitters, exists in two forms (A and B) whose role has not yet been elucidated.

3.7.2.2 *Reductions*
Metabolic reduction is also an important pathway in the biotransformation of xenobiotics, notably being a major route of metabolism for aromatic nitro and azo compounds as well as for a wide variety of aliphatic and aromatic *N*-oxides which are reduced to tertiary amines. Reduction of sulphoxides and sulphones is not considered to be a major metabolic pathway, however.

Metabolic reduction has been shown to occur within the endoplasmic reticulum and cytosol of the cell, but the enzyme systems concerned have not yet been identified. Reductions may also be carried out by anaerobic bacteria within the GI tract, and nonenzymatic reactions may also occur. Bacterial NADH or NADH-dependent flavoproteins can reduce flavins which in turn reduce azo compounds nonenzymatically.

3.7.2.3 *Hydrolysis*
The vast majority of esters and amides may be hydrolysed in the animal body, the extent and rate of hydrolysis being dependent upon the chemical reactivity of the functional group. Aromatic esters and amides are, in general, more stable than their aliphatic counterparts, although hydrolysis is a minor metabolic route even for simple aliphatic amides, other functionalities being more amenable to metabolic degradation. A number of enzymes and nonenzymatic catalysts, such as serum albumin, cause hydrolysis of a wide variety of esters, and the stomach is responsible for extensive acid catalysed reactions. Hydrolysis occurs in all mammalian tissues with the liver and blood and GI tract being the most important metabolic organs; however, significant differences do occur between individuals.

3.7.3   Phase II or conjugation reactions

3.7.3.1   Glucuronic acid conjugation
The conjugation reactions used by mammalian organisms to metabolise xenobiotics have well defined roles in the metabolism of endogenous substrates and biosynthesis in the organism. Whereas, however, the transferase enzymes concerned exhibit a high specificity for their endogenous substrates, they have a much broader applicability for xenobiotics. Each reaction entails the synthesis of a new energy requiring bond which may result in two ways. The endogenous conjugating agent is usually activated first (usually as a nucleotide), but occasionally the xenobiotic itself is activated before

its conjugation. The endogenous roles of the principal conjugation reactions and the related functional groups are summarised in Table 3.3.

Glucuronic acid conjugation is the most versatile reaction and accounts for the major proportion of the metabolites found in the excreta, Glucuronic acid is derived from glucose, and the presence of the four hydroxyl groups confers great aqueous solubility on its derivatives. Glucuronidation entails uridine diphosphate glucuronic acid, UPDGA (9), which is synthesised in a two-stage process from glucose-1-phosphate via uridine triphosphate.

UDPGA reacts with groups containing active hydrogen such as alcohols, thiols, amines and acids in the presence of glucuronyl transferase (e.g. 10). The different types of compounds forming conjugates with glucuronic acid are listed in Table 3.4.

As well as their enhanced water solubility glucuronides are more acidic, and hence are ionised at physiological pH, when the lipophilicity of the parent molecule is drastically reduced. In general, conjugation thus facilitates detoxification and facile elimination of a drug substance. Elimination occurs predominantly via the kidneys although certain high molecular weight glucuronides are excreted via the bile into the gastrointestinal tract where subsequent hydrolysis may result in reabsorption of the drug or metabolites (biliary recirculation) or excretion in the faeces. UDPGT is present in the endoplasmic reticulum of the liver and many other tissues. A large number of isozymes have been isolated from the liver of various animal species including man.

3.7.3.2 Glutathione conjugation

Glutathione (11) is a nucleophilic tripeptide which is able to undergo conjugation via its thiol function with electrophilic centres in a wide variety of xenobiotics. Conjugation with glutathione usually results in detoxification of the electrophile by preventing its reaction with nucleophilic centres in macromolecules such as proteins and nucleic acids. The substrate is usually eliminated as a mercapturic acid after further metabolism of the S-substituted glutathione. The electrophilic substrate for glutathione may be generated by prior metabolism of the xenobiotic, or by displacement of suitable electron withdrawing groups in nitro or halo-alkanes, benzenes and sulphonic acid esters by the sulphur atoms of glutathione. Glutathione also reacts by Michael addition across appropriately substituted double bonds.

The glutathione conjugations are catalysed by the glutathione-S-transferases which occur in the cytosolic fractions of the liver and most other organs, and more than eight isozymes have been characterised from the rat liver. The distribution of the isozymes varies from organ to organ and is dependent on exogenous chemicals and the sex hormones. Glutathione conjugates are usually extensively excreted via the bile owing to their molecular and physicochemical properties, and are extensively metabolised by the enzymes of the gut flora. The resultant intermediates are transformed by a number of chemical reactions including transamination, S-oxidation, carbon sulphur bond cleavages and N-acetylation.

Glutathione conjugation is a widely used protective mechanism against the potential toxic effects of internally generated electrophiles, and glutathione levels of the system are a measure of challenge and exposure to potentially toxic xenobiotics.

Table 3.3. Classification of the major conjugation reactions

Reaction	Conjugating agent	Functional groups involved	Endogenous roles
Reactions involving activated conjugating agents			
Glucuronidation	UDP glucuronic acid	OH, CO_2H, NH_2, NR_2, SH, CH	Biosynthesis, detoxication, e.g. bilirubin
Sulphation	PAPS	OH, NH_2, SH	Biosynthesis, e.g. chondroitin, steroid metabolism, detoxication, e.g. indoxyl
Methylation	S-Adenosyl-L-methionine	OH, NH_2	Biosynthesis, detoxication, e.g. catecholamines
Acetylation	Acetyl CoA	OH, NH_2	Biosynthesis, intermediary metabolism
Reactions involving activated foreign compounds			
Glutathione	Glutathione	Arene oxide, epoxide, alkyl and aryl halide	Maintenance of intracellular redox potential, leukotriene synthesis
Amino acid conjugation	Glycine, glutamine, ornithine, taurine	CO_2H	Detoxication of endogenous acids, especially in amino acidurias

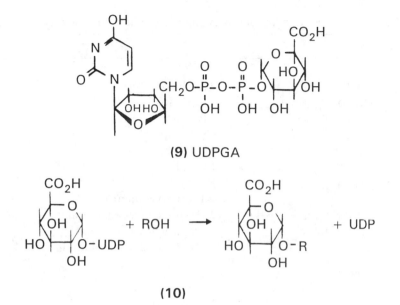

(9) UDPGA

(10)

2.7.3.3 Amino acid conjugation

Amino acid conjugations result from the reaction of the carboxylic acid group of a xenobiotic with one of a number of amino acids, and the extent of conjugation is very dependent on the steric availability of the xenobiotic carboxylic acid. A relatively small group of substrate structures such as aromatic, heteroaromatic, cinnamic and arylacetic acids are susceptible to amino acid conjugation.

Conjugation occurs mainly with glycine, glutamine, taurine and ornithine but also other amino acids such as alanine, and histidine have also been implicated in amino acid conjugations of xenobiotics. The nature of the amino acid depends on the animal species, with the most common being glycine. Amino acid conjugations enhance elimination and decrease toxicity of the parent acid but are not as effective as the conjugation reactions. The acid is initially activated by the formation of an acyl adenylate, and this is converted to a high energy acyl CoA thioester which subsequently reacts with the amino acid liberating free CoA.

3.7.3.4 Acetylation

Whilst acetylation of a primary amino group function in a number of xenobiotics is a widely occurring metabolic process, the corresponding acetylation of hydroxyl and thiol groups do not appear to take place. The acetyl group transferred is derived from acetyl CoA which is present in all living cells, and the reaction is catalysed by N-acetyl transferase.

Acetylation of xenobiotics reduces their polarity and frequently reduces aqueous solubility, processes not obviously commensurate with facile elimination. N-acetyl metabolites of a number of drugs retain the biological activity of the parent compounds and, only in rare cases, are the conjugates further metabolised. The role of acetylation in the metabolic pathways is, consequently, somewhat unclear.

Table 3.4. Types of compounds giving rise to glucuronic acid conjugates

Functional group	Example
Hydroxy	
Primary alcohol	Trichloroethanol
Secondary alcohol	Propranolol
Tertiary alcohol	*t*-Butanol
Alicyclic alcohol	Cyclohexanol
Terpenoid alcohol	Menthol
Phenol	Phenol
Terpenoid phenol	Eugenol
Enol	4-Hydroxycoumarin
Aliphatic hydroxylamine	*N*-Hydroxychlorphentermine
Aromatic hydroxylamine	2-Naphthylhydroxylamine
Hydroxamic acid	*N*-Hydroxy-2-acetamidofluorene
Carboxylic acid	
Alkyl	2-Ethylheanoic acid
Aromatic	Benzoic acid
Heterocyclic	Nicotinic acid
Arylacetic	Indole-3-acetic acid
Arylpropionic	Hydratropic acid
Aryloxybutyric	Clofibric acid
Carbamic acid	Tocainide carbamate
Amino functions	
Aromatic	Aniline
Azaheterocyclic	Sulphisoxazole
Carbamate	Meprobamate
Sulphonamide	Sulphadimethoxine
Hydroxylamine *N*-	*N*-Hydroxy-2-acetamidofluorene
Tertiary aliphatic	Cyproheptadine
Urea	Dulcin
Sulphur functions	
Thiol	2-Mercaptobenzothiazole
Dithiotic acid	*N*,*N*-Diethyldithiocarbamic acid
Carbon centres	
Pyrazolone ring	Phenylbutazone
Selenium centres	
Selenium	2-Selenobenzanilide (metabolite of Ebselen)

3.7.3.5 *Methylation*

Methylation of the hydroxyl, catechol, thiol and various nitrogen functions in xenobiotics occurs extensively. Whereas methylation is of great significance in the

$$
\begin{array}{l}
\text{CONHCHCONHCH}_2\text{CO}_2\text{H} \\
\quad\;\, | \qquad\;\; | \\
\quad\;\, \text{CH}_2 \quad\; \text{CH}_2\text{SH} \\
\quad\;\, | \\
\quad\;\, \text{CH}_2 \\
\quad\;\, | \\
\quad\;\, \text{CHNH}_2 \\
\quad\;\, | \\
\quad\;\, \text{CO}_2\text{H}
\end{array}
$$

(11)

metabolism of endogenous materials it is of little significance in the disposal of xenobiotics. Methylation, like acetylation, tends to increase the lipophilicity and decrease water solubility of the parent substance.

The transferred methyl group is derived from the nucleotide S-adenosyl-L-methionine and the reaction is carried out by a member of the methyl transferase group of enzymes. Little is known about the zoological distribution of methylation and the relevant isozymes.

3.7.3.6 Sulphation

Sulphate conjugation results in esterification of a hydroxyl group of a xenobiotic by sulphate ion to give a very polar, highly ionised, conjugate. The source of inorganic sulphate used in the conjugation is the high energy 3-phosphoadenosine-5-phospho-sulphate (PAPS), and sulphate transfer entails a sulphotransferase. The enzymes taking part in activation and transfer are closely related and are present in the cytosol of the liver and many other tissues.

All hydroxyl groups of xenobiotics including alcohols, phenols, catechols and hydroxylamines give rise to sulphate conjugates (Table 3.5), whilst certain aromatic amines give rise to sulphamic acids. Thiols are not sulphated, whereas many of the substrates may also undergo glucuronidation. Sulphation is an alternative to glucuronidation, and the relative extent of these conjugations depends on the chemical structure of the xenobiotics. Sulphation is favoured for small, hydrophilic molecules which are sterically unhindered and often preferentially distributed in the cytosol. Sulphate conjugation is of limited capacity, the proportion of sulphation decreasing

Table 3.5. Xenobiotic substrates for sulphate conjugation

Functional group (hydroxy)	Example
Primary alcohol	Ethanol
Secondary alcohol	Butan-2-ol
Phenol	Phenol
Catechol	α-Methyl-DOPA
Alicyclic alcohol	Dehydroepiandrosterone
Heterocyclic alcohol	3-Hydroxycoumarin
Hydroxyamide	N-Hydroxy-2-acetamidofluorene
Aromatic hydroxylamine	2-Naphthylhydroxylamine
N-oxide	Minoxidil

with increasing concentration of the xenobiotic. Sulphate conjugation is significant at low doses of administered substances but decreases very significantly at high doses, owing to the limited availability of PAPS for conjugation. Saturability of the process is thought to arise to some extent from the kinetic properties of the sulphotransferases rather than restricted availability of inorganic sulphate.

Sulphate conjugates of xenobiotics are highly polar and water soluble, resulting normally in the rapid detoxification and excretion of metabolites. Certain hydroxylated metabolites are sulphated, however, to generate toxic electrophilic intermediates as a result of the ready elimination of the O-sulphate leaving group with concomitant formation of carbonium and nitrenium ions.

4

The pharmacodynamic phase

4.1 INTRODUCTION

The interaction of a drug with its site of action in the biological system takes place during the *pharmacodynamic phase*. The very existence of potent, structurally specific drugs must mean that there exist specific sites at which they act, and this can be readily shown by a simple calculation. 1 mg of a drug of molecular weight 200 contains approximately 1×10^{18} molecules. The human body is composed of about 1×10^{13} cells each of which contains at least 1×10^{10} molecules, thus every drug molecule could react randomly with one of some 10^5 molecules, a gross and incompatible imbalance. This fact was first recognised by Langley at the end of the 19th century who consequently proposed that drugs react at "specific reactive sites" i.e. molecules or parts of molecules within the body. Shortly afterwards Ehrlich refined the concept and postulated that reactive sites were portions of biological macromolecules and that the biological effect was consequent upon binding to this site. Thus the idea of a "receptor" was born. This chapter will consider some of our current understanding of biological receptors, their interactions with a variety of ligands, and the biological consequences of this interaction. The use of this information to design new drugs will be discussed further in Chapter 5. As Ehrlich proposed, receptors are biological macromolecules either proteins or nucleic acids. Ligand interaction with one class of protein, the enzymes, forms the second part of this chapter, whilst the first part will focus on interactions with nonenzymatic proteins and nucleic acids. Protein receptors are predominantly found in the outer membrane of cells, although some, particularly those for steroids, are located in the interior of the cell. Before we consider the interaction of ligands with receptors, it will be helpful to consider in brief the structure of the cell.

4.2 CELL STRUCTURES

The human body is a highly complex, multicellular organism formed from approximately 1×10^{13} individual, specialised but cooperating and communicating cells.

These vary enormously in function, size and in shape, as indicated in Figure 4.1. However, the key elements of cellular structure are common to most cells although there are some exceptions, notably the red blood cell (erythrocyte) which lacks a nucleus. Figure 4.2 shows a schematic representation of an idealised cell with its major constituents. These include:

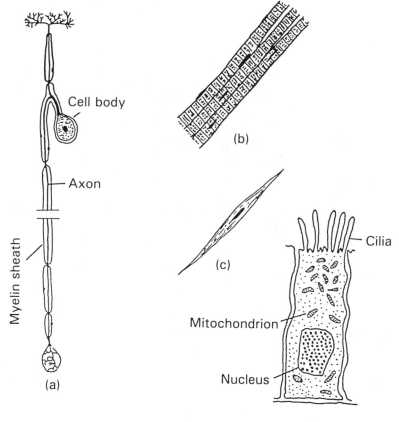

Fig. 4.1.   Structures of representative body cells (not drawn to scale). (a) Sensory nerve cell showing the very long axon. (b) Skeletal muscle cell. (c) Visceral muscle cell. (d)·Ciliated columnar cells from the nasal respiratory epithelium.

(i)   The cellular (plasma) membrane — the membrane which defines the outer surface of the cell and controls the flow of material in and out of the cell. It is the site of many of the cell's receptors and, owing to its relevance to this chapter, its structure will be considered in greater detail below.

(ii)   The nucleus —. the volume of the cell delineated by the nuclear membrane in which is found the genetic material DNA (deoxyribonucleic acid) and its associated proteins.

(iii) The cytoplasm — this comprises all the space between the nuclear and plasma membranes. It is filled with a fluid, the cytosol, and a number of organelles

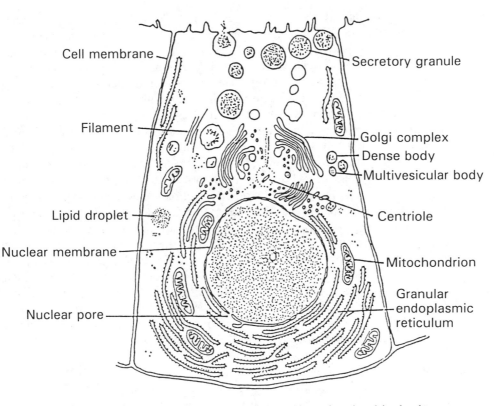

Fig. 4.2. Diagram of a cell as it would appear in a thin section viewed in the electron microscope. This is in fact a secretory cell, but the major components are common to all cells.

which conduct specialised functions. It is a highly structured domain in which a large number of proteinaceous fibres (microtubules, intermediate filaments and actin filaments) of different sizes, structures and complexities anchor the organelles and provide the inner structure of the cell.

(iv) The mitochondrion — this is a small, hard capsule of dimensions $1–10\ \mu \times 1.5\ \mu$ which is responsible for the production of much of the cell's energy. Food in the form of sugars and fatty acids entering the cell is initially broken down to pyruvic acid which enters the mitochondrion and is then further degraded ultimately to carbon dioxide and water via the Krebs or citric acid cycle. This is a highly organised stepwise process in which the oxidative steps are used to produce adenosine triphosphate (ATP) the hydrolysis of which to adenosine diphosphate (ADP) is highly exothermic, and this is used to drive other endothermic reactions. As might be expected, the greatest number of mitochondria is found in heavy energy users such as muscle cells.

(v) The endoplasmic reticulum — a highly convoluted inner membrane which permeates the whole of the cytoplasm and forms the endoplasmic reticulum. It exists in two types, the rough and the smooth, with the former attaining its

appearance because of the presence of granular particles, the ribosomes, on its surface. This is the site of much of the cell's protein synthesis, whilst the smooth variety,
which lacks the ribosomes, performs the same function for lipid biosynthesis.
The use of a vast surface area carrying enzymes catalysing consecutive
reactions in close proximity makes these processes extremely efficient.

(vi)   The Golgi apparatus — this is another complex membranal structure arranged
around a central core of four to six flattened cisternae which have a plate-like
appearance. These are joined together by a series of peripheral tubules, and
closely associated with the structure are found large numbers of small vesicles
and a smaller number of larger, secretory vesicles. Vesicles formed from lipid
bilayers are used in the cell to carry materials while preventing their exposure
to the cytoplasm. By fusing with other membranes the contents can readily
pass through the membrane into the region beyond. The Golgi apparatus
contains enzymes responsible for the final assembly of proteins prepared on the
endoplasmic reticulum. These proteins arrive in the small vesicles, are modified
largely by alterations to the carbohydrate portions of glycoproteins or by
cleavage of peptide fragments to give the final active form, and are then
transported to their site of action or even outside the cell by the larger vesicles.

(vii)   Lysosomes — these are a group of small vesicles of various shapes and sizes
containing a potentially lethal concoction of enzymes whose function is to digest
all unwanted material in the cell. This includes both materials absorbed by the
cell and unwanted fragments of the cell itself.

(viii) Centrioles and centrosomes — are formed by the coming together of two groups
of microtubules in the cytoplasm with two of these in association forming a
centriole. This body plays a crucial role in the initiation of cell division.

(ix)   Microbodies — not all enzymatic degradation of foodstuffs takes place in the
mitochondria; some also occurs in microbodies. These are small ($<0.5\ \mu$m diameter), single membranal vesicles packed with degradative enzymes. However,
in contrast to the mitochondria, no ATP is produced by them and the final product is not water but hydrogen peroxide. As this is toxic to the cell, the enzyme
catalase which decomposes this to oxygen and water is invariably present.

All of these cell structures are obviously important in the functioning of the cell, and
ultimately the whole organism, but the cell membrane, the boundary of its interaction
with the external world, will now be considered in greater detail.

4.3   THE CELL MEMBRANE

As stated above, the limits of the cell are defined by its outer plasma membrane.
Many organelles are surrounded by similar membranes, many vital processes take
place on or in membranes, and there is a constant traffic of material through
intracellular membranes with exchange between the cell and its environment.

Three elements constitute mammalian membranes, proteins, lipids and carbohydrates, the relative proportions of which vary with the function of the cell. Thus
myelin, the membrane which surrounds and insulates nerve cells, has less than 25%

of its mass as protein, while in membranes involved in energy transfer the proportion of protein can be as much as 75%. More usually, the relative proportion of lipid to protein is 50:50 which means that because of their smaller mass there are some 50 lipid molecules present for each protein molecule.

4.3.1 Membrane lipids

Three major types of lipids are found in biological membranes. The most abundant of these are phospholipids. The structures of four representatives, phosphatidylcholine (1), sphingomyelin (2), phosphatidylserine (3), and phosphatidylethanolamine (4) are shown in Figure 4.3. All of these molecules have in common a polar hydrophilic head and a long hydrophobic nonpolar chain. Only phosphatidylserine (3) carries a net negative charge, and thus this phospholipid will have different properties from the others.

Two other lipids are cholesterol (5) and a group of carbohydrate derived glycolipids, e.g. galactocerebroside (6), in which the sugar nucleus carries long fatty acid side chains.

$CH_2OCOC_{15}H_{31}$
|
$CHOCOC_{15}H_{31}$
|
$CH_2OP(O)_2OR$
     +
(1) $R = CH_2CH_2 \overset{+}{N}Et_3$ +
(3) $R = CH_2CH(CO_2^-) \overset{+}{N}Et_3$
     +
(4) $R = CH_2CH_2 \overset{+}{N}H_3$

$CH = CHC_{13}H_{27}$
|
$CHOH$
|
$CHNHCOR$
| +
$CH_2OP(O)_2OCH_2CH_2 \overset{+}{N}Me_3$

(2)

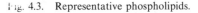

Fig. 4.3. Representative phospholipids.

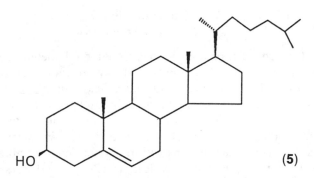

HO   (5)

As a result of their amphipathic character any phospholipid placed in water will form either a bilayer or a micelle (Figure 4.4) in which the polar heads aggregate together and interact with the water while the hydrophobic chains interact with each other. Within each layer, lipid molecules can readily diffuse laterally with a diffusion coefficient of approximately 10^{-8} cm^2 sec^{-1}. However, diffusion between the layers is much more difficult because the polar head of the lipid has to find its way through the hydrophobic heart of the membrane. This uncatalysed process, which has been given the colourful designation of "flip-flop" (Figure 4.5), occurs on average less frequently than once a month.

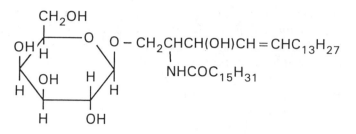

(6)

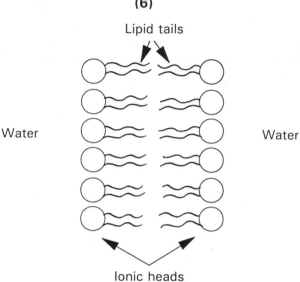

Fig. 4.4.   Phospholipids in water.

Thus a picture emerges of a two-dimensional fluid membrane in which lipid molecules can readily diffuse. The fluidity of the system can be affected by a number of factors, particularly the nature of the fatty acid side chain. For instance, the introduction of a single double bond in this chain can have a significant effect because the resultant change in conformation increases its bulk and fluidity.

The slow rate of the "flip-flop" motion means that any asymmetry of the membrane introduced as it is synthesised remains with the functioning membrane, and this has profound effects on its mode of action, effects which will be discussed below. One of the clearest examples of this asymmetry is provided by the glycolipids which are exclusively found in the outer layer where they comprise approximately 5% of the content. Their precise structure differs markedly from species to species and tissue to tissue but in mammalian cells they are exclusively derived from ceramide (**7**). The polar head groups in all cases are formed from sugars and can contain from 1 to 15 neutral sugar residues. One example is galactose found in galactocerebroside (**6**) a major constituent of myelin; other more complex structures are gangliosides, derived from sialic acid (**8**), which are found in the membranes of neurons. It is assumed that the presence of these glycolipids in the external layer with the sugars in the

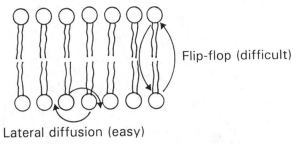

Fig. 4.5. Motion available in a lipid bilayer.

$$CH = CHC_{13}H_{27}$$
$$|$$
$$CHOH$$
$$|$$
$$CHNHCOC_{15}H_{31}$$
$$|$$
$$CH_2OH$$

(7)

(8)

extracellular environment means that they play a role in cell–cell signalling. Indeed, one ganglioside acts as a cell surface receptor for cholera toxin, and it seems likely that other more important roles exist.

4.3.2 Membrane proteins

Most of the specific functions of the membrane are performed by proteins. These proteins lie in the fluid bed of the lipids (Figure 4.6) either as transmembranal proteins or in association with only one of the layers (Figure 4.7). This arrangement is known as the "fluid mosaic" model. As their name suggests, transmembrane proteins have part of their structures outside the cell, part spanning the membrane and part inside the cell, and are asymmetric, the extra- and intra-portions performing different functions. The section of the protein passing through the (hydrophobic) membrane adopts an α-helical conformation to maximise internal hydrogen bonds between the amino and carbonyl groups which places the hydrophobic side chains on the outside of the helix. The number of passes through the membrane varies from one to several. Proteins associated solely with the outer layer do so by being covalently bound usually via oligosaccharides to the minor phospholipid, phosphalidylinositol, the fatty acid chains of which are embedded in this layer. Those associated with the cytoplasmic face can be either covalently bound to a fatty acid immersed in this layer or noncovalently bound to a transmembranal protein.

Receptors are mainly (but not entirely) components of membranal proteins. The process of ligand binding to a receptor causes a conformational change in the protein which initiates a change in the functioning of the cell. This process is discussed in much greater detail later.

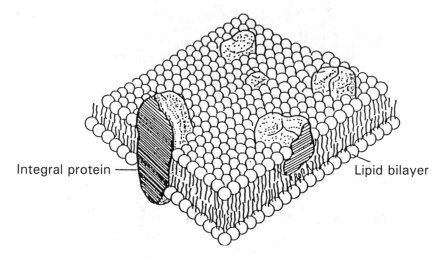

Integral protein ———   Lipid bilayer

Fig. 4.6.   The fluid mosaic model of the membrane.

EXTRACELLULAR SPACE

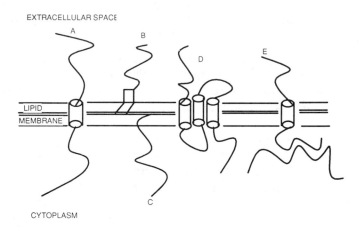

LIPID
MEMBRANE

CYTOPLASM

POSSIBLE MODES OF ASSOCIATION OF PROTEINS WITH PLASMA
MEMBRANE

A. PROTEIN WITH A SINGLE TRANSMEMBRANAL REGION
B. PROTEIN ONLY ASSOCIATED WITH OUTER MEMBRANE LAYER
C. PROTEIN ONLY ASSOCIATED WITH INNER MEMBRANE LAYER
D. PROTEIN WITH MULTIPLE TRANSMEMBRANAL REGIONS
E. CYTOPLASMIC PROTEIN NONCOVALENTLY ASSOCIATED WITH A
TRANSMEMBRANAL PROTEIN

Fig. 4.7.

4.3.3   Membrane carbohydrates

The total carbohydrate protein of the cell membrane represents between 2% and 5%
of its total weight. Most of this is present either as glycolipid or as poly- or
oligosaccharides covalently bound to asparagine, serine, or threonine residues of
membrane proteins. Whilst most proteins are glycosylated and only one in ten lipid
molecules are, in absolute numbers more lipid molecules carry sugars than do

proteins. However, the combination of greater polysaccharide chain lengths and multiple oligosaccharides found on proteins means that the greater carbohydrate mass is nevertheless protein bound. This carbohydrate probably plays a role in cell signalling processes.

4.4 RECEPTOR THEORIES

As described at the beginning of this chapter the concept of "specific receptor substances" with which structurally specific drugs interact was introduced in the late 19th century by Ehrlich and Langley. Most often these "specific receptor substances" are, in fact, proteins which in the majority of cases are found in the plasma membrane.

In view of the importance of this interaction it is not surprising that a number of attempts have been made to describe the process mathematically. Perhaps in view of the complexities it is also not surprising that none of the theories advanced so far has been able to account for all the subtleties.

The basic drug–receptor interaction can be summarised as:

$$\text{RECEPTOR (R) + LIGAND (L)} \underset{k_{-1}}{\overset{k_1}{\rightleftharpoons}} \text{RL} \overset{k_2}{\longrightarrow} \text{R + effect} \tag{1}$$

Many theories have taken this process as being similar to the familiar ligand enzyme expression (equation (2)), but there are very important differences. Enzymes catalyse reactions whose starting materials and products can be measured and the kinetics solved for k_1 and k_2. In the case of receptors the "effect" is not so readily measured because, as will be examined in greater detail later the drug–receptor interaction actually initiates a chain of events which, at a distance, produce the measurable biological response. In between interaction and response there are numerous opportunities for the signal to be modulated and thus prevent the response from being a true measure of the original ligand–receptor interaction. Recent work which provides complete pictures of the structures of a number of molecular receptors will be described later, but a quantitative model of the action of a receptor is still awaited.

$$\text{ENZYME (E) + SUBSTRATES (S)} \underset{k_{-1}}{\overset{k_1}{\rightleftharpoons}} \text{ES} \overset{k_2}{\longrightarrow} \text{E + PRODUCTS} \tag{2}$$

A further difference from enzymes lies in the fact that the diffusion of a ligand to its receptor may be limited and thus drug concentrations in the vicinity of the receptor may not reach equilibrium values instantaneously as required by the mathematical approach.

Before outlining the mathematics of the drug–receptor interaction it is useful to define some of the terms which are used when discussing receptors. The dissociation constant k_D (or its inverse, the association constant k_A) is a measure of the affinity of a receptor for a given ligand. B_{max} is the density of binding sites on a concentration/weight basis and is a measure of the total number of receptors in a tissue. The k_D has units of concentration whilst B_{max} is concentration per mg of protein. *Agonists* are ligands which invoke a response; full agonists give, in sufficient concentration, a full response; partial agonists can give only a partial response irrespective of concentration. *Antagonists* bind to a receptor giving no biological response of their own but are capable of preventing a true agonist from binding and electing a response. Competitive antagonists bind to the same receptor as agonists while noncompetitive antagonists exert their effect by binding to a different but related receptor. The two antagonists result in different dose–response curves as will be shown later. Very recently the agonist–antagonist spectrum has been widened by the discovery of *inverse agonists* in the benzodiazepine series. In this case the agents have pharmacological activities opposite to those of agonists and again both partial and full inverse agonists have been identified. In all cases "biological response" can refer to whole animal or human data or a much simpler tissue preparation with the latter being a preferred measurement as the response is less likely to be affected by post-receptor modification.

The first attempt to quantify the interaction of ligands with their receptors was the "occupancy theory" of Clark which was proposed in 1926. He suggested that the Langmuir isotherm for the absorption of gases onto metal surfaces could be used as an expression for the mass action relationship between a drug and its specific receptor sites. The underlying assumptions of the model are that the law of mass action can be applied to the drug–receptor interaction, that one drug molecule occupies one receptor site and that the concentration of the drug in the medium is sufficiently large that it remains effectively constant during the binding process. Clark was studying the effect of the agonist acetylcholine on the contraction of strips of cardiac and abdominal muscle and found that if he plotted the biological response against the logarithm of the concentration of the agonist, a curve such as that shown in Figure 4.8, curve a, was produced. Eventually a maximum response was produced and addition of further agonist produced no further effect. Presumably under these conditions either all the receptors are occupied or the tissue has been stimulated to the limit of its capacity. A partial agonist produces a curve such as (b) in Figure 4.8.

When the experiments were repeated in the presence of an antagonist, e.g. atropine, the dose–response curves were shifted to the right (Figure 4.9 curves b–e reflecting increasing concentrations of the antagonist). What these curves are showing is that to give a certain level of response more of the agonist is required than in the situation where no antagonist was present. Further, provided that sufficient agonist is added the same maximal response is achieved. In this situation the agonist and antagonist are competing for the receptor, with the agonist eventually able to dominate provided that enough of it is present to prevail by a mass action effect. Curve f represents a different case as here no maximal response is achieved whatever level of agonist is added. In this case the agonist and antagonist are not competing for the same receptor and the law of mass action will not apply.

Clark's explanation of these data came by writing equation (1) in the simplified form, equation (1a).

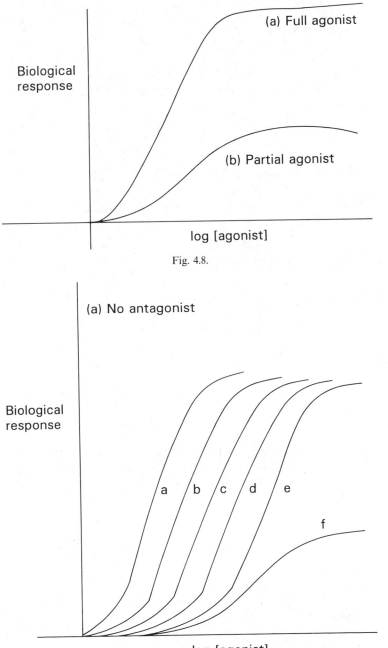

Fig. 4.8.

Fig. 4.9.

$$R + D \underset{k_2}{\overset{k_1}{\rightleftharpoons}} RD \overset{k_3}{\longrightarrow} E \tag{1a}$$

Where R is receptor, D is drug, k_1, k_2 are, respectively, the rates of association and dissociation and E is the effect. Occupancy theory assumes that the effect, E, will be proportional to the number of sites occupied, i.e.

$$E = k_3 [RD] \tag{3}$$

where k_3 is a rate constant
Thus at equilibrium, equation (4) will be generated

$$\frac{[R][D]}{[RD]} = \frac{k_2}{k_1} = K_D \tag{4}$$

Where K_D is the dissociation constant.
Alternatively, K_A the affinity constant can be defined as:

$$K_A = \frac{[RD]}{[R][D]} \tag{5}$$

The total number of receptors R_t, will be given by:

$$[R_t] = [R] + [RD] \tag{6}$$

giving

$$K_D = \frac{[R_t - RD][D]}{[RD]} \tag{7}$$

Since the biological effect depends on the number of receptors occupied, the maximal effect will be given when [RD] in equation (3) is equal to $[R_t]$, i.e.

$$E_m = k_3[R_t] \tag{8}$$

and

$$\frac{E}{E_m} = \frac{[RD]}{[R_t]} \tag{9}$$

Reworking equations (7) and (9) gives:

$$E = \frac{E_m[D]}{[D] + K_D} \tag{10}$$

This has the form of curve a (Figure 4.9). The validity of this approach depends on the following assumptions:

(i)   RL complex is reversible,
(ii)   association is bimolecular while dissociation is unimolecular,

(iii) all receptors of a given type are identical and act independently of one another,
(iv) the binding of the ligand to the receptor does not alter either the free concentration of the drug or the affinity of the receptor for the ligand,
(v) the response elicited by receptor occupation is directly proportional to the number of receptors occupied,
(vi) the biological response depends on attaining an equilibrium between R and D, and
(vii) the receptor, in its role as a transducing element, does not modify the ligand but is itself shifted from an inactive to an active state.

The limitations of the theory relate to its inability to define the relative concentrations of both the free receptor and the receptor ligand complex and to its inability to account for partial agonists. Nevertheless, it has played an important role in the development of molecular pharmacology and medicinal chemistry.

To overcome these difficulties the concept of "intrinsic activity" (E) was introduced. This is the quantal stimulus received by a receptor on interaction with a drug molecule. The total response of a tissue will then be the summation of these quantal responses over all the occupied receptors. At any time the fraction of receptors bound by a drug (RD) is given by the Hill equation reworking equations (4) and (6).

$$\frac{[RD]}{[R]} = \frac{[D]}{[D] + K_D} \tag{11}$$

Thus the stimulus to the tissue per receptor (S_R) is given by

$$S_R = \frac{E[D]}{[D] + K_D} \tag{12}$$

and the tissue will receive a net signal which is the summation of those quantal stimuli for the receptor density $[R_t]$ i.e.

$$S = [R_t] = \frac{E[R_t]}{1 + K_D[D]} \tag{13}$$

The final response (E) will be an unspecified function (f) of the stimulus

$$E_2 = f \frac{E[R_t]}{\left(1 + \dfrac{K_A}{[D]}\right)} \tag{14}$$

Thus the response of a tissue to a drug can now be seen to be dependent upon four, and not two, factors. As well as the original ones of receptor density and drug–receptor equilibrium dissociation constant there are efficacy which is a measure of how well the ligand induces the receptor to react and the amplification factor which is a measure of how a post-receptor cascade of reactions modulates the original interaction and converts it into the tissue response.

The term "efficacy" was introduced by Stephenson; an alternative concept of "intrinsic activity" was introduced by Ariens at about the same time. Ariens proposed that ligands have a modifying factor varying in value between 0 (antagonists) and 1 (full agonists) with partial agonists having fraction values. Intrinsic activity is thus a proportion of the maximal response (effect = intrinsic activity × [RD]) whilst efficacy is a proportionality factor with no meaning on the molecular level.

A further complication was uncovered when it was shown that on guinea pig ileum strip, a maximum response to the agonist, histamine, was still possible even when 99% of all the histamine receptors had been blocked by an irreversible competitive antagonist. This was explained by the concept of "spare receptors" (or "receptor reserve") which were defined as the fraction of the total receptor pool which is not required for a maximal tissue response. While the concept can explain some experimental findings, its biochemical rationale is more difficult to envisage. To summarise, drug-related responses depend on four factors:

(a) the density of receptors,
(b) the efficiency of the tissue in translating the binding of the ligand to the receptor into a pharmacological response,
(c) the equilibrium dissociation constant of the RL complex,
(d) the intrinsic efficiency of the binding interaction of the drug with the receptor.

Faced with the difficulties of the occupancy theory, Paton introduced the "rate theory" of ligand–receptor interaction in which the response is determined by the rate of the ligand–receptor complex formation. In other words, this is a kinetically controlled situation rather than an equilibrium one and stable receptor complex is not required for initiation of a biological response whose magnitude will be proportional to the rate of association and dissociation of the drug with the receptor. Mathematically, rate theory is expressed as:

$$E = \theta V_{eq} \tag{15}$$

where E is the effect, θ reflects the processing of the receptor–ligand complex and includes an efficacy component, and V is the velocity of the response. The rate of receptor–drug formation is measured in terms of discrete "all-or-none" changes in receptor-mediated events within the cell or tissue. Agonists have rapid rates for both association and dissociation, while antagonists have rapid rates of association but only slow rates of dissociation.

The spectrum of activity from agonist to antagonist is then explained by the decreased rates of dissociation of the drug–receptor complexes. Whilst the rate theory does explain the data found in the experiments on guinea pig ileum, there are many other cases where the theory does not apply. For example, if the post-receptor stimulus process is the major rate-limiting step then the kinetics of the receptor–ligand response may not reflect the tissue response.

As with occupancy theory, the rate theory has difficulty in explaining the subsequent molecular events in the tissue's response to a ligand.

The above discussions have considered that a ligand binds to a receptor at one site and that this provokes a series of events which ultimately results in the biological response. Allosteric modulators differ from these "classical" ligands in that they bind to a distant site. This binding causes a conformational change in a receptor, a change which affects the primary binding site and thus the affinity of this latter site for a ligand.

Two models of this behaviour have been proposed and both of these envisage that the receptor is a multicomponent oligomer. In the concerted model of Monod the oligomer comprises a finite number of identical subunits symmetrically arranged which have a single binding site for the ligand. The whole receptor exists in two conformational states, one of which has preference for the ligand, and a conformational state transition includes a simultaneous shift in the state of all subunits. No hybrids can exist.

In the induced fit model of Koshland the oligomer is formed from symmetrically arranged protomers each with a single binding site. Each of these protomers can exist in two conformational states with transition between them being induced by the ligand while the binding of the ligand removes the receptor symmetry.

Isolation and cloning of receptors by the techniques of molecular biology have shown that many are multi-unit species, which would fit in with the allosteric concept, but precisely how these function and particularly how subtle differences in function arise, is unclear.

The current situation as regards the theory of drug–receptor interaction is still unresolved. In a sense the issue is held in abeyance as the structures of actual receptors are being elucidated by molecular biology (as will be described shortly), and it is hoped that these studies will provide a molecular explanation for their activities. In the meantime the use of radioligand receptor binding studies which will be described in section 4.6 has perhaps provided a better method of discovering new receptor ligands and optimising their structures. Nevertheless, as will be explained, it is still necessary to evaluate potential ligands in tissues, or whole animals, to obtain a full picture of their functional activity.

4.5   TYPES OF BINDING IN DRUG–RECEPTOR INTERACTIONS

There is nothing exceptional about the particular interactions between a drug and its receptor, the forces available to control this interaction being the same as those experienced by all interacting organic molecules. Table 4.1 shows the binding forces involved and gives an indication of the free energy changes consequent to their formation.

4.5.1   Covalent bonds

Covalent bonds are very strong and, unless a specific enzyme is present to break this bond, covalently bound complexes between drugs and receptors are unlikely to be dissociated. This would be a great disadvantage for potential pharmacodynamic agents where an "on-off" response is required, but is not for chemotherapeutic agents where an irreversible blockade of the receptor essential for some aspect of the functioning of the cell is an effective way of destroying an invading organism. The covalent interaction of a drug with enzymes, particularly those in parasitic infections, will be discussed in greater detail in the section on enzymes.

However, covalent binding of an agent to a receptor is known, some anticancer alkylating agents work by alkylating purine and pyrimidine bases in DNA, thus interfering with its replication. The α-adrenergic antagonist, phenoxybenzamine (**9**), is also thought to act on the receptor by directly alkylating the active site. Benextramine (**10**) another α-adrenergic antagonist is also believed to react with its receptor by disulphide interchange with sulphydryl groups on the receptor.

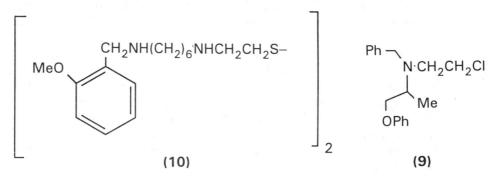

(10)   (9)

An established technique is to covalently label receptors by photolytic generation of an active centre on a ligand, such as a nitrene or carbene, thus aiding its identification or isolation. In general, however, covalent bonding of ligands to their receptors is not a significant factor in ligand binding.

While the major drug–receptor interactions are due to a combination of the bond types shown in Table 4.1 the relative importance of the different bonding interactions is still a subject of much debate. On the one hand it is argued that strong ionic interactions dominate, but others counter this by claiming that the large solvation energies of the free ions in water largely negate the overall free energy change involved in binding. For these scientists hydrophobic and dispersion forces are the dominating ones in forming the drug–receptor complex. The issue is as yet unresolved and solely the nature of these forces is described here. It should also be noted that the values quoted in free energy changes for these forces are very approximate, all being dependent on direction and distance and consequently will be highly variable from one ligand and receptor to another.

4.5.2   Electrostatic interaction

Opposite charges attract and this attraction leads to three main types of noncovalent bonds, ion–ion, ion–dipole and dipole–dipole. The first of these is the most important since at physiological pH a number of amino acids, especially lysine and arginine, are protonated whilst aspartate and glutamate are ionised, thus proteins containing these amino acids will have respectively positively and negatively charged centres. Thus drugs containing ionised carboxylic acid or protonated amino groups can interact strongly with these proteins, and from simple electrostatic theory the strength of this interaction is strongly dependent upon the distance between the charges, and the dielectric constant of the medium separating them. While the bond is strong when the distance is small, aqueous solvation of the separated ions greatly reduces

Table 4.1. Interaction energies of bond types

Bond type	Interaction energy (kcal/mol)
Covalent	$-(40-110)$
Electrostatic	
Ion–ion	$-(4-8)$
Ion–dipole	$-(1-7)$
Dipole–dipole	$-(1-7)$
Hydrogen bond	$-(1-5)$
Charge redistribution	
Polarisation	$-(1-3)$
Charge transfer	$-(1-3)$
Non-polar (van der Waals)	$-(0.5-1)$
Entropy-based	
Loss of rotational/ Translational entropy	$-(1-3)$
Hydrophobic interactions	-0.7 per CH_2 group

the total free energy change on association and means that the interaction is freely reversible. Such strong, but readily reversible bonds, are conceptually ideal for pharmacodynamic agents which should bind to the receptor, initiate a biological response and then dissociate. As a result of the electronegativity difference between oxygen, sulphur or nitrogen and carbon, bonds between these elements are polarised with an increased electron density on the heteroatom and a reduced electron density on the carbon atom. Consequently, an uneven electron distribution is established throughout the molecules and ion–dipole and dipole–dipole interactions between the centres of excess or reduced electron density in the drug and the converse in the receptor provide many opportunities for binding. Indeed, although the strength of each interaction is less for ion–dipole and dipole–dipole than it is for ion–ion interactions, they are much more prevalent and therefore overall may be more significant for the binding process.

Hydrogen bonding is a particular example of an electrostatic bond formed between the hydrogen atoms of OH and NH bonds and the electronegative atoms oxygen, nitrogen and sulphur. The strongest hydrogen bonds are those formed between groups with the greatest electrostatic character, i.e. carboxylates are better acceptors than amides, ketones or unionised carboxyls. Since OH and NH bonds are common constituents of proteins and many drugs contain electronegative atoms, hydrogen bonds would be expected to play a significant part in the binding process. However, water is a strong hydrogen bonding agent itself as both a donor and acceptor and thus any such drug will be strongly hydrogen bonded in the free state. Thus, as was the case above for ion–ion interactions, the overall energy change for the binding may not be favourable.

4.5.3   Charge redistribution

During a drug–receptor interaction some charge redistribution usually takes place. When this process occurs within a molecule, either that of the drug or the receptor, it is known as polarisation; when it involves both molecules it is referred to as charge distribution. Interactions due to polarisation occur when a temporary dipole is induced in a group or bond by the field owing to a charged group which can be either an ion or a dipole. Charge transfer interactions occur when an electron donor makes a sufficiently close contact with an electron acceptor to allow electron transfer from a high-energy occupied molecular orbital of the donor to a low-energy molecular orbital of the acceptor. This type of bonding is particularly important with large aromatic molecules and may be especially concerned in the interaction of intercalating agents with DNA.

4.5.4   Van der Waals' forces

These are the most universal forces of attraction that arise between atoms and result from the natural polarisation in electron clouds induced by atoms as they approach one another. This polarisation disturbs the electron clouds and consequently the nuclei of each atom are attracted to the electrons of the other atom. Van der Waals' forces operate in all types of molecules, both polar and nonpolar, and occur over very short periods, $c.\ 10^{-6}$ seconds. While they are weak and short-acting their ubiquitous nature means that overall they add up to an important element of the binding process. In fact, they are possibly more important in maintaining protein structure than hydrogen bonding or ionic interactions simply because of the cumulative effect of many such interactions.

4.5.5   Entropy-based forces

The formation of a drug–receptor complex results in considerable loss of rotational and translational degrees of freedom by the drug molecule. Although some of this is replaced by vibrational degrees of freedom in the complex there is usually a considerable entropy loss entailed in the binding process, the more rigid the drug molecule the less will be this entropy loss.

When a nonpolar molecule is exposed to water, strong water–water interactions around the solute lead to an ordering of the structure of the solvent and a subsequently negative entropy of dissolution. When the nonpolar solute binds to a nonpolar region of a receptor the total nonpolar surface area of the system will also be reduced. Consequently, the amount of structured water will be reduced and the total entropy of this system will be increased; the resultant free energy change provides the driving force for this hydrophobic bond. In view of the large amounts of nonpolar regions available to proteins and many drugs this bonding is of considerable importance in the binding of small molecules to biological macromolecules.

4.6   THE USE OF RADIO-LABELLED LIGANDS

Ever since the concept of receptors was first advanced much of the work of pharmacology and medicinal chemistry has been directed towards their understanding and the nature of the interaction with ligands. At first this required investigating the

behaviour of tissues, or derived fragments, with putative ligands in the
other modifying agents. Whilst such studies provided much information
in the development of significant numbers of novel therapeutic agents, t
objective is the actual isolation of a receptor. It has been estimated, ho
all the receptor proteins in brain tissue amount to only about one millic
total protein mass, and thus the task of isolating sufficient pure single re....p...r by
classical means to fully characterise its properties would be very difficult to say the
least. In section 4.7.3 the techniques of molecular biology which are making this aim
reality are described, but an alternative, and extremely useful, approach has been to
use radio-labelled ligands.

It had been recognised for some time that a useful strategy would be to use a
ligand specific to one type of receptor to identify these receptors in a tissue, provided
that the extremely small amounts of bound ligand could be identified. Radio-labelling
provides the obvious method whereby the extremely low levels of bound material
could be detected, but it required significant technical advances before ligands with
specific activities greater than 20 Ci/mmol became available whereupon the concept
could be validated. Suitable isotopes available to provide these levels of radioactivity
are tritium [^{3}H], iodine [^{125}I] and sulphur [^{35}S].

Experimentally the technique is very straightforward. Approximately one milligram
of a tissue rich in the receptor under investigation is incubated in buffer solution
with labelled ligand until equilibrium is reached. The temperature and time for this
incubation depend on the receptor and the tissue being investigated but are commonly
4°C and 15–20 minutes. Excess ligand is then removed by washing and either
filtration or centrifugation. The precise technique varies with the chosen receptor but
the filter method is much faster and permits a greater throughput of assays. The
amount of labelled ligand bound to the tissue can then be measured by standard
liquid scintillation counting of the whole sample. Not all the ligand held by the
sample will be bound to the specific receptor however; nonspecific binding to other
biopolymers in the tissue, to the filters and to the test tubes can also take place, and
it is essential to differentiate between them. The number of specific receptor sites will
be limited while the nonspecific sites are essentially unlimited in number. The binding
experiment is therefore repeated in the presence of a very large excess (100-fold) of
nonradiolabelled ligand under which conditions it is unlikely that any radio-labelled
ligand will bind to the specific sites while nonspecific binding will be unaffected. The
difference in the binding values for the two experiments then measures the amount
of specific binding. While the amount of specific binding can vary between 40% and
98% of the total binding, specific binding of less than 30% in practice gives results
of limited utility. Repeating the binding experiments with a range of labelled ligand
concentrations allows a plot to be drawn such as that shown in Figure 4.10. The
extent of specific binding reaches a limit which is not exceeded whatever the
concentration of ligand, providing clear evidence for the existence of a limited finite
number of receptor sites. This, of course, is exactly what would be expected if the
experiment was really measuring only receptor sites specific for the ligand under
investigation. The data in Figure 4.10 can be reworked to give a Scatchard plot
using:

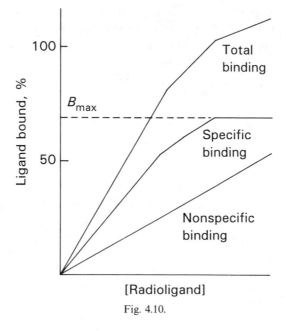

Fig. 4.10.

$$\frac{B}{F} = -\frac{1}{K_d}B + \frac{B_{mas}}{K_d} \tag{16}$$

where B is the amount specifically bound, B_{max} is the maximum bound, F represents the free ligand and K_d is the dissociation constant. Using this equation and plotting B/F against B gives a straight line plot (Figure 4.11) from which B_{max} and K_d can be obtained. B_{max} is the density of binding sites on a concentration/weight basis and is a measure of the total number of receptors in a tissue.

The purpose of these studies and the reason for their great popularity with medicinal chemists working in certain therapeutic areas is to repeat the binding experiments in the presence of a putative ligand for the receptor. Varying amounts of the compound under investigation are added to the incubation medium containing a fixed amount of the labelled ligand, the amount of specific binding is then plotted against the concentration of added compound and from the curve IC_{50} values can be determined. This is the concentration of the added compound which reduces the specific binding of the ligand to 50% of its maximal value. This figure is a direct measure of the potency of binding of the compound relative to the labelled ligand on the specific receptor. In practice, values of IC_{50} greater than 10^{-4} M are deemed to be inactive. The great value of IC_{50} values determined in this way is that they are a direct measure of the potency of a compound at the receptor, unaffected by transport or metabolic processes found *in vivo*, and they are also unaffected by post-receptor modulation effects encountered in studies in tissues.

The method is rapid, needs only milligram quantities of material to determine IC_{50} values and provides a screening process whereby the activity of a large number of compounds may be compared on a specific receptor. The method is routinely used

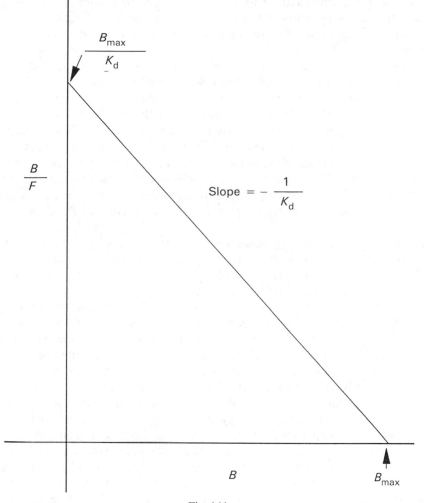

Fig. 4.11.

when searching for a new lead structure in a series of molecules not hitherto tested on a certain receptor or when attempting to modify a basic structure to increase the binding potency. There are, however, a couple of caveats since results obtained *in vitro* cannot be directly extrapolated to the *in vivo* situation where metabolism and transport effects may prevent the drug ever reaching the appropriate receptor. In addition, such studies cannot indicate whether the new ligand is an agonist or an antagonist at the receptor (the labelled ligand can be either). This is unlike the situation with experiments on isolated tissues where the tissue response shows the agent to be an agonist or antagonist. In fact, for a number of systems where both agonists and antagonists are available in labelled form it is found that single putative ligands often have markedly different IC_{50} values depending on which labelled ligand is used. Use of a labelled agonist results in other agonists binding more strongly to the receptor than antagonists and vice versa, leading to the conclusion that the two agents are binding to different receptors (or to the same receptor in significantly different ways).

As well as aiding medicinal chemists in the search for more potent drugs, binding studies have been used for a number of other purposes. Thus they have been used to investigate fundamental malfunctions in a number of disease states. An early example of such a study by a major pioneer in the field (Snyder) showed that haloperidol, a drug widely and successfully used to control the devastating mental illness called schizophrenia, acted on a physiological dopamine receptor. This suggested the involvement of the dopamine system in the disease; stronger evidence came from a series of experiments where he was able to show that a whole range of antischizophrenic drugs also acted on the dopamine receptor; furthermore, that the strength of their binding to the receptor was directly related to the clinical dosage of the drug.

Another use of receptorology arises from the extreme potency of many drugs (IC_{50} values are usually in the nanomolar range) so that displacement studies can be used as a highly sensitive quantitative measure of the drug in the body fluids for kinetic measurements and appropriate dosage titration.

While many of the technical problems of the methodology have been solved, it is worth pointing out some of the inherent reservations. A number of criteria have been devised which must be satisfied before it can be concluded that a specific receptor is being measured; the binding of the ligand must be saturable (a finite number of sites exist); binding constants must be high with IC_{50}s in at least the nM region; the binding must be reversible; the distribution of the binding sites both between tissues and within cells must be compatible with the proposed physiological role of the natural ligand; the pharmacology of the binding site should have similar agonist/antagonist properties to those observed for the natural ligand in functional test procedures, and a corresponding correlation of binding with biological dose/concentration curves in the corresponding tissue preparation should be generated.

The potential for misinformation resulting from use such studies is well illustrated by the stereoselective binding of the opiate antagonist naloxone to talc and the binding of phencyclidine to filter discs!

4.7 ISOLATION OF RECEPTORS

4.7.1 Separation of specific receptors from membranes

Expressed simply, the problem of isolation of a given receptor from its membrane is one of identification and separation of a specific protein from all the other proteins. Recent developments in chromatographic techniques have greatly increased the potential for the successful execution of such studies.

The first stage is to tease a complex mixture of proteins out of a membrane with as little damage to them as possible which is relatively easy when the protein is only loosely bound (peripheral membrane proteins) and usually only needs removal of cations such as Ca^{2+} and Mg^{2+} from the medium by washing or chelation. In these cases the protein is usually released into the solution essentially free from lipid fragments.

The situation is much more difficult with integral proteins, however, which extend through the membrane and have three distinct regions: an extracellular one projecting into the environment surrounding the membrane; one which passes through the membrane; and an intracellular one protruding into the cell. Such proteins are integral components of the cell membrane and interact with it much more strongly, and, moreover, their tertiary structure and adopted conformation may be directed by its presence in the membrane. Release of such a protein from the membrane can severely affect conformation and hence its ligand binding ability. More severe conditions are required to release such proteins, and the detergents, Triton X-100, Lubrol and CHAPS-(3-cholamidopropyl-dimethylammonio-1-propane sulphate) or the choatropes, urea, sodium thiocyanate and medium chain length alcohols are extensively used to disrupt the membrane and release the target protein.

4.7.2 Purification of target protein

The isolation of a target protein from the complex mix of released proteins necessitates the use of very sophisticated chromatographic separation techniques. Of these, the most commonly used is affinity chromatography, the basic concept of which is simple enough, although the practice is more complex. The basic concept is that the receptor binds strongly to its ligand such that this interaction can be used to discriminate the required protein. Thus the ligand is covalently bonded to a solid support via a linking chain such that its binding ability is essentially unaffected, when passing a solution of various peptides over the column results in the receptor required being preferentially retained. When the other proteins have been washed off, the receptor can be liberated by passing through the column a concentrated solution of the ligand. Radio-labelled ligand can be used subsequently to detect in which tubes the receptor is located (Figure 4.12).

Stage one
Soluble receptors are freed from guinea pig lung by centrifugation in presence of digitonin

Stage two
Affinity column separation over alphenolol-Sepharose
(i)   Receptors bind to alprenolol on the inert support
(ii)   All other proteins are washed off column, thus leaving a pure preparation of receptor on
       column
(iii) The receptor is eluted off column by alprenolol solution

Stage three
Further purification of receptors takes place using:
(i)   DEAE ion exchange chromatography
(ii)   Size exclusion HPLC
(iii) Preparative SDS-PAGE

Fig. 4.12.   Separation of mammalian β-adrenergic receptors (schematic).

Related techniques rely on immunoaffinity chromatography or immunoprecipitation where mono- or poly-clonal antibodies are used to provide the highly selective interaction needed to separate the required protein. Recent advances in high-performance liquid chromatography (HPLC), particularly size-exclusion HPLC, ion-exchange HPLC, and reverse phase HPLC have significantly extended the methodology to allow many receptor proteins to be isolated. It should be pointed out that all these methods are invariably complicated and require great technical skill by the experimentalist to prevent the appearance of artefacts and the generation of subsequently specious results.

The primary proof that the appropriate receptor has been obtained is provided by its high affinity binding to its ligand. Another way of ensuring that the correct protein is isolated is via photoaffinity labelling of the receptor. In this case a radio-labelled ligand is prepared containing a suitable functional group which, on photolysis, releases a reactive entity such as nitrene or carbene which covalently binds to the receptor. The β-adrenergic receptor, for example, has been labelled by using iodocyanopindolol diazine and the dopamine receptor with azido-N-methyl piperone. Treatment of a membrane with these reagents followed by photolysis leaves the receptor permanently labelled by the radioactive ligand enabling it to be readily detected throughout subsequent manipulations.

4.7.3   The use of molecular biology
While significant progress has been made in developing the techniques for isolating receptors these are obviously inherently limited by the small amounts of receptor present in any membrane as well as the practical difficulties inherent in determining protein structures. The use of molecular biology, however, provides alternative methods which overcome these limitations. A typical study (Dixon, Lefkowitz *et al.*) on the β-adrenergic receptor illustrates the power of the method.

This receptor obtained from hamster lung was isolated and purified by the techniques of sequential affinity chromatography and molecular sieve HPLC described above. In practice, the complete protein could not be sequenced by normal techniques, and so it was fragmented by treatment with cyanogen bromide. The corresponding fragments could be readily sequenced, and an oligonucleotide corresponding to the DNA encoding for one 34 amino acid fragment was synthesised and used to isolate the gene for the receptor. The sequence of the gene could be readily determined and provided the primary amino acid sequence of the protein with all the fragments from the original cyanogen bromide cleavage being accounted for. The structure of the receptor was thus established, and in subsequent work it was expressed from the isolated gene. Many such studies on a plethora of receptors have been carried out.

4.8   PRIMARY AND SECONDARY MESSENGERS

So far receptors and their interactions with agents loosely described as "ligands" have been discussed without describing in any detail what is meant by this term and what the function of these ligands or the consequences of their binding with the receptor might be. Primary messengers are present throughout the body to control its functioning, whereas secondary messengers are released inside the cells subsequent to the binding of a primary messenger to its receptor. The secondary messengers are thus responsible for translating a macrophysiological signal external to the cell into an intracellular biochemical one.

4.8.1   Primary messengers

Two distinct and very different systems, the endocrinal and the nervous, control all the functions of the body. The endocrinal system comprises a number of specialised organs which secrete the chemicals known as hormones into the bloodstream where they are transported to the appropriate target organs. The nature of the control exercised by this system is essentially long term, responsible as it is for *inter alia*, growth, the initiation and modulation of sexuality, the rate of metabolism, and the level of blood glucose. In addition the immune system, which controls the body's response to infection, and rejects tissues which it perceives as being foreign to it, operates through a system of highly specialised tissues and cells via a family of protein messengers, the cytokines. The nervous system is quite different in that it uses a network of specialised cells, the neurons, to communicate throughout the body by a combination of electrical and chemical transmission. It is the system which controls rapid movement, produces near-instantaneous reflex response to physiological threats, controls heart rate and blood pressure, lung function, digestion, and monitors and reacts to changes in the external environment.

Anatomically, the nervous system is divided into the central and peripheral sections: the central nervous system (CNS) comprises the brain and spinal cord and is the thought and control centre of the body; the peripheral system permeates all the organs of the body. Since an understanding of the nervous system is so important for drug action and subsequent drug design it is necessary to consider its structure in more detail. Two major classes of cells, the neurons and the glia, constitute the nervous system along with the necessary blood supply system. The glial cells appear to act in a supportive role to the neurons and are not directly involved in electrical transmission, and as they have not, to date, been shown to be sites of action for drugs will not be discussed further. Attention will be focused on the neuron, which is the fundamental building block of the nervous system.

4.8.1.1   The neuron

The neuron is a highly specialised cell which appears in a number of different forms, two of which, the spinal motor and sensory neurons, are represented in Figure 4.13. Despite the diversity of shape and size, all neurons possess three distinct regions, the cell body, the dendrites, and the axon. The cell body contains the nucleus whilst the dendrites and axon are spiky processes growing out from its surface. Dendrites are short highly branched processes of irregular diameter whose function is to transmit impulses to the cell body. Whereas a neuron may have a number of dendrites it usually has only one axon. This is much longer than the dendrites, is sparsely branched, has a regular diameter, and its function is to transmit impulses from the cell body to a target muscle or organ. In some motor nerves the axons can reach one metre in length, making these neurons the longest cells in the body. The axons are covered not only by a normal membrane but also by another cell, the Schwann cell, which envelops it. A long axon will have a number of associated Schwann cells each covering several millimetres of its length, and in some places the Schwann cell is wrapped repeatedly round the axon until it is covered by a multiple layer of membrane. This covering forms the "myelin sheath", and junctions between adjacent stretches of multiple layers where the axon is covered only by a single Schwann cell layer are known as the nodes of Ranvier. The essential purpose of the myelin sheath is to increase the protective insulation around the neuron, improving the electrical transmission along it; the purpose of the node of Ranvier is to facilitate this transmission.

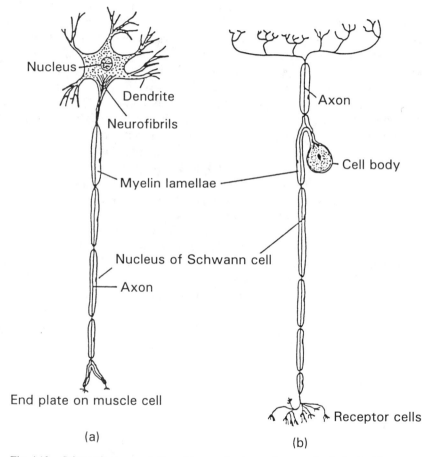

Fig. 4.13.   Schematic representation of two major types of neuron in the body: (a) a motor neuron, (b) a sensory neuron.

The junction between an axon and another axon, a dendrite, a cell body, or a muscle cell is known as a synapse. This junction consists of a gap of some 200–500 Å across which the information carried by the neuron is transmitted via the release of a neurotransmitter from one side of the synapse. The released transmitter permeates the synaptic cleft and reacts with its receptor on the other side, thus provoking a further response, the nature of which will depend on the precise location of the synapse. Between two neurons the response may be to initiate or inhibit a subsequent nerve impulse, whereas between a neuron and a muscle cell the response will ultimately be the physical contraction or elongation of the cell. The biochemical consequences of this interaction are considered in section 4.8.2.

The role of the synapse is to allow a graded response of the system to stimulation or ennervation with a finite time to occur. As will be described in the next section, an electrical transmission is an all or nothing procedure whereas response to a neurotransmitter will be directly related to the amount of it interacting with the receptor. Moreover the existence of a finite number of receptors prevents the receptor system from being overloaded. It must be noted that overall transmission can take place only in one direction which is an essential organisational aid controlling the functioning of the neuronal network.

4.8.1.2 Electrical transmission in neurons

Because cell membranes are not equally porous to all cations and anions, most cells of the body have concentrations of ions inside the cell which are different from those found in the extracellular fluids. The membranes of most cells appear to be quite permeable to potassium and chloride ions, but a specific mechanism, the "sodium-potassium ion pump", exists to keep the intracellular sodium ion concentration considerably lower (about nine times) than that on the outside. Since the larger potassium ions remain inside the cell where they are electrostatically attracted to large electronegative nonpermeating proteins, there is an imbalance in electrical charges, which results in the interior of the cell being electronegative relative to the exterior. The electrical potential thus generated which is around 70 mV is known as the resting membrane potential.

Electrical transmission within neurons begins with a sudden localised and transient increase in membrane permeability to sodium ions, an increase which is believed to arise from the loss of calcium ions from pores in the membrane. This increase in permeability leads to a diffusion controlled influx of sodium ions. Some potassium ions are consequently displaced, but as the rate of efflux of potassium ions is very much slower than the rate of influx of sodium ions the membrane potential is reversed as the inside of the cell becomes positive relative to the outside. In this condition, the neuronal membrane is said to be depolarised. As the sodium pump reasserts itself the sodium ions are pumped out and the polarity reverts to normal. Figure 4.14 summarises the resultant changes in membrane potential with time, the maximum change in electrical potential being known as the action potential.

The action potential moves down the axon because along the length of a nonmyelinated axon there are channels which are selectively permeable to either sodium or potassium ions. The action potential is triggered by a signal from the cell opening a sodium channel which allows sodium ions into the cell, thus reversing the polarity. The existence of the action potential then closes the sodium channel, opens the potassium channel, and reverses the ion flow. Moreover, the presence of an action potential in one part of the axon opens sodium channels in an adjacent part, and this propagates the action potential along the axon. After a suitable period the process can be repeated. In myelinated neurons the exchange of ions takes place only

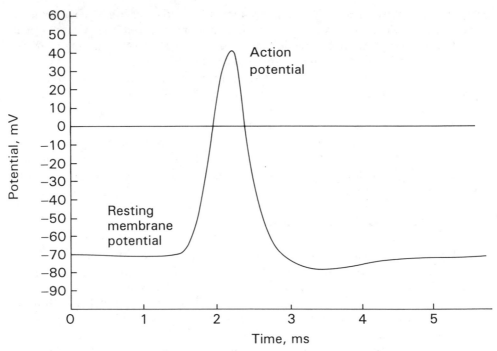

Fig. 4.14. Changes in membrane potential during the development of an action potential.

at the nodes of Ranvier, and the action potential has to jump between adjacent nodes.

Since the value of the action potential is essentially controlled by the molecular properties of the neuronal membranes this cannot be altered for a given system, and the only mechanism for varying the degree of response is by altering the number of impulses generated in a finite period. The arrival of the action potential at the synapse causes release of the neurotransmitter. It is tempting to draw an analogy between nerve transmission and that of electrical transmission through electrical wiring, but this is an imprecise analogy. Electrical currents in conducting wires travel essentially at the speed of light, while nerve impulses travel at speeds varying from less than 3 mph to 200 mph. Moreover, nerve fibres themselves are very poor electrical conductors and the impulse is transmitted only because it is being continually replenished, which requires expenditure of considerable amounts of energy.

4.8.1.3   *The organisation of the nervous system*
The central nervous system consists of the brain and the spinal cord and contains about 10^{11} neurons and, since each of these cells forms synapses with up to one thousand other neurons, the extreme complexity of the system can be appreciated. More than 80% of the brain comprises a deeply grooved walnut-like mass which is known as the cerebral cortex in which all the control, sensory, and creative functions of the body are coordinated (Figures 4.15 and 4.16). From above, the cerebrum appears to be symmetrical—an impression reinforced by the existence of a deep

fissure running from back to front. Although the brain is anatomically symmetrical, however, and many of its functions are bilateral, one side tends to dominate the other for different functions, the centres controlling speech, for example, are predominantly in the left hemisphere. A consequence of this differential dominance is that similar amounts of brain damage to the two hemispheres can lead to remarkably different overt consequences to the casualty.

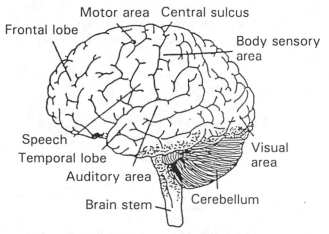

Fig. 4.15.   Major areas of the human brain.

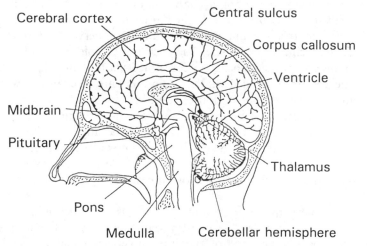

Fig. 4.16.   Sectional view showing major regions of the brain.

Pasteur, for example, suffered a stroke which a post-mortem examination showed years later had severely damaged the right hemisphere of his brain. Despite this injury Pasteur had suffered only mild paralysis of one side of his body and he was able to complete much of his most important work. Had this damage occurred in the other hemisphere the consequences for him and society would have been much more serious. A further complexity is the fact that the right-hand side of the brain controls the functioning of the left-hand side of the body and vice versa. Whilst scientific understanding of the functioning of the brain is still in its infancy, significant progress is being made in identifying and modulating the neurotransmitters involved in the chemistry of the brain. The discussion of these neurotransmitters forms the substance of section 4.8.1.4.

The peripheral nervous system is much less complex than the CNS and comprises two main arms, the sensory and motor functions (Figure 4.17), with the motor functions being further divided into the voluntary and autonomic sections. The autonomic system itself is subdivided into the parasympathetic and sympathetic nervous systems

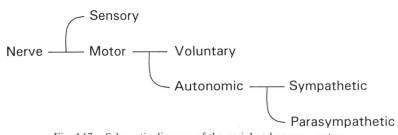

Fig. 4.17.   Schematic diagram of the peripheral nervous system.

Sensory nerves run from the receptors at the skin surface which detect heat or cold, pressure and pain, to the spinal cord from which information can be transmitted to the appropriate region of the brain. The voluntary motor nerves run in the reverse direction, namely from the spinal cord to the muscle fibres. Conscious decisions taken within the brain control the impulses through these nerves and thus affect the movement of the specific target muscle. The decisions to hold this book and to move the eyes to follow the printed words are controlled via the voluntary motor nerves. Whilst these nerves are controlled via the brain there are mechanisms which permit even faster involuntary implementation of responses such as the knee-jerk response to mild pressure which is familiar to anyone who has undergone a medical examination. This reflex reaction occurs so rapidly because the nervous system is able to bypass the brain pathways. A small neuron, known as the internuncial neuron, lying as shown in Figure 4.18 in the spinal cord between a sensory neurone and a motor neuron, is able to relay such sensory impulses directly to the motor neuron implicated.

The autonomic nervous system primarily controls the functioning of the major body organs such as the heart, the intestines, and blood vessels and is concerned essentially with the maintenance of the internal environment of the body. The definition "autonomic" is really a misnomer which was introduced when it was felt that these functions of the body were not under conscious control of the brain, although it is now appreciated that many people are able to control their heart rate, blood pressure, and metabolic rate to some extent.

The autonomic nervous system is divided into the sympathetic and parasympathetic areas as shown in Figure 4.17 with both arms usually impinging on the same organ with opposing effects. Sympathetic nerves have the role of preparing the body for

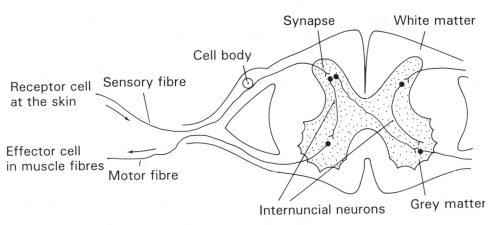

Fig. 4.18.   Diagrammatic view of the reflex arc showing the presence of internuncial neurons in the spinal cord.

"fight or flight", and thus the expenditure of energy, whilst the parasympathetic system is concerned with conserving or restoring energy. The various physiological effects induced by the activation of the two systems on a number of organs of the body are shown in Table 4.2.

4.8.1.4 Neurotransmitters
In view of the crucial importance of the synapse to body functioning, it is obviously of great significance to establish the neurotransmitters implicated in the activity of various synaptic clefts. This is by no means a simple task, and a number of scientific criteria have been identified which must be met before a molecule can be regarded as a neurotransmitter. The major criteria are:

(1) a true transmitter is released only when the nerve is stimulated,
(2) an enzymatic system must exist in the neuron itself capable of synthesising the neurotransmitter together with a further mechanism capable of rapidly removing it,
(3) an antagonist must be capable of blocking the biological response produced both by natural stimulation and the putative transmitter,
(4) introduction of the putative transmitter into the appropriate tissue preparation must induce the appropriate biological response.

Criterion (1) follows from the discussion above in which it was pointed out that neurotransmitter release in a neuron results from the action of an action potential at its synaptic membrane. Criterion (2) recognises that the quantity of neurotransmitter needed for nerve transmission can only be present if it is synthesised locally within the neuron since uptake of a transmitter from the bloodstream would be a very much less efficient process. Furthermore, a transmitter has to be released from its receptor and subsequently efficiently removed from the synaptic cleft since otherwise stimulation of the receptor would never cease. Criteria (3) and (4) establish that the putative transmitter and the natural transmitter interact with the same receptor.

Table 4.2   Effects of stimulation of sympathetic and parasympathetic nerves on organs of the body

Organ	Sympathetic	Parasympathetic
Blood vessels	Constriction, except coronary vessels which are dilated	Usually nil
Heart	Acceleration and augmentation	Inhibition
Eye: Iris	Contraction of radial muscle	Contraction of circular muscle
Ciliary muscle	Nil	Contraction
Skin: Sweat secretion	Augmentation	Nil
Erection of hairs	Increased	Nil
Salivary glands	Slight secretion	Free secretion and vasodilation
Stomach: Contractions	Inhibition	Augmentation
Secretions	—	Increase
Sphincters	Contraction or relaxation	Relaxation or contraction
Intestinal movements	Inhibition	Augmentation
Gall bladder	Relaxation	Contraction
Liver	Glycogenolysis	Nil
Spleen	Contraction	Nil
Pancreatic secretion	—	Increase
Bronchial muscle	Relaxation	Contraction
Bronchial secretion	Nil	Increase
Ureter	Relaxation	Contraction
Bladder: Fundus	Relaxation	Contraction
Sphincter	Contraction	Relaxation
Uterus	Contraction and relaxation	

In accordance with these criteria acetylcholine and noradrenaline have been identified as the two major neurotransmitters in the peripheral nervous system, with dopamine, noradrenaline, acetylcholine, histamine, γ-aminobutyric acid, glutamic acid and glycine important transmitters in the central nervous system. Within the peripheral nervous system, it can be seen that in four of five synapses found in the three arms of the peripheral nervous system acetylcholine is the exclusive neurotransmitter, and only at the neuromuscular function in the sympathetic autonomic nervous system is noradrenaline, in addition, responsible for nervous transmission (Figure 4.19). However, acetylcholine does not have the same effect at each synapse. In the neuromuscular junction of the voluntary system and the ganglia of the autonomic system its effects are immediate, brief, and localised, such properties being those required for facilitating fine, precise nervous control. At the post-ganglionic nerve ending in the parasympathetic system, however, the effects are slower in onset, less localised, and more prolonged in action, the appropriate properties required here for maintaining muscle tone.

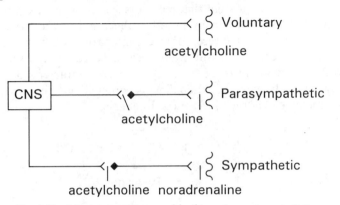

Fig. 4.19.   Neurotransmitters used in the motor nervous system.

Not only are its effects at the different synapses different but also the agonists which can mimic these actions of acetylcholine are different. Thus, in the first case, nicotine (**11**) is a potent agonist, and these synapses are defined as "nicotinic", while in the second case muscarine (**12**) is a potent agonist, and these receptors are characterised as "muscarinic". These simple findings are very profound as they clearly show that not all receptors bind with the same ligand in the same way and that, as a consequence, agonists and antagonists can bind to different receptors with different potencies. This is the basis of the principle of selectivity discussed in Chapter 1 and historically such studies were conducted on strips of muscle tissue where the activity of putative agents on the cholinergic receptor could be readily measured.

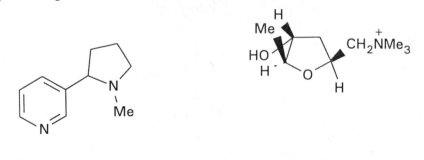

(11)   **(12)**

Similar affects are seen in the adrenergic system where noradrenaline (**13**) is the established transmitter at the synapse in the sympathetic nervous system (Figure 4.19). Adrenaline and noradrenaline are biosynthesised from tyrosine as shown in Figure 4.20, whilst adrenaline (**14**), the *N*-methylated derivative of noradrenaline, is not thought to be a peripheral neurotransmitter. Adrenaline is produced by the adrenal medulla, a gland located near the kidneys, and can interact with the same receptors as noradrenaline. Whereas noradrenaline functions to maintain smooth muscle tone and the blood circulation, adrenaline acts as an "activator" to prepare the body for fight or flight. From the early pharmacological studies on the adrenergic nervous system it became apparent that receptors existed which gave rise to different effects in response to stimulation by noradrenaline, and it was postulated that α-receptors were excitatory and β-receptors were inhibitory. With the development of other agonists, however, the classification became based on the sensitivity of the receptors to these new agonists, and α-receptors were characterised by an order of agonist activity, noradrenaline $\simeq$ adrenaline $>$ isoprenaline (**15**) and β-receptors by the order isoprenaline $>$ adrenaline $>$ noradrenaline.

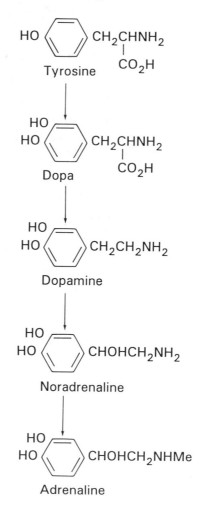

Fig. 4.20.   Synthesis of noradrenaline and adrenaline from tyrosine.

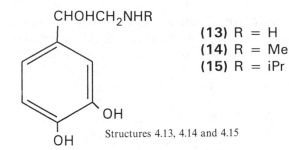

CHOHCH$_2$NHR

(13) R = H
(14) R = Me
(15) R = iPr

Structures 4.13, 4.14 and 4.15

Further work resulted in subdivision of the β-receptors into β$_1$ and β$_2$ types where, in pharmacological terms, agonism of β$_1$ receptors leads to cardiac stimulation and fat breakdown whilst β$_2$ stimulation gives rise to bronchodilation and vasodepression. The various effects due to different receptor stimulation on the different organs are summarised in Table 4.3. The diversity of these effects has made possible the discovery of agents selective for particular organs: the antiasthmatic salbutamol (β$_2$ stimulant) produces bronchodilation with no significant cardiac effects, whilst the antihypertensive prazosin (16) (postsynaptic α-blocker) is devoid of side effects on the respiratory system. Selective β-antagonists which can selectively reduce heart rate are extremely important in modern medicine owing to the high prevalence of cardiovascular problems in Western society. Thus from hundreds of synthetic derivatives of general structure Ar CH(OH)CH$_2$NHiPr propranolol (structure 54, Chapter 1) was found to be a pure β-blocker with no sympathomimetic activity.

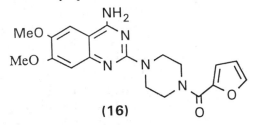

(16)

These data clearly illustrate that, even when the body uses the same transmitter system in different synapses, subtle differences in receptor shape exist so that it is possible to design agonists and antagonists which are specific for the same receptors in different tissues and thus to selectively affect a single target organ.

Within the central nervous system the number of known transmitters is much larger and because of the complexity of the organ it is less easy to identify their precise activities. Despite this, spectacular progress has been achieved in some areas. The major motor disorder Parkinson's disease results from atrophy of dopamine-containing neurons in the basal ganglia, a large mass of neurons found in the cerebellum, and a variety of mental disorders ranging from anxiety to schizophrenia appear to be linked to the production of deficiencies or excesses of neurotransmitters in specific areas of the brain.

The development of the radio-labelled ligand binding studies previously described has done much to elucidate the complexities of the system. As might be expected, it is found that multiple subtypes of most identified neurotransmitters exist and a list of these and other subtypes is shown in Table 4.4. The receptor for the opium alkaloids was the first to be identified within the CNS, although its function remained a mystery until the natural ligands the enkephalins (**17**) were discovered. More recently receptors for the benzodiazepines and cannabinoids have also been discovered, but as yet their natural endogenous ligands have not been defined.

Table 4.3   Receptors mediating adrenergic effects

Effector organ	Response	Receptor
Heart	Increase in rate, contractility, excitability	$\beta1$
Blood vessels (coronary, pulmonary, skeletal muscle, abdominal viscera)	Dilation	$\beta2$
(to skin)	Contraction	α
Lungs	Relaxation of bronchial muscle	$\beta2$
Uterus	Relaxation	$\beta2$
Kidney	Stimulation of renin release	$\beta1$
Gastrointestinal tract	Relaxation of smooth muscle	β
	Contraction of stomach and intestine	α
Eye	Relaxation of ciliary muscle	β
	Contraction of radial muscle	α
Skeletal muscle	Decreased tension and degree of fusion of incomplete tetanic contractions of slow muscle	$\beta2$
	Stimulation of glycogenolysis, lactate production	$\beta2$
Adipose tissue	Stimulation of lipolysis	'$\beta1$'
Pancreas	Increased insulin secretion	$\beta2$
Blood	Increase in factor 8 levels and fibrinolysis and decrease in whole blood clotting time. Increase in platelet aggregation	$\beta2$

From W. G. Richards, *Quantum Pharmacology*, 2nd edn, 1950, p.50.

4.8.1.5   *Other transmitters*

Table 4.4 also lists a number of receptors, such as those for bradykinin and the leukotrienes whose ligands are not neurotransmitters. Some of these ligands, notably the prostaglandins, leukotrienes, a variety of proteins such as bradykinin and the cytokines are hormones released into extracellular fluids from a number of cells and tissues which are then transported to the target cells and tissues where they act via specific receptors. The further differentiation of many of these into subtypes necessi-

Table 4.4   Examples of receptors showing multiple subtypes

Receptors for	Subtypes
adenosine	A_1, A_2
adrenaline-α	$\alpha 1_a$, $\alpha 1_a$, $\alpha 2_A$, $\alpha 2_B$.
adrenaline β	β_1, β_2, β_3,
-aminobutyric acid	A, B
bradykinin	β_1, β_2,
cholecystokinin and gastrin	CCK_A, CCK_B
dopamine	D_1, D_2
excitatory amino acids	N-methyl-D-aspartate, D,L-α-amino-3-hydroxy-5-methyl-4-isoxalone propionic acid, L-amino-4-phosphonobutanoate, kainic acid
histamine	H_1, H_2, H_3
leukotriene	LTB_4, LTC_4, LTD_4
muscarinic	M_1, M_2, M_3
nicotinic	muscle type, neuronal type
opioid	μ, , K,
P2-purinoreceptors	P_{2X}, P_{2Y}, P_{2Z}, P_{2T}
serotonin (5HT)	$5HT_{1A}$, $5HT_{1B}$, $5HT_{1C}$, $5HT_{1D}$, $5HT_2$, $5HT_3$
tachykinin	NK_1, NK_2, NK_3
vasopressin and oxytocin	V_{1A}, V_{1A}, V_2, OT

Table 4.5   Neuropeptidic transmitters

Neuropeptides
Cholecystokinin
Substance P
Neurotensin
β-Endorphin
Leu-enkephalin
Met-enkephalin
Oxytocin
Vasoactive intestinal polypeptide (VIP)
Neurotensin
Antiotensin II
Somatostatin
Thyrotropin releasing hormone (TRH)
Luteinizing-hormone releasing hormone (LHRH)
Carnosine
Bombesin
Vasopressin
Corticotropin

Tyr-Gly-Gly-Phe-Met

Tyr-Gly-Gly-Phe-Leu

(17)

tates the discovery of specific agonists and antagonists as pharmacological tools to demonstrate selective effects on target organs.

4.8.1.6 *Neuromodulators*

In addition to the small molecule neurotransmitters there also exists a steadily increasing list of peptides which have been demonstrated to act as neuromodulators (Table 4.5). Neurotransmitters characteristically act very locally and very briefly and, after release from the receptor, are either taken up by the neuron or surrounding cells or deactivated by specific enzymes. They are thus ideal in affecting only transient changes in cellular communication or nervous transmission whereas the neuromodulators, on the other hand, have a much more diffuse action which is slower in onset and longer acting. Memory consolidation is one process which is thought to use neuromodulation. Neuromodulators include adenosine and a number of neuroactive peptides including cholecystokinin, α-melanocyte stimulating hormone, β-endorphin and neuropeptide Y. Studies using fluorescent antibodies to such peptides have shown that in many neurons two transmitters can exist concurrently. Thus cholecystokinin has been found with dopamine and neuropeptide Y with catecholamines. To date four types of multiple transmitter neurons have been identified:-

(i)   two nonpeptide transmitters present,
(ii) one nonpeptide and one peptide transmitter,
(iii) two peptidic transmitters derived from the same gene,
(iv) two peptidic transmitters derived from different genes.

The purpose of having two (or more) transmitters in a neuron is presumably to mutually affect their activities, and there are a number of ways in which this might be done. Both transmitters could affect the same receptor at different sites with the combined activity being different from that with either alone, both transmitters could affect the same receptor, and both could affect different receptors either on the same or different neurons. Clearly the use of more than one neurotransmitter greatly increases the sophistication and potential of the synaptic processes.

4.8.2 **Secondary messengers**

It has long been an aim of scientists interested in drug action to better understand the molecular and biochemical events which follow the interaction of an agonist with its receptor. As well as the intellectual challenge posed by such an objective, its importance, of course, lies in the possibility of uncovering fresh targets for drug intervention. In recent years, inspired "classical" biochemical studies allied to the newer molecular biological techniques have begun to uncover some of the extraordinary details of these processes.

An example is the simplest and fastest reacting system the "ligand-gated ion channel", of which the nicotinyl acetylcholine receptor is a good example. This receptor is made up of a ring of five protein subunits formed around a central waterfilled core. The binding of acetylcholine to two high-affinity sites located on one of the subunits causes a conformational change in the receptor such that small inorganic ions, particularly Na^+, K^+ and Ca^{2+} can freely pass through it. This diffusion causes membrane depolarisation which leads, eventually, to muscle contraction, action potential generation or hormone release, depending on the nature of the target tissue. In this case no other species acts between binding of the agonist and the ion channel response, and the system is ideal for triggering rapid, brief effects at precise targets.

In a more complicated situation, the receptor may be an enzyme which becomes activated after binding of the agonist. Insulin and a number of growth factors work through such receptors which are tyrosine-specific protein kinases. A kinase is an enzyme which transfers the terminal phosphate group from adenosine triphosphate (ATP) to either a serine or threonine amino acid in the target protein. Such phosphorylation usually activates the enzyme which then reacts with its substrate. In this way the action of the agonist binding to its receptor initiates a process leading to phosphorylation of an enzyme and activation of the synthesis of other agents which complete the target cell response. Increasing complexity is provided by the large number of agonists which are known to exert their effects via another group of proteins known as guanosine-5'-triphosphate (GTP) binding proteins or G-proteins. These are glycoproteins of which at least six different types have so far been identified, and their generalised structure is shown in Figure 4.21, while Table 4.6 shows a list of agonists which have so far been established to function via these G-proteins.

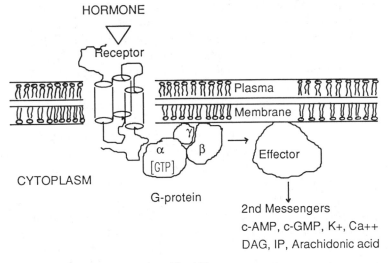

Fig. 4.21.

Stimulatory G-protein (Gs) comprises three polypeptide subunits referred to as α, β and δ. The α subunit Gsα binds and hydrolyses GTP and activates adenyl cyclase;

Table 4.6   G-protein coupled receptors

Small molecule	Peptide	Sensory
Adrenergic	Enkephalin	Rhodopsin
	Endorphin	Olfactory
Muscarinic, cholinergic	Cholecystokinin	
Dopamine	Bombesin	
Histamine	Substance K	
Adenosine	Substance P	
Serotonin	Neuromedin	
Prostaglandin	Bradykinin	
Leukotriene	fMetLeuPhe	
Thromboxane	C5a,C3a	
Prostacyclin	Thrombin	
PAF	Vasopressin	
cAMP	Oxytocin	
	Angiotensin II	
	VIP	
	Parathyroid hormone	
	Calcitonin	
	Neurotensin	
	TRH	
	Somatostatin	

the β and δ units form a tight, noncovalent complex which anchors the G-protein to the plasma membrane. Initially, the α unit binds guanosine diphosphate (GDP); as the receptor is activated Gs is modified with the result that GTP replaces GDP, but the nature of the interaction between the receptor and Gs is not clear. The binding of GTP causes further changes in Gs because the complex then breaks up, Gsα moves away from the β and δ units interacting with the enzyme adenyl cyclase, which catalyses the synthesis of cyclic adenosine monophosphate (cAMP) (**18**) from ATP. The binding of Gsα to adenyl cyclase stimulates the enzyme for some 10–15 seconds before the GTP is hydrolysed back to GDP and causes the Gsα-enzyme complex to dissociate with the enzyme now being deactivated and Gsα recombining with β and δ to reform the G-protein complex and set up further interaction with its receptor (Figure 4.22).

It was mentioned above that there is more than one class of G-proteins, the inhibitory G-protein Gi inhibiting adenyl cyclase and, contrary to the effect of Gs, reducing the amount of cAMP present inside the cell. Interestingly, it has been found that the β-adrenergic receptor couples with Gs while the α_2-adrenergic receptor couples to Gi; findings which may begin to explain their different activities.

The catastrophic effects which can result from pharmacological interference with the G proteins are illustrated by the effects of cholera and pertussis toxins. Cholera toxin is an enzyme which catalyses a reaction of the α-subunit of Gs with ADP-

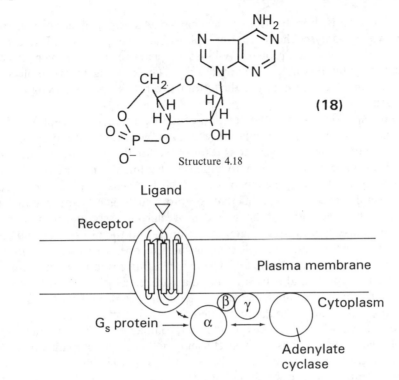

Structure 4.18

(18)

Association of ligand-receptor complex with G_s-protein activates it for GTP–GDP exchange.

↓

GTP displaces GDP; subunit dissociates from G_s; and binds to, and activates adenylate cyclase.

↓

Adenylate cyclase releases many molecules of cAMP.

↓

Hydrolysis of GTP by α-subunit causes conformational change and dissociation of subunit from adenylate cyclase thus inactiving enzymes. α-subunit reassociates with βγ-complex.

↓

Process is repeated until loss of ligand from receptor stops activation of G-protein complex.

Fig. 4.22.   Representation of G-protein coupled activation processes.

ribose resulting in the unit being no longer able to hydrolyse its bound GTP. Thus the Gsα cannot be deactivated, adenyl cyclase remains activated, and the intracellular levels of cAMP rise enormously causing a massive efflux of Na^+ and water from intestinal epithelial cells into the gut, giving rise to the severe diarrhoea which is characteristic of this disease. Pertussis toxin produced by the bacterium responsible for whooping cough has a similar effect on Giα, but here the result is to prevent the complex from binding to the receptor and, since this Gi-protein normally inhibits adenyl cyclase, the result is again for the cAMP levels to rise dramatically.

   The effects of fluctuating cAMP must be considered before returning to consider other G-proteins. Normal levels of cAMP in the resting cell are less than 10^{-6} M, but upon stimulation this level can rise five-fold in as many seconds. This effect of cAMP is to activate a number of specific proteins mainly by allosteric interactions, but the major effect is the activation of one enzyme cAMP-dependent protein kinase (A-kinase), which catalyses the transfer of a phosphate group from ATP to serine or threonine residues on target proteins. A-kinase appears to be a tetramer formed by two regulatory subunits and two catalytic units. The binding of two molecules of cAMP to each regulatory unit causes the tetramer to break open, releasing the active catalytic units.

To take the specific example of activation of the β_2-adrenergic receptor, A-kinase phosphorylates the enzyme phosphorylase kinase which in turn phosphorylates glycogen phosphorylase. This enzyme is responsible for the first stage in the process whereby glycogen is broken down to glucose, the further metabolism of which provides energy for the contraction process. In other cells different consequences ensue from similar effects on the different receptors such as cortisol secretion from the adrenal cortex, resorption in bone, and progesterone secretion in the ovary. In nerve cells A-kinase can phosphorylate ion channels and the G-proteins and cAMP can react directly with these channels causing them to open or close. This process is a slower, more diffuse, more complex and longer lasting response than occurs with channel-linked receptors and is used to modulate the effect of these rapid receptors.

The other major intracellular messenger is the Ca^{2+} ion, and its levels are also influenced by G-proteins although in a different way. Normal intracellular levels of Ca^{2+} are very low ($\sim 10^{-7}$ M) whilst in the extracellular fluid they are much higher ($> 10^{-3}$ M). The cell has thus evolved efficient methods of pumping Ca^{2+} against concentration gradients. The cell has also evolved a special intracellular calcium-sequestering compartment in which high levels of calcium are held loosely bound to a protein calsequestrin. The opening of ion channels to either of these sources of Ca^{2+} will result in a rapid rise in intracellular Ca^{2+} concentrations which then leads to a whole range of responses dependent on the function of the cell. Thus in nerve cells depolarisation of the plasma membrane, as described above, causes the Ca^{2+} ion channel to open and the influx of Ca^{2+} ions stimulates the release of the relevant neurotransmitter.

In other cells the Ca^{2+} is released internally via the action of another secondary messenger, inositol triphosphate. In this case the receptor is coupled to a different G-protein (Gp) which activates another enzyme phospholipase C. The inositol phosphates (Figure 4.23) are minor constituents of the plasma membrane and are found carrying none, one, or two phosphate groups as, respectively, phosphatidylinositol (PI), phosphatidylinositol phosphate (PIP), and phosphatidylinositol bisphosphate (PIP$_2$). The last cited is the most crucial despite its being the least abundant since it is cleaved by the enzyme phospholipase C following activation by Gp to inositol triphosphate (InsP$_3$) and diacylglycerol, both of which have second messenger activities. InsP$_3$ acts on the ion channels releasing Ca^{2+} from the internal sequestering component, whilst diacylglycerol has two other signalling roles. It can activate another kinase, protein kinase C (C-kinase), and, as with A-kinase, this enzyme phosphorylates serine and threonine residues in target enzymes and proteins including some ion channels. The modified proteins are thus activated or deactivated and the functioning of the cell is subsequently modified. The other signalling role of diacylglycerol arises during its hydrolysis by phospholipase A$_2$ to give arachidonic acid, the precursor of the prostaglandins and leukotrienes which play major cell recruiting roles in a variety of inflammatory processes. Amongst the cells known to use the inositol–phospholipid signalling pathway are liver cells in response to vasopressin, smooth muscle with acetylcholine, and blood platelets in response to thrombin. Lithium ions are widely used in cases of severe depression, and it appears that they have a number of inhibitory effects on the enzymes active in the inositol phosphate pathway, which may be the source of their activity.

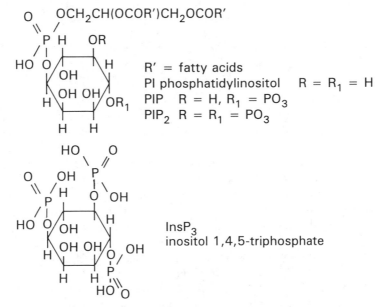

Fig. 4.23. Inositol phosphates

A final family of G-proteins are the ras proteins so called because they are produced by ras genes that were first found in viruses which cause rat sarcomas. These are coupled to a variety of receptors for growth factors and take part in the signalling processes which lead to cell division and growth in response to these factors. All of this is highly complex and so prompts the question of why it is used. The simple answer is because of the opportunity which is provided by such processes to amplify the original signal which arises at each stage. Thus one molecule of an agonist reacts with a receptor, but this can interact with more than one G-protein each of which can activate a different adenyl cyclase, and during the time these enzymes are activated they may produce many cAMP molecules. Each pair of these can act on a kinase, each of which can produce many molecules of the final product (Figure 4.24) and thus one molecule of agonist has provoked the production of very many molecules of final product. For the medicinal chemist each of these steps provides the opportunity for selective interference as a potential target for the design of new drugs.

4.9 INTRACELLULAR PROTEINACEOUS RECEPTORS

The vast majority of known receptors are situated in or on the plasma membrane presumably to alleviate the need for the ligand to have to penetrate into the cell.

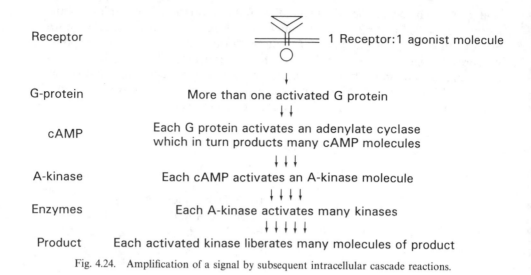

Receptor   1 Receptor:1 agonist molecule

G-protein   More than one activated G protein

cAMP   Each G protein activates an adenylate cyclase
                           which in turn products many cAMP molecules

A-kinase   Each cAMP activates an A-kinase molecule

Enzymes   Each A-kinase activates many kinases

Product   Each activated kinase liberates many molecules of product

Fig. 4.24.   Amplification of a signal by subsequent intracellular cascade reactions.

However, a number of hormones, notably vitamin D, thyroxine and the steroidal hormones, interact with receptors that are found either in the cytosol or within the nuclear membrane. All these ligands have in common the feature that binding to their receptors results in the receptor–ligand complex interacting with DNA, promoting the new synthesis. Vitamin D (**19**) is crucial to the proper development of bone, and the deficiency of it or of its receptor leads to the disease rickets, which is characterised by a bow-legged appearance. Vitamin D is active as its metabolite, 1, 25-dihydroxyvitamin D_3 (**20**), and its main activity is to raise the blood levels of calcium and phosphate ions to the levels necessary for mineralisation of the organic matrix of bone. Of a number of proteins whose synthesis is known to be induced by vitamin D, only one, a calcium binding protein of molecular weight of 9000, has been identified.

The thyroid hormone T3 (**21**) stimulates body oxygen consumption, affects heart rate and force, plasma cholesterol and triglyceride levels, and aids brain development in the early days of life. In this case the receptor is a chromatin-bound nonhistone protein, and amongst the proteins whose synthesis is induced by the receptor–ligand complex is growth hormone. The steroids are a complex class of compounds responsible for a wide variety of physiological effects including sexual development, maintenance of pregnancy, growth, and certain malignancies. In this case the receptors appear to be rather unstable, and whilst their primary amino-acid sequences are known the secondary and tertiary structures are not. For all these receptors their distribution in either cytosol or nucleus is difficult to determine, and the full subtleties of their actions are still to be elucidated.

4.10   DNA AS A RECEPTOR

The final type of macromolecular receptor to be described is DNA itself and a significant number of drugs are known which act via binding to it. In addition, as

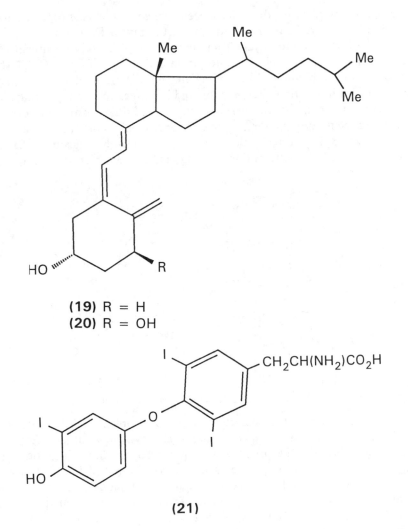

(19) R = H
(20) R = OH

(21)

mentioned above, a significant number of proteins bind to specific sections of DNA and act either as promotors or repressors of gene expression.

The structure of DNA is highly ordered and well characterised and thus is an attractive target for drug design. Indeed recent work has begun to produce agents capable of binding to specific segments of DNA thus providing the possibility that these could be used to influence gene expression. However, the only therapeutic agents which today can be shown to work by interacting with DNA are certain antibiotics and anticancer agents which do so by intercalating the agent between adjacent base-pairs in the DNA helix. As a result of such intercalation the functioning of its DNA is affected to the detriment of the bacterium or cancer cell. However, the exact mechanism by which the intercalating agent affects the target DNA in terms of its subsequent functioning is unclear.

Three types of intercalating drugs have been defined on the basis of their directional entrance into the DNA helix. The antibiotic actinomycin D enters from the minor groove, the antitumour daunomycin from the major groove, and the anticancer agent, ellipticine, appears to be able to enter from either site. Figure (4.25) shows a representation of the binding of the mutagenic aminoacridine dye, proflavine. Such intercalation is an interesting phenomenon and is important therapeutically. Striking improvements to binding have been achieved by adding substituents designed to interact with specific groups; for example 9-hydroxyellipticine may be more active because its hydroxyl group is able to bind to a phosphate group. The greatest challenge, however, lies in attempting to design molecules which will bind to specific sequences of DNA.

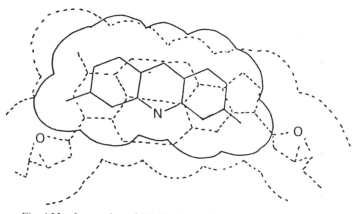

Fig. 4.25.   Interaction of 3,6-diaminocridine (proflavine) with DNA.

Dewan and Hurley have focused attention on the problems faced in attempting to design DNA-specific agents. Thus according to Hurley the overall problem of design of nonprotein DNA-effective molecules can be broken down into three phases: learning the rules of DNA sequence specific recognition and identification of key sequences to target for modulation of gene expression, amplification, or recombination; design and synthesis of appropriate compounds; development of cell-specific delivery systems. These are all formidable problems but they will be aided by work which identifies and characterises the biologically important lesions in DNA produced by significant DNA-active drugs such as bleomycin and aflatoxin, thus giving considerable information on the interaction processes. Such drugs can also act as templates upon which substitution could be made to further examine binding characteristics. None of this is easy, but already a number of agents such as the natural product netropsin (**22**) and the synthetic compound CC 1065 (**23**) are known which do interact directly with DNA, and one can predict that this will become an increasingly important area for rational drug design.

4.11   ENZYMES

Enzymes are the biological macromolecules which catalyse essentially all of the chemical reactions in the body, thus allowing them to proceed at the appropriate

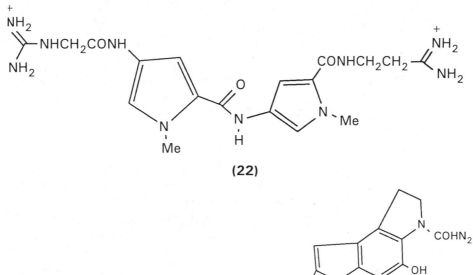

(22)

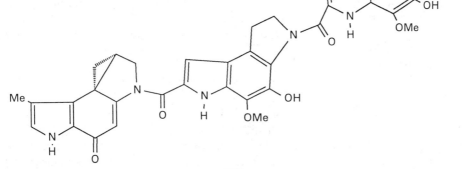

(23)

rate under physiological conditions of pH, temperature and concentration. Until the early 1980s all enzymes were considered to be proteins, but it was then discovered that some ribonucleic acids (RNA) also possess enzymatic activity. This section will focus on proteinaceous enzymes, leaving discussion of RNA enzymes (ribozymes) until the final section.

4.11.1 Definitions
The list of identified enzymes currently stands at 2477 classified into six major types dependent on the chemical reactions that they catalyse:

Reaction type	Description
• oxidation–reduction reactions	oxidoreductases
• group transfer reactions	transferases
• hydrolytic reactions	hydrolases

- elimination reactions giving double bond and the   lyases
  converse, addition to double bonds

- isomerisation reactions   isomerases

- bond-forming reactions joining two molecules, the ligases or synthetases
  energy for which is supplied by the simultaneous
  cleavage of nucleoside triphosphates to nucleoside diphosphates

---

The nomenclature of enzymes has been fraught with confusion and complexity arising from a desire to reconcile scientific exactness with convenience. The International Union of Biochemistry established an Enzyme Commission which proposed a systematic name for each enzyme for which the reaction being catalysed is well characterised and which could be written as a formal equation. They then recommended both a trivial name and a unique four figure code for each enzyme. Thus, for example, the enzyme which catalyses the transfer of an amino group from L-aspartic acid to 2-oxo-glutaric acid has the systemic name L-aspartate: 2-oxoglutarate aminotransferase; the recommended name aspartate aminotransferase and the Enzyme Commission number 2.6.1.1. The name clearly indicates that the enzyme is a transferase.

The number is unique to this enzyme, and the code which enables one to describe the enzyme from its number is given both in the International Union of Biochemistry publication *Enzyme Nomenclature* (Academic Press, New York 1984) and in a briefer tabular form, in *Comprehensive Medicinal Chemistry* volume 2, ed P. G. Sammes, p 38 (Pergamon Press, Oxford, 1990). Using this table and presented with an enzyme numbered, such as 1.14.11.1, one can readily deduce that it is an oxidoreductase (1...) that it acts on paired donors with incorporation of molecular oxygen (1.14....), and that it uses 2-oxoglutarate as one donor and incorporates one atom each of oxygen into both donors (1.14.11...). The last number then identifies the individual enzymes of this class.

4.11.2 Isoenzymes and isofunctional enzymes

A considerable number of enzymes are present in the same organism, and even on occasion in the same cell, which catalyse the same reactions and which show close similarity of structure and function but which are nevertheless distinguishable. Differences found for these isoenzymes include the effects of inhibitors, their electrophoretic mobilities, temperature stability, and kinetic parameters. A typical enzyme is lactate dehydrogenase which is found in five different isoenzymatic forms depending on which particular set of subunits makes up the tetramic functional enzyme.

Isofunctional enzymes perform the same reaction but have much greater structural differences than those found in isoenzymes. Isoenzymes are formed from different combinations of the same gene products, but isofunctional enzymes arise from different genes and the different structures of such enzymes provide rich opportunities for selectivity. One of the most important examples is the enzyme dihydrofolate reductase which in bacteria is much more susceptible to the effect of the antibiotic trimethoprim than is the equivalent enzyme in the host. This example will be referred to again later in this chapter.

4.11.3 Enzyme catalysis

Because enzymes are present in much greater quantities in the organism than receptors, studies of their properties have been more advanced. Thus a cell-free extract with enzymatic properties was prepared by Büchner in 1897, the first crystallation of an enzyme was achieved for urease by Summer in 1926, and the first enzyme structure to be determined by X-ray crystallography, that of lysozyme, was reported by Phillips in 1965. The fact that enzymes catalyse recognisable reactions on defined substrates has meant that even before they could be isolated and purified the specificity and kinetics of such reactions could be readily studied. Enzyme kinetics is a very large and important field of biochemistry, and the results have been used to deduce much about the possible mechanisms of such transformations. However, it should be noted that usually more than one mechanism can fit a particular kinetic profile, and thus such studies do not provide definitive answers.

4.11.3.1 Kinetics

The simplest representation of an enzyme catalysed reaction involving a single substrate is given by:

$$\text{E} + \text{S} \underset{k_{-1}}{\overset{k_1}{\rightleftharpoons}} \text{ES} \xrightarrow{k_2} \text{EP} \longrightarrow \text{E} + \text{P} \tag{17}$$

in which E is the enzyme, S the substrate, ES the enzyme–substrate complex, P the product, and k_n the various rate constants. The enzyme–substrate complex, ES, is a noncovalent complex which is formed rapidly and reversibly before decomposing to give the product.

The consideration of the kinetics can be much simplified if we consider only the initial stages of the reaction before any significant amount of products has been formed. Under these circumstances the formation of ES from the product is essentially zero and then the constant k_{-2} can be ignored. It is also assumed that the concentration of the enzyme is negligible compared with that of the substrate, an assumption that is logical given the high catalytic efficiency of enzymes.

Under these conditions it is found that the initial rate (v) follows saturation kinetics with respect to the concentration of the substrate. At low concentrations of S the rate increases with increasing concentrations of S but eventually becomes independent of S at higher concentrations, that is, the rate increases to a maximum above which it cannot go whatever the concentration of S.

A plot of v against S has the general appearance of the curve in Figure 4.26.

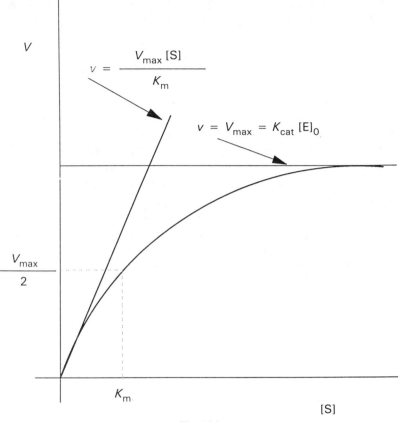

Fig. 4.26.

Initial approaches to quantifying enzyme kinetics assumed that ES was in equilibrium with E and S — an equilibrium which was almost instantaneously established — and that the breakdown of ES to products was too slow to disturb this equilibrium. This leads to:

$$k_1[E][S] = k_1[ES] \tag{18}$$

From this, K_s, the dissociation constant for the enzyme–substrate complex, can be defined as:

$$\frac{[E][S]}{[ES]} = \frac{k_{-1}}{k_1} = K_s \tag{19}$$

The total amount of enzyme $[E]_o$ must be the sum of the free enzyme E and that bound in the enzyme–substrate complex:

$$[E]_o = [E] + [ES] \tag{20}$$

Thus substituting equation (20) into (19) gives:

$$K_s = \frac{\langle[E]_0 - [ES]\rangle[S]}{[ES]} \tag{21}$$

leading to:

$$[ES] = \frac{[E]_0[S]}{K_s + [S]} \tag{22}$$

The rate of the reaction, v, is given by:

$$v = k_2[ES] \tag{23}$$

and substituting equation (21) into equation (23) leads to:

$$v = \frac{k_2[E]_0[S]}{[S] + K_s} \tag{24}$$

The maximum rate of the reaction v_{max} will be given when all the substrate is contained in the enzyme–substrate complex and this leads to:

$$v_{max} = k_2[E]_0 \tag{25}$$

The derivation of equation (24) was criticised because of its assumption that an equilibrium must exist, and in its place the concept of the steady state was introduced. This assumes that the ES will break down as rapidly as it is formed either to product or back to starting material. This is an assumption which is justified as the amount of enzyme is so small compared with substrate that the amount of ES formed will be determined by the amount of enzyme, but this applies only in the very first stages of the reaction before significant amounts of product have been formed. Under these conditions, equation (26) holds:

$$k_1[E][S] = k_{-1}[ES] + k_2[ES] = \langle k_{-1} + k_2\rangle[ES] \tag{26}$$

This leads to:

$$K_m = \frac{k_{-1} + k_2}{k_1} = \frac{[ES][S]}{[ES]} \tag{27}$$

and, as above this leads to:

$$v = \frac{k_2[E]_0[S]}{[S] + K_m} \tag{28}$$

Here, K_m, is known as the Michaelis constant and is in fact the concentration of the substrate at which the initial reaction rate is half the maximal rate.

Comparison of equations (19) and (27) leads to:

$$K_m = K_s + \frac{k_2}{k_1} \tag{29}$$

thus showing that K_m will equal K_s when k_2 is very small, but in all other situations K_m will be greater than K_s.

The Michaelis–Menten scheme can also be applied to more complex situations in which a number of intermediates are produced between the substrate and the product. In this case K_m and k_{cat} are combinations of various rate and equilibrium constants.

$$E + S \underset{}{\overset{K_s}{\rightleftharpoons}} ES \underset{}{\overset{K}{\rightleftharpoons}} ES' \underset{}{\overset{K'}{\rightleftharpoons}} ES'' \underset{slow}{\overset{K_4}{\longrightarrow}} E + P \tag{30}$$

Here

$$[ES'] = K[ES] \tag{31}$$

and

$$[ES''] = K'[ES'] \tag{32}$$

Then

$$K_m = \frac{K_s}{1 + K + KK'} \tag{33}$$

and

$$k_{cat} = \frac{k_4 KK'}{1 + K + KK'} \tag{34}$$

Note that in the simplest Michaelis–Menten situation of a single enzyme–substrate complex and in which all the binding steps are fast, k_{cat} is the first-order rate constant for the conversion of ES to EP. In more complicated situations k_{cat} will be a function of all first-order rate constants and cannot then be so easily defined.

Additionally, k_{cat} is known as the turnover number, being the maximum number of substrate molecules converted to product per active site per unit time.

4.11.3.2   Graphical representation

Equations (23) and (24) can be rewritten as:

$$\frac{1}{V} = \frac{1}{V_{max}} + \frac{K_m}{V_{max}[S]} \tag{35}$$

A plot of $^1/_V$ against $^1/_{[S]}$ gives a straight line plot known as the Lineweaver–Burke plot (Figure 4.27). An alternative rewriting (equation (36) gives the Eadie–Hofstee plot (Figure 4.28).

$$v = V_{max} - \frac{K_m v}{S} \tag{36}$$

Both of these plots are widely used in enzyme studies and have their adherents, but the Eadie–Hofstee plot is generally considered to be more accurate. The Lineweaver–Burke plot compresses the data points at high concentrations into a

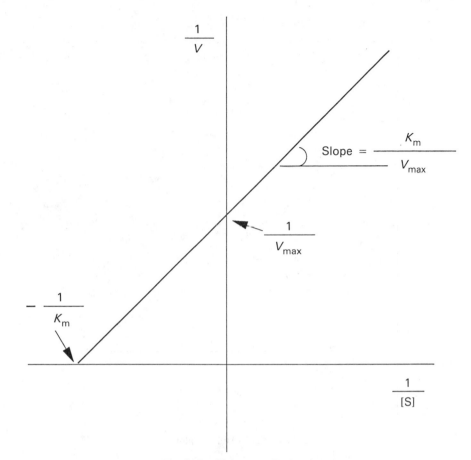

Fig. 4.27.   Lineweaver–Burke plot.

small region while emphasising the points at lower concentrations, but it does have the advantage that values of v at a given value of [S] are easy to read. The Eadie–Hofstee plot does not compress the higher concentrations but the values of v against [S] are more difficult to determine rapidly.

4.11.3.3   The nature of enzymatic catalysis

Enzymes vastly increase the rate of chemical reactions over their noncatalysed equivalents. Thus, for example, the apparently simple isomerisation of dihydroxy-acetone phosphate (DHAP) to D-glyceraldehyde-3-phosphate (GAP) (Figure 4.29) proceeds some 10^{10} times faster when catalysed by the enzyme triose phosphate isomerase rather than by a simple base such as the acetate ion.

Clearly this represents a profound interference with the reaction, and an explanation for the effect has been sought by many researchers. In fact one author has claimed that at least twenty-one theories have been advanced to explain the observed rate-enhancing effects. However, the simplest and probably most correct explanation was

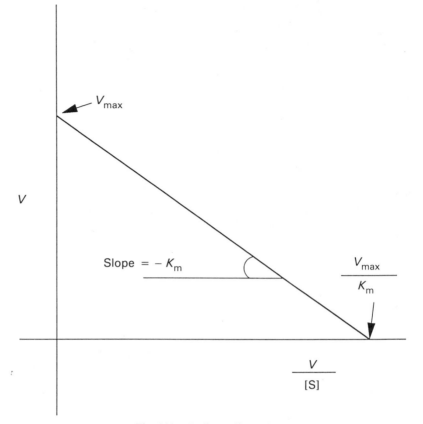

Fig. 4.28.   Eadie–Holfstee plot.

produced by Linus Pauling in the late 1940s when he wrote

> ... the only reasonable picture of the catalytic activity of enzymes is that which involves an active region of the surface of the enzyme which is closely complementary in structure not to the substrate molecule itself in its normal configuration, but rather to the substrate molecule in a strained configuration, corresponding to the "activated complex" for the reaction catalysed by the enzyme.... .

Despite the simplicity and clarity of this assertion it was not immediately widely acknowledged or accepted but has recently been well espoused by Kraut. He has shown that the theory results from a combination of two fundamental principles of physical chemistry: absolute reaction rate theory and the thermodynamic cycle. Expressed more simply, if the energy of the transition state is reduced the reaction goes more rapidly. So, expressed very simply, reaction rate (transition state) theory depends on two assumptions: that the reaction rate is controlled by decomposition of an activated transition state complex and that the system can be treated as though the transition state complex is in equilibrium with the reactants. This leads to

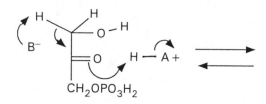

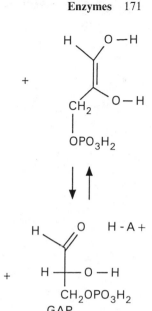

Fig. 4.29. Isomerisations of DHAP to GAP.

equation (37) to define the rate of the reaction.

$$k = K \upsilon K^{\neq} \tag{37}$$

where k = the observable reaction-rate constant, K = transmission coefficient, υ = frequency of normal mode oscillation of the transition state complex along the reaction coordinate, and $K^{\neq}$ = equilibrium constant for the formation of the transition state complex from reactants.

Figure 4.30 describes a thermodynamic cycle relating substrate and transition state binding. The upper line represents the uncatalysed reaction, the lower the enzyme catalysed one. (The superscript $\neq$ defines transition states.) The comparison of first-order rate constants for an elementary single substrate enzyme catalysed reaction following equation (37) leads to:

$$\frac{k_e}{k_n} = \frac{K_e \upsilon_e K_e^{\neq}}{k_n \upsilon K_n^{\neq}} \tag{38}$$

This can be simplified very approximately to:

$$\frac{k_e}{k_n} = \frac{K_s}{K_T} \tag{39}$$

which in effect relates the rates of reaction to the ratio of dissociation constants for the substrate, K_s, and for the transition state, K_T. This effectively says that the transition state must bind enormously more strongly to the enzyme E than does the substrate S in its ground state (i.e. than the substrate binds in the Michaelis complex ES) by a factor roughly equal to the enzymic rate acceleration. This also formalises

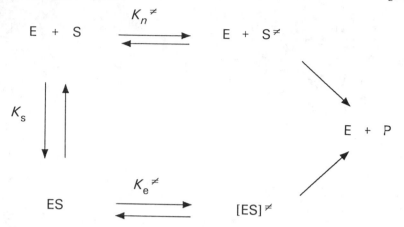

Fig. 4.30.   Thermodynamic cycle relating substate and transition state binding.

the Pauling concept by clearly relating the rate enhancement of the enzyme catalysed reaction to the extra binding of the transition state over that of the substrate.

The energy changes associated with the reaction are shown diagramatically in Figure 4.31 which depicts an enzyme catalysed reaction proceeding through a single Michaelis–Menten complex. It is important to note that this complex is not the same as the maximum energy transition state; in fact it is not immediately clear why the complex should be such a feature of enzymatic catalysis. It must be that an enzyme which strongly binds to a transition state can also bind to a structure which is not greatly different. This will be especially true of a large molecular weight substrate where the binding will not only involve the atoms undergoing reaction but also very many more in other fragments of the molecule. The same considerations presumably account for the fact that many enzymes catalyse the reactions of a wide range of substrates; the endopeptidases, for example, cleave terminal amino acids from a large number of peptides. The binding to the group undergoing reaction is highly specific but in addition there are a very large number of nonspecific interactions with the rest of the substrate.

The applications of these ideas to the design of transition state analogue inhibitors will be discussed later in this chapter.

4.11.4   Cooperativity and allosterism

The basic Michaelis–Menten equation (equation (18)) describes enzymatic reactions in which a substrate reacts with a single centre on an enzyme. Two further quantities, the fractional saturation, Y, and the binding constant, K_b, can be defined according to equations (40) and (41):

$$Y = \frac{[ES]}{[E]_0} \tag{40}$$

$$Y = \frac{K_b[S]}{K_b[S] + 1} \tag{41}$$

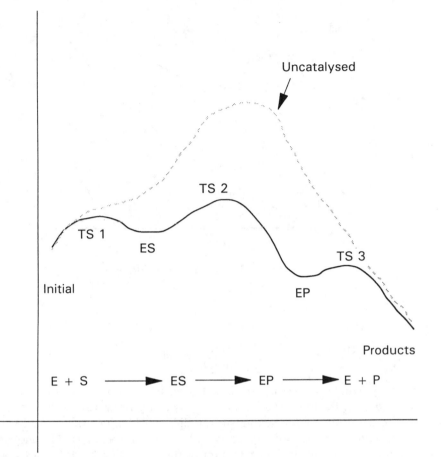

K_b is equal to the reciprocal of the dissociation constant K_s. A plot of Y against [S] at constant $[E]_0$ gives the hyperbola shown in Figure 4.32 (curve a).

It was shown by Bohr in 1904 that if the fractional saturation of myoglobin with oxygen was plotted against the oxygen partial pressure, the resultant curve was indeed a hyerbola. However, when myoglobin was replaced by haemoglobin the curve became sigmoidal (curve b in Figure 4.32), and the explanation for this difference was provided by Hill in 1906, and again by Adair in 1925. They proposed that the haemoglobin was composed of a number of subunits each of which could bind one molecule of oxygen and that the binding of one molecule affected the subsequent binding of others. Hill did not know how many subunits were present, but Adair fitted the experimental curve with four such units and established the binding constants as 0.024, 0.074, 0.086 and 7.4 mm 1 Hg (at 25°C, pH 7.4 and 0.1 M NaCl):

$$\text{Hb} \underset{\longleftarrow}{\overset{K_1, O_2}{\rightleftharpoons}} \text{HbO}_2 \underset{\longleftarrow}{\overset{K_2, O_2}{\rightleftharpoons}} \text{Hb(O}_2)_2 \underset{\longleftarrow}{\overset{K_3, O_2}{\rightleftharpoons}} \text{Hb(O}_2)_3 \underset{\longleftarrow}{\overset{K_4, O_2}{\rightleftharpoons}} \text{Hb(O}_2)_4 \qquad (42)$$

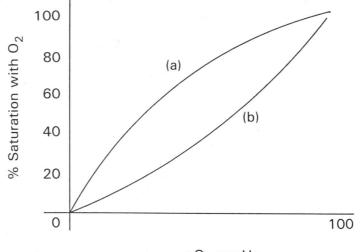

Fig. 4.32.

where

$$K_1 = \frac{[HbO_2]}{[Hb][O_2]} \qquad K_2 = \frac{[Hb(O_2)_2]}{[HbO_2][O_2]} \, etc.$$

The really remarkable feature of these figures is the enormous rate enhancement for the binding of the fourth molecule of oxygen. This result cannot be explained by the existence of four noninteracting sites of different affinities since in that case the high affinity site must be saturated first. Rather, the binding of the first molecules of oxygen must so change the conformation of the remaining binding sites that their affinity is positively affected. This is an example of one of four types of cooperativity in ligand building which have been identified:

(a) *positive cooperativity* where the binding of one molecule of a substrate or ligand increases the affinity of the protein for other molecules of the same or different substrate or ligand;

(b) *negative cooperativity* where the binding of one molecule of a substrate or ligand decreases the affinity of the protein for other molecules of the same or different substrates or ligands;

(c) *homotropic cooperativity* where the binding of one molecule affects the subsequent binding of the same substrate;

(d) *heterotrophic cooperativity* where the binding of one molecule affects the subsequent binding of molecules of a different ligand or substrate.

Allosterism is the name given to the special case of heterotrophic cooperativity which was originally proposed by J. Monod in the early 1960s to explain the phenomenon whereby the products of a biosynthetic pathway could exercise feedback control in the earlier phases of the synthetic sequence. For example, in the biosynthesis of isoleucine the first enzyme threonine deaminase is inhibited by isoleucine but activated by valine; the significant differences in structures between the ligand and the inhibitors and activitors strongly suggest that they act on different sites.

Two theories, the Monod–Wyman–Changeux (MWC) concerted mechanism and the Koshland–Némethy–Filmer (KNF) sequential model have been proposed to explain these effects. The MWC model is based on the assumptions that:

(a) The proteins are oligomers.
(b) The protein exists in two conformational states which are in equilibrium. The predominant form in the unligated state is called the T (or tense) state and the other, the R (or relaxed) state. The two states differ in their energies and the bonding between the subunits with the result that the T state is more constrained than the R state.
(c) The T state has lower affinity for ligands.
(d) All the binding sites in each state are equivalent and have identical binding constants for a given ligand. This is the symmetry assumption and is the feature of the model which is most open to criticism.

The allosteric constant, L, is defined as the ratio of T to R in the unligated state (equation (43)) whilst K_T and K_R are the dissociation constants for each site in the T and R states respectively.

$$L = \frac{[T]}{[R]} \tag{43}$$

Figure 4.33 gives a diagrammatic representation of the MWC model as applied to a tetramic protein.

In this system an activator would function by binding to the R state, thus increasing its concentration, whilst an inhibitor would act likewise on the T state. In the extreme situation, the activator will displace the equilibrium to such an extent that the R state predominates, and cooperativity is abolished and "normal" Michaelis–Menten kinetics result.

The MWC model can account for the sigmoidal binding curve even though the binding of one molecule of ligand does not affect the affinity for the ligand of other binding sites on the molecule. This is because of the affect of the ligand on the allosteric constant, L. When L is large, the equilibrium favours the T form and, therefore, when low levels of the ligand are present there will not be enough to react with the small amount of R. As the amount of ligand increases this will steadily displace the equilibrium towards R by reacting with R. Thus the T form acts as a reservoir for the R form, a reservoir which is available only when the ligand concentration is high enough to cause appreciable amounts of the ligand–protein complex to be produced. This effect will be manifested by a surge in the binding curve in the region of the critical ligand concentration. Beyond this concentration all of the protein will eventually be fully saturated with ligand. By this means the sigmoidal curve can be explained.

It was mentioned above that a weakness of the MWC model is the assumption of symmetry. The KNF sequential model avoids this but assumes that the progression

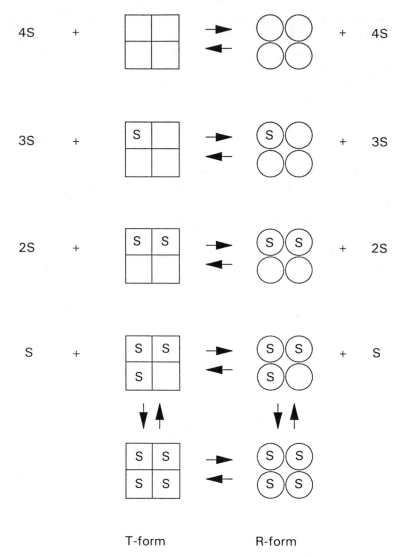

T-form   R-form

Fig. 4.33.

from T to the ligand bound R state is sequential (Figure 4.34). The conformation of each subunit changes as it binds to a ligand and there is no sudden dramatic switch from one state to another. The great difference from the MWC model is the existence of hybrid forms containing the two conformation of the subunits in the same oligomer of the protein. The two basic assumptions of the KNF model are:

(a) in the absence of a ligand the protein exists in one conformation;
(b) on binding the ligand induces a conformational change in the subunit to which it is bound—a change which may be transmitted to the neighbouring vacant subunits via their interfaces.

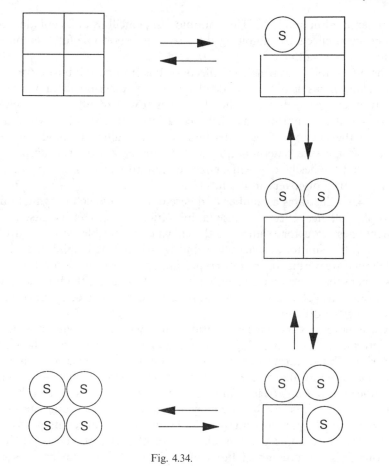

Fig. 4.34.

This model does allow more complex allosteric modifications than were seen in the MWC case. Thus the modifier could bind to the same form of the enzyme as the substrate and cause the same, or different, conformational change, and furthermore, the binding of the modifier could affect subsequent ligand binding either positively or negatively. The possible consequences can, therefore, be seen to be quite extensive.

An interpretation of allosteric control in molecular terms has recently been achieved, most notably for haemoglobin and some of its mutant forms. The interested reader is referred to the recent authoritative review by Perutz cited in the bibliography.

4.11.5 Enzyme inhibition

A large number of biologically active molecules exert their effects by the inhibition of one or more enzymes crucial to the functioning of the target. For example, aspirin inhibits the cyclooxygenase enzyme responsible for the oxidative transformation of arachidonic acid, the unstable products of this reaction being further transformed into thromboxanes and prostaglandins which manifest physiological effects such as fever, inflammation and pain. The antiobiotics, penicillins and cephalosporins, exert their beneficial effects by inhibiting the enzymes responsible for the construction of the bacterial cell wall.

In these examples the beneficial effects of the enzyme inhibitors were discovered before the mechanisms of their mode of action were determined, and the same is true for many other agents. However, the situation is now changing as increased knowledge of biochemical mechanisms has identified a large number of enzymes as potential targets for therapeutics. When this information is allied to modern sophisticated methods of structure determination and computer aided drug design it becomes apparent that the design of specific enzyme inhibitors promises to play an increasing role in new drug discovery in the future.

Figure 4.35 illustrates a number of different ways in which enzyme inhibition can lead to physiological effects. In case (a) inhibition leads to an increase in levels of A. Acetylcholinesterase, for example, is the enzyme responsible for the hydrolysis of the major neurotransmitter acetylcholine, and if this enzyme is inhibited when levels of acetylcholine are normal the result is rapid, fatal paralysis. In the condition myesthenia gravis, where the levels of acetylcholine are much reduced, the use of inhibitors such as physostigmine (**24**) enables the small residual levels to be maintained much longer, ameliorating the disease.

Case (b) represents the typical situation found where a biosynthetic sequence leads to the production of a physiologically active material. Any one of the steps could in theory be inhibited but, in practice, it is important to choose one which cannot be readily overcome by alternative pathways or one where the build-up of intermediate does not lead to unwanted effects. For example, the last two stages in the mammalian metabolism of purines involve the enzyme xanthine oxidase and the final product, uric acid, causes the painful joint disorder gout when produced in excessive amounts. An inhibitor of xanthine oxidase, allopurinol (**25**), is used to control this disease. Situation (c) is more complex but can be illustrated by means of the antibiotic trimethoprim (**26**). This antibiotic inhibits the enzyme dihydrofolate reductase which normally catalyses the conversion of dihydrofolate to tetrahydrofolate, a cofactor essential for the functioning of the enzyme thymidylate synthetase, which is essential for the survival of the target organisms. In case (e) a combination of inhibitors leads to more effective inhibition than either would alone; trimethoprim, for example, is widely used in combination with sulphamethoxazole which inhibits dihydropteroate synthetase. An inhibitory cofactor may also be given in combination with a drug to prevent its metabolism as, for example, in the use of clavulanic acid (**27**) to inhibit the lactamase enzyme which metabolises and deactivates the penicillins.

4.11.5.1   Types of inhibition
Two types of enzyme inhibition are possible, namely reversible or irreversible, depending on whether the binding is either noncovalent (weak) or covalent (strong).

4.11.5.1.1   Reversible inhibition
Reversible inhibitors bind noncovalently to the enzyme and are classified into four main types: competitive, noncompetitive, uncompetitive, and mixed. These can be

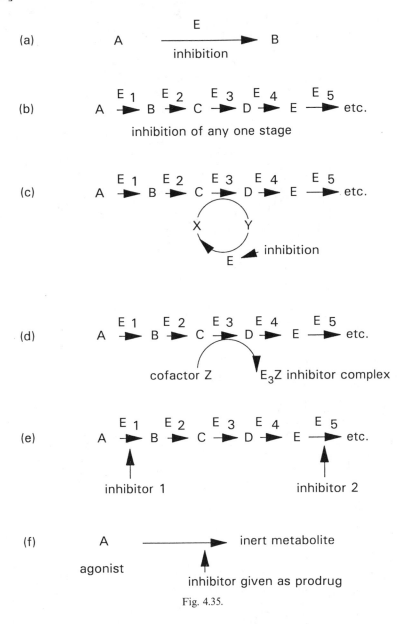

Fig. 4.35.

distinguished by their effects on the measured kinetics, but it should be remembered that kinetic studies do not clarify the actual mechanism of the inhibition.

Competitive inhibition results when an inhibitor I competes with the substrate S for the same site, thus preventing S from undergoing productive binding. In these circumstances equation (17) must be rewritten to include a new term, EI, the enzyme inhibitor complex, and gives:

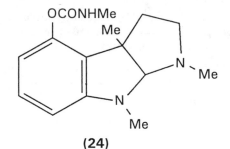

(24)

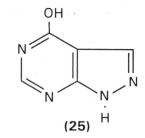

(25)

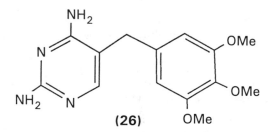

(26)

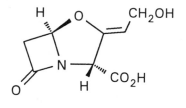

(27)

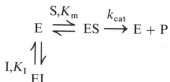

$$(44)$$

Equally equation (20) must be rewritten as:

$$[E]_0 = [ES] + [EI] + [E] \tag{45}$$

and (23) as:

$$v = \frac{[E]_0[S]k_{cat}}{[S] + K_m\langle 1 + I/K_I\rangle} \tag{46}$$

Thus K_m is increased by a factor of $(I + I/K_I)$ i.e. an increased concentration of substrate is required to reach half the maximum rate of the reaction. In contrast,

V_{max} will not be affected since the use of a sufficiently large concentration of S will swamp the effect of I. Equation (46) will hold for all mechanisms which obey the Michaelis–Menten equation and the resultant Eadie–Hofstee and Lineweaver–Burke plots are shown in Figure (4.36).

Noncompetitive (Figure 4.37), uncompetitive (Figure 4.38) and mixed inhibition result when I and S bind simultaneously to the enzyme but do not compete for the same site. In these situations the basis equation is modified to:

$$
\begin{array}{ccc}
 & S,K^1_{\mathrm{m}} & k_{\mathrm{cat}} \\
\mathrm{E} & \rightleftharpoons & \mathrm{ES} \longrightarrow \\
\mathrm{I},K_{\mathrm{I}} \updownarrow & \mathrm{I} \updownarrow \mathrm{K}^1_{\mathrm{I}} & \\
 & & k^1 \\
\mathrm{EI} & \rightleftharpoons & \mathrm{ESI} \longrightarrow \\
S,K_{\mathrm{m}} & &
\end{array}
\tag{47}
$$

Clearly the complexity of this situation will depend on the relative values of the equilibrium and catalytic constants. In the simplest case the dissociation constant of S from EIS is the same as that from ES ($K_{\mathrm{m}} = K_{\mathrm{I}}$) but ESI does not react ($k_{\mathrm{I}} = 0$) and the rate is given by:

$$
v = \frac{k_{\mathrm{cat}} \langle 1 + 1/K_{\mathrm{I}} \rangle}{[S] + K_{\mathrm{m}}}
\tag{48}
$$

4.11.5.1.2 *Reversible inhibitors: transition state analogues*
If enzymes function by stabilising the transition state of a reaction then a stable molecule which resembles that transition state but which cannot undergo the reaction catalysed by the enzyme could be an inhibitor of the system. Of course a transition state is a high-energy one in which the bond lengths, angles and charge distribution are unlike those of any isolable molecule, so it will be difficult to get an exact match. In addition, the enzyme also probably undergoes conformational changes on binding to the substrate such that ground and transition state geometries may not be identical.

These caveats notwithstanding, the concept has led to the discovery of a number of potent inhibitors. For example, the hydrolysis of amide groups in peptides is presumed to proceed via a tetrahedral intermediate (**28**), and Bartlett has shown that the stable phosphinic acid group (**29**) can represent the transition state and because it does not decompose can result in inhibition. The potent inhibitor (**30**) of the enzyme thermolysin has been confirmed by X-ray crystallography to indeed bind to the active site of the enzyme. Perhaps in a way more remarkable is the finding that the natural product phosphoramidon (**31**) is a potent inhibitor of a number of peptidases including thermolysin, enkephalinase and elastase, demonstrating that nature had already exploited the potential of the phosphorus group.

An alternative stable tetrahedral structure is provided by the α-difluoroketone group (**32**) which exists in aqueous solution largely as the 1,1-diol (**33**). Phospholipase A_2 is a hydrolytic enzyme which removes the acyl group from the 2-position of

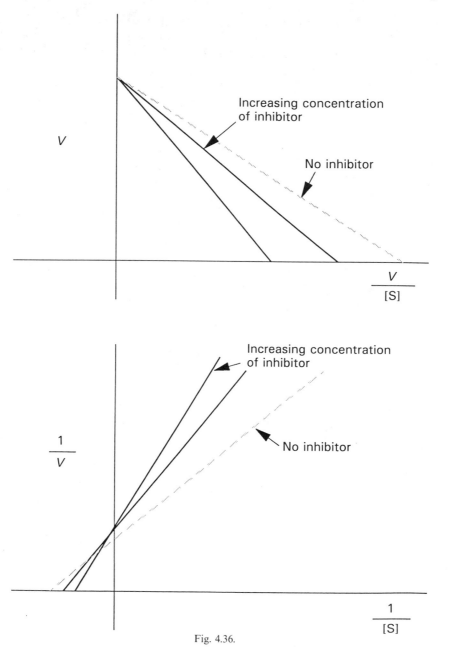

Fig. 4.36.

glyceryl phospholipids (**34**), and Gelb has prepared a range of difluoroacyl derivatives, such as (**35**), many of which are potent inhibitors of this enzyme.

4.11.5.1.3   *Reversible inhibitors: multisubstrate analogues*
A considerable number of enzymes bring together more than one molecule to

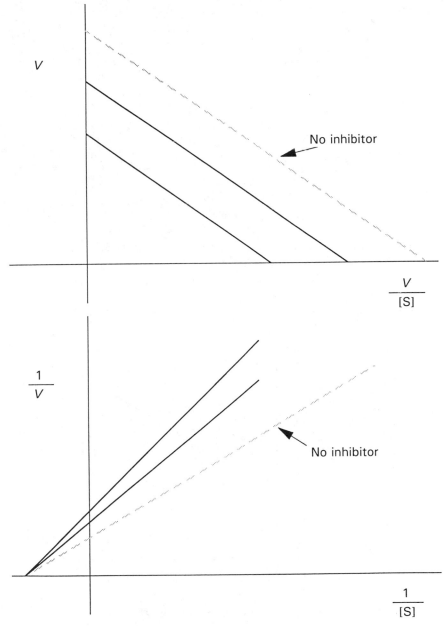

Fig. 4.37.   Noncompetitive inhibition.

complete a required transformation. Thus transaminases catalyse the conversion of α-keto acids to α-amino acids using pyridoxal 5′-phosphate (36) as the cofactor:

$$R\ CO\ CO_2^- \longrightarrow RCHNH_2CO_2^- \tag{49}$$

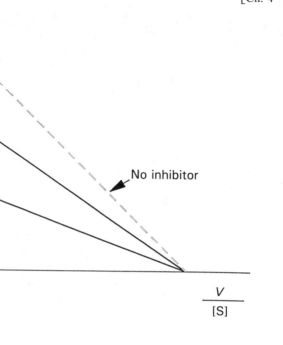

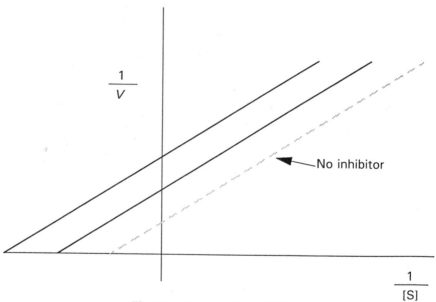

Fig. 4.38.   Uncompetitive inhibition.

To bring together three small molecules simultaneously onto the surface of the enzyme causes a tremendous loss of rotational and translational entropy. Combining two or more of the small molecules into a single structure will much reduce this entropy loss, and this has been the basis of the design of a number of inhibitors. The result can be made even more effective if the linking chain contains a group which

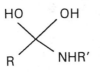

(28)

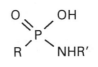

(29)

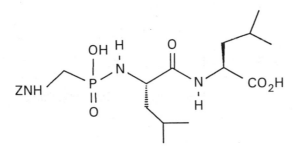

(30)

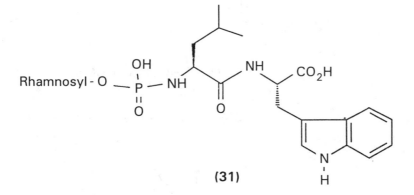

(31)

can act as a transition state analogue. Examples of multisubstrate analogues are pyridoxylalanine (**37**) a potent inhibitor of pyridoxamine-pyruvate transaminase and P'(adenosine-5')-P^5-(adenosine-5') pentaphosphate (**38**). The former enzyme catalyses the transfer of an amino group from alanine to pyruvic acid via the aldimine (**39**). (**37**) clearly contains both structural elements of the substrate and the cofactor, which can bind to their appropriate centres on the enzyme, but because it lacks the double bond (**37**) cannot undergo the transaminase reaction. The entropy loss for the single molecule in such a case will be less than that for the two substrates.

Similar considerations apply to (**38**) but in this case the linking chain possibly also acts as a transition state analogue of the enzymatic reaction (**40**).

4.11.5.1.4   Irreversible enzyme inhibitors

Irreversible enzymes are not removed from the enzyme by dialysis, gel filtration or dilution, and this definition includes both covalently bound and slowly dissociating,

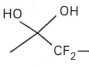

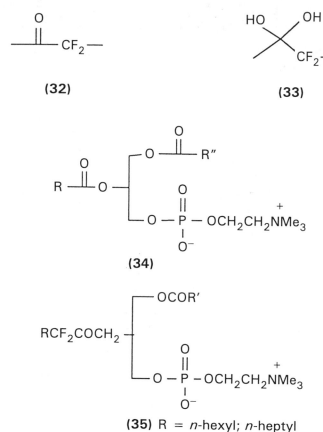

(32)

(33)

(34)

(35) R = *n*-hexyl; *n*-heptyl

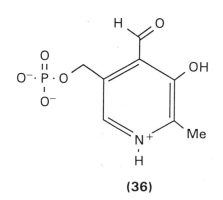

(36)

tightly bonded noncovalent compounds. In the former case, the initial interaction may be noncovalent with the covalent bond forming subsequently.

The kinetics of such inhibition is extremely complex and depends on concentrations, competition with the substrate, the rate of dissociation and the rate of reaction.

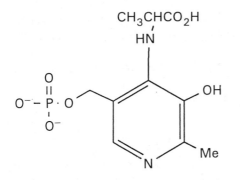

(37)

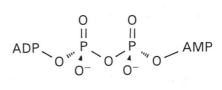

(38)

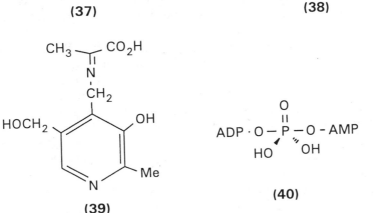

(39)

(40)

4.11.5.1.5   *Irreversible enzyme inhibitors: active site directed inhibitors*

Generally such inhibitors show time-dependent inhibition and form covalent bonds in a stoichiometric manner with (usually) nucleophilic groups on the enzyme close to or in the active site. To make a good, specific inhibitor, the molecule should have the reacting site bound to a recognition site specific for the enzyme. For example serine proteases are inhibited by organophosphates ($ROO_2PO(X)$) (X is a leaving group) which react with the hydroxyl group in the active site of the enzyme to give (**41**), which does not readily hydrolyse to release the active enzyme.

$$Enz\text{-}O\text{-}PO(OH)_2$$

(41)

Other inhibitors of this class include aspirin in which the salicylic acid binds to the cycloxygenase enzyme which is then acetylated by the acetyl group. Penicillins and cephalosporin work because the highly electrophilic β-lactam structure reacts with nucleophilic groups in the enzyme D-alanyl-D-alanine transpeptidase which normally functions by a transamination reaction in which the terminal D-alanine of one pentapeptide sidechain is replaced by an amino group from an adjacent chain thus forming a crosslinked structure in the bacterial cell wall. Acylation of the nucleophilic group in the enzyme by the β-lactam prevents the construction of the bacterial cell wall thus leading to its death. It will be appreciated that in this particular case the desirable inhibition arises because the enzyme is found only in the parasites and not the host organism.

A potential problem with such systems is that if the electrophilic group is too reactive it may well react with many other structures before it reaches its target. A second class of inhibitors attempts to overcome this problem.

4.11.5.1.6   Irreversible enzyme inhibitors: mechanism-based inhibitors

These inhibitors were initially called by the more evocative name of "suicide inhibitors" on the basis that an unreactive molecule is converted by an enzyme into a reactive species which then irreversibly inhibits the enzyme thereby invoking its own destruction.

For example 6-β-halopenicillins (**42**) are potent inhibitors of β-lactamase because the intitial ring opened structure (**43**) formed by enzymatic attack on (**42**) contains a very reactive halogen atom which is readily displaced by the nucleophilic thiol atom giving (**44**). Since (**44**) is a relatively stable–acyl–enzyme complex the enzyme is inhibited. Another such inhibitor is the fungal metabolite gabaculine (**45**), a structural analogue of the inhibitory amino acid γ-aminobutyric acid (**46**), which inhibits γ-aminobutyric acid transaminase. This is another pyridoxal-based enzyme the reaction of which proceeds via an imine intermediate of structure (**47**) which rapidly and irreversibly aromatises to inhibit the enzyme. This type of inhibition thus provides many challenges to the ingenuity of the medicinal chemist in order to exploit the mechanisms of enzymatic reactions to produce new selective agents.

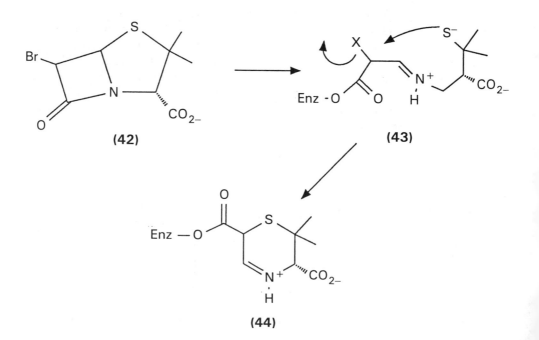

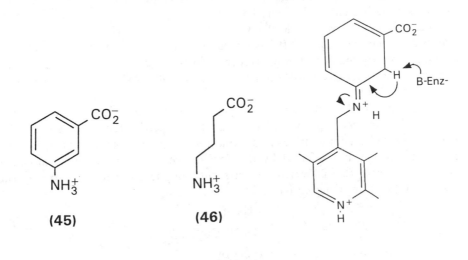

Structures 4.45, 4.46 and 4.47   **(47)**

4.11.6   Resistance and tolerance

From the very earliest days of antibiotic therapy it was realised that microorganisms varied in their sensitivities to such drugs. This also applied to different strains of the same organism, and tolerant strains were defined as those which are totally resistant to the agent. Resistant strains are defined as being susceptible only to concentrations of drug many times greater than those which are normally lethal, and such varying susceptibilities must be the result of differences in the structures of the enzymatic targets of the antibiotics.

The appearance of these strains is not a new phenomenon. Strains resistant to naturally occurring antibiotics have appeared throughout evolution, but it is only following the widespread use of such agents in modern therapy that the pressure for such selection has really been intense. In 1941 very nearly all pathogenic strains were sensitive to antibiotics whereas today the situation is totally different. There have been major outbreaks of antibiotic-resistant diseases such as dysentery in Central America and India caused by resistant *Shigella dysenteriae*, of typhoid due to chloramphenicol-resistant *Salmonella typhi* and of gonorrhoea due to pencillin-resistant strains of *Nesseria gonorrhoea*. There is absolutely no doubt that the situation will continue, that more resistant strains will appear in future, that new antibiotics will be required to counteract these, and that the discovery of such agents will continue to challenge the medicinal chemist and microbiologist.

The molecular reason for the appearance of resistance is perhaps most easily seen in the penicillins. As mentioned earlier these bind to a number of enzymes, transpeptidases and D,D-carboxypeptidases involved in cell wall synthesis. In resistant strains this resistance can arise from three different causes, namely a decrease of affinity for the pencillin, an alteration in the quantity of binding protein produced, and an increased rate of breakdown of the pencillin–protein complex. All of these obviously involve major changes in the structure of the protein, changes which are presumably intitiated at the gene level. Alternatively, the organism produces the enzyme β-lactamase which cleaves the reactive β-lactam ring in the penicillin to produce an inactive product. It has proved possible to neutralise the effects of this enzyme either by modification of the penicillin side chain to prevent binding to the lactamase, or by co-administration of a specific inhibitor of the enzyme, such as clavulanic acid (**27**).

Chloramphenicol (**48a**), a major antibiotic used to treat typhoid and meningitis, acts by inhibiting the peptidyl transferase centre located on the 50 ribosomal subunit which is responsible for peptide bond formation during polypeptide chain elongation. Resistance is largely conferred by the appearance of an enzyme chloramphenicol acetyl transferase (CAT) which converts chloramphenicol stepwise to the totally inactive 1,3-diacetoxy derivative (**48b**).

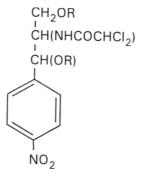

CH_2OR
$CH(NHCOCHCl_2)$
$CH(OR)$

NO_2

(**48a**)   R = H
(**48b**)   R = Ac

These are but two examples of the way in which microbial agents have overcome attack by antibiotics and thus been able to survive and flourish to the detriment of mankind. Many other systems exist but all present potential targets for drug discoveries which could prolong the clinical effectiveness of a number of drugs.

4.11.7 Specific enzymes

There are so many different classes of enzymes operating on such a number of different substrates that detailed coverage in this chapter is not possible. Instead the interested reader is referred to any one of the many excellent specific texts published on enzymes, and only a selection of enzymes particularly relevant to drug discovery will be discussed further.

4.11.7.1 Oxygenases

Many oxidases contain complexes of iron, copper or, in the case of xanthine oxidases, both molybdenum and iron, and use as a cofactor flavin (**49**), a heterocyclic base which readily undergoes reversible redox reactions. The iron-dependent oxygenases usually have an iron-protoporhyrin IX cofactor as a tightly bound prosthetic group. The initial complex binds the organic substrate and then undergoes one electron reduction to give a high spin Fe^{2+} oxidation state. This reacts with oxygen and another electron to generate a highly reactive oxygen species $Fe^{3+} = 0$ which catalyses substrate oxidation followed by release of water and oxidised substrate (Figure 4.39).

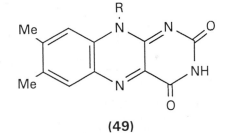

(49)

Among such enzymes are the monoamine oxidases (MAO) which catalyse the oxidation shown in equation (50) and which are grouped into two classes, type A and B, with different inhibitors.

$$RCH_2NHR^1 + O_2 + H_2O \rightarrow RCHO + H_2O + H_2NR^1 \tag{50}$$

MAO Type A selectively deaminates 5-hydroxytryptamine and noradrenaline while type B works best on phenylethylamines. As might be expected from such different substrate specificities the two types are inhibited by different ligands, and clorgyline (**50**) potently inhibits type A whereas L-deprenyl (**51**) inhibits type B. Centrally active inhibitors of monoamine oxidase are potent antidepressants although their use is limited by the risk of hypertension crisis following concomitant tyramine ingestion in food.

Perhaps the most important range of oxidases are the mixed function oxidases, cytochrome P-450, which are responsible for the majority of metabolic oxidations of xenobiotics in the liver. These enzymes are capable of oxidising a remarkable range of substrates including the hydroxylation of unactivated C–H bonds, sulphide and tertiary amines to sulphur and nitrogen oxides and double and triple bonds to aldehydes and carboxylic acids.

The extremely complex enzyme xanthine oxidase may be mentioned as a final example of important oxidases. It is responsible for the final stages of the mammalian metabolism of purines and, when excessive amounts of uric acid are produced, gives rise to the disease of gout. It is also important in ischaemia when the lack of oxygen in a tissue results in the catabolism of ATP to hypoxanthine, and on readmitting oxygen to the system a burst of xanthine oxidase activity leads to the production of hydrogen peroxide, superoxide ion and hydroxyl radicals which cause significant tissue damage. Inhibition of this process for instance by allopurinol (**25**) could be of great significance in limiting such damage.

4.11.7.2   *Reductases*

Folic acid (**52**) is a water soluble vitamin which after reduction to a tetrahydro form accepts single carbon units. These are subsequently transferred enzymatically from cofactors to precursors of the purines, pyrimidines and methionine. The reduction of folic acid is catalysed by dihydrofolate reductase, an enzyme inhibited by a number of significant therapeutic agents. Methotrexate (**53**) inhibits dihydrofolate reductase

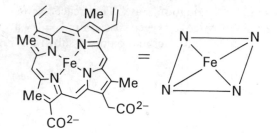

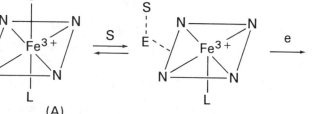

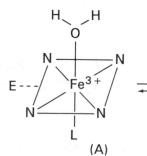

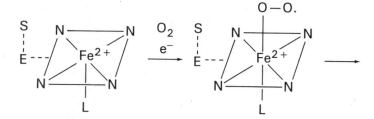

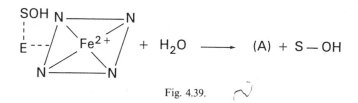

Fig. 4.39.

in neoplastic tissue, trimethoprim (**26**) in bacteria, and pyrimethamine (**54**) in protozoal diseases, and the crucial fact underlying the use of these agents is that the dihydrofolate reductases from mammalian, protozoan and bacterial sources have sufficient structural differences that it is possible for them to show selective inhibition. In cancer chemotherapy the relative toxicity shown by methotrexate results from a combination of differences in uptake, glutamylation, cellular excretion and cellular metabolic balance. The identification of these agents and the clinical importance of these enzymes provided the central theme of the extensive work of Hitchings and Elion which resulted in their Nobel Prize for physiology or medicine in 1988.

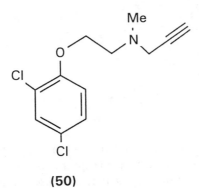

(50)

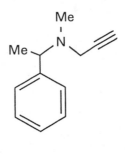

(51)

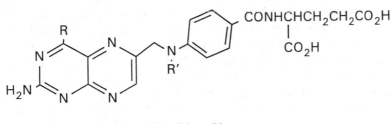

(52) R = OH, R′ = H
(53) R = NH2, R′ = Me

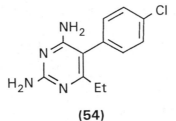

(54)

4.11.7.3 *Hydrolases*

These enzymes catalyse the cleavage of bonds between carbon and a number of other atoms with the addition of water, and include acetylcholinesterases, peptidases, lipases, phospholipases and phosphatases.

Acetylcholinesterase, as mentioned previously, hydrolyses the neurotransmitter acetylcholine following its release from the cholinergic receptor in the synaptic cleft and thus limits its activity. Potent irreversible inhibitors of acetylcholinesterase such as tabum (**55**) are nerve gases which rapidly lead to death; more usefully, carbamates such as physostigmine (**24**) are used in the muscle weakening disease myasthenia gravis to preserve the reduced stocks of acetylcholine and thus maintain neuron function.

$$Me_2N - \overset{\displaystyle O}{\underset{\displaystyle Et}{\overset{\|}{P}}} - CN$$

(55)

4.11.7.4   *Peptidases*

Peptidases cleave amide bonds in peptides and are subdivided into exopeptidases which cleave chain ends and endopeptidases which cleave internal bonds. In view of the biological importance of proteins it is not surprising that proteases, a generic term covering all enzymes hydrolysing proteins and peptides, are a very significant class of enzymes responsible for, *inter alia*, release of peptide hormones, neuromodulators and enzymes from inactive precursors, and the termination of biological responses by the degradation of transmitter peptides. Clinically important peptidase inhibitors include captopril (**56**) which inhibits angiotensin converting enzyme (ACE), the enzyme responsible for the generation of the hypertensive angiotensin II from its precursor angiotensin I. The lowering of levels of angiotensin II leads to a reduction in blood pressure, and captopril, along with the subsequently discovered ACE inhibitors, represents the latest class of agents effective against various forms of heart disease.

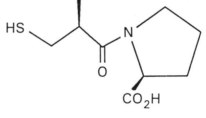

(56)

   The discovery of captopril by Ondetti and Cushman represents one of the earliest cases of intelligent drug design. ACE was known to be a zinc-containing enzyme but the structure of its active site was unknown. However, it was reasoned that the mechanism of action should resemble that of carboxypeptidase, whose active site structure is known, since they are both endopeptidases. The role of zinc was envisaged to coordinate with the amide carbonyl group rendering it more susceptible to aqueous hydrolysis. Acidic and basic groups in the enzyme backbone assist the proton transfer in the process. Based on what was known about the selectivity of ACE it was proposed that a dipeptide, such as (**57**), should bind into the active site, and this did indeed do so. Further, replacement of the carboxyl group by a more strongly zinc chelating thiol group gave (**56**). The binding interactions of (**56**) with ACE as proposed by Ondetti are shown in (**58**). Many other inhibitors based on this reasoning have been designed, and a steadily increasing number of ACE inhibitors confirm the hypothesis.

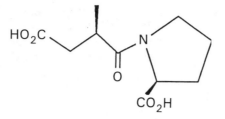

(57)

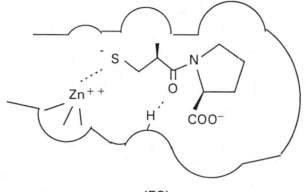

(58)

Another peptidase enzyme which has been the subject of extensive rational drug design efforts, although with less therapeutic success, is collagenase. This also is a zinc metalloproteinase which cleaves the major structural protein collagen at specific peptide bonds, and its inhibition could be of use in various arthritic conditions. From what is known of their preferred site of action a number of potent inhibitors, such as (59), have been designed. It will be noted that this compound contains a hydroxamic acid group to coordinate the zinc atom and a methylene group in place of the susceptible amide group. Whilst these inhibitors have nanomolar effects *in vitro*, to date no potent compounds *in vivo* have been described, however.

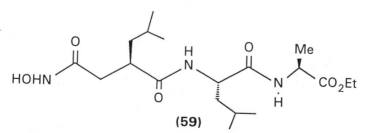

(59)

A potentially important proteinase which is the target of much drug design is the viral protease found in the human immunodeficiency virus (HIV), the causative agent of acquired immune deficiency syndrome (AIDS). This protease cleaves a polyprotein to yield smaller proteins which form the structural proteins of the virus core. Based on the mechanism of action and the crystal structure of the enzyme very selective inhibitors of the enzyme have been designed. Thus, for example, the Roche compound (**60**) shows potent *in vitro* inhibiting activity with little cellular toxicity. A considerable number of similar agents have been described and clinical results are awaited with interest.

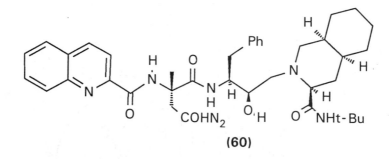

(60)

4.11.7.5   *The enzymes in cholesterol synthesis*

In recent years a causal relationship between high blood levels of cholesterol and heart disease, particularly atherosclerosis, has been determined. Cholesterol circulates in blood as a fatty acid ester within a lipoprotein particle known as a "low-density lipoprotein" (LDL). This particle is taken up into liver cells by means of a specific LDL receptor which is then internalised when the ester is hydrolysed and free cholesterol released. The biosynthesis of cholesterol has a sequence of 26 steps from acetyl Co-enzyme A, and in this pathway the conversion of hydroxymethyl-glutaryl-Co-enzyme A to mevalonate catalysed by HMG-CoA reductase is the rate-limiting step (**61**). Inhibition of this enzyme reduces the amount of cholesterol produced and, since a supply of cholesterol is essential, e.g. in membrane synthesis, the only way that this can be obtained is by increased uptake of LDL which leads to reduced blood cholesterol levels.

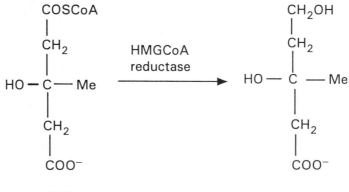

(61)

During screening of microbiological extracts, compactin (**62**) was isolated from *Penicillin citrinum*, and mevinolin (**63**) was found in *Aspergillis terreus*. Both of these compounds are potent inhibitors of HMG-CoA reductase and lower blood cholesterol levels in dogs and primates including man. Mevinolin is now in widespread clinical use for controlling cholesterol levels and a number of other synthesis inhibitors are in clinical development.

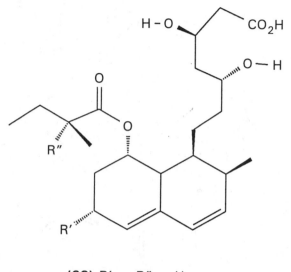

(62) R′ = R″ = H
(63) R′ = Me R″ = H

4.11.7.6   Cell wall biosynthesis

Bacteria are different from mammalian cells in that they have an additional cell wall which lies outside the cell membrane. Damage to this wall leads to osmotic pressure bursting and destruction of the bacterium. The cell wall and more particularly the enzymes responsible for its construction consequently represent attractive targets for antibiotic therapy via selective actions. The β-lactam antibiotics react with peptidases responsible for the synthesis of the peptidergic structure of the cell wall, as previously mentioned. Tunicamycin (**64**) inhibits the formation of undecaprenyl-P-P-N-acetylmuramoylpentapeptide synthesis, while vancomycin (**65**) acts by tightly binding the acyl-D-alanyl-D-alanine terminus of the growing peptide chain and preventing the addition of other amino acids to it. Inside the cell wall is a cycloplasmic membrane which is the target for a number of antibiotics including the gramacidins, a group of 15 amino acid linear peptides. These form helical structures which create open, waterfilled pores through the membrance through which protons and inorganic ions can diffuse to the detriment of the organism. Polyene antibiotics, such as amphotercin B (**66**), alter the permeability of the cell membrane to protons and specific ionophores, e.g. valinomycin (**67**), induce specific K+ for H+ exchange by rendering the bacterial membrane selectively permeable to cations. This causes a depletion of potassium levels in the cell and results in the inactivation of cellular macromolecular synthesis.

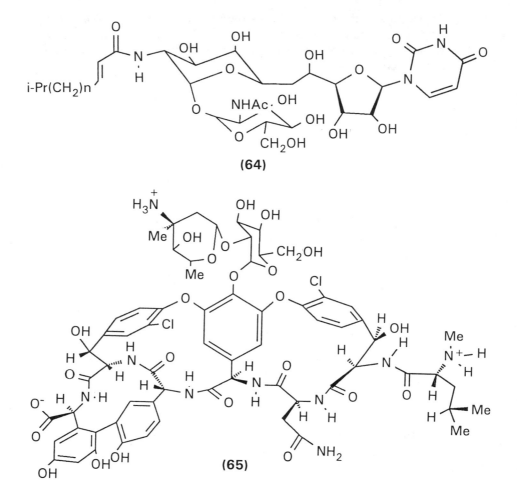

(64)

(65)

4.11.7.7   *Enzymes affecting DNA replication*

The conceptually simple process of unwinding of the DNA helix, transcription to RNA, and reformation of the double helix actually requires the assistance of a considerable number of enzymes. Interference with these enzymes provides an attractive target for the action of antibiotics and anticancer agents since selectivity might be expected to arise from structural differences in the first instance and more rapid turnover in the latter.

The quinolone antibacterials, e.g. **(68)**, have successfully exploited this strategy as they are potent inhibitors of the bacterial enzyme topoisomerase II (DNA gyrase) but are only weak inhibitors of the human enzyme. The consequently wide therapeutic index confers good clinical usefulness on this class of antibiotics. The topiosomerases break transiently one or both DNA strands along with the formation of an enzyme–DNA covalent bond, altering the topology of the DNA chain and causing the chains to separate. Thus DNA replication, gene expression and cell proliferation are crucially

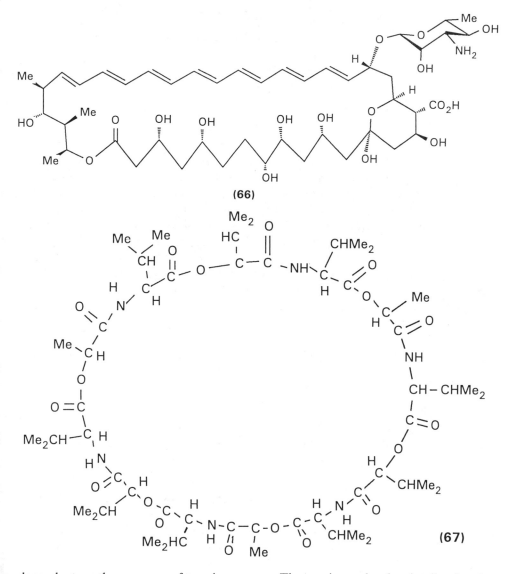

(66)

(67)

dependent on the presence of topoisomerases. The precise molecular details whereby (**68**) and its analogues inhibit DNA gyrase and prevent reforming of the broken DNA duplex are not clear.

Unfortunately, the clear structural differences which obviously exist between bacterial and mammalian enzymes are not seen between tumour and normal cells. Thus cytotoxic agents work only because of the greater proliferation rate of malignant cells and thus are much less effective against slowly developing tumours. The discovery of differences between such cells and normal ones which can be exploited beneficially remains a major goal of drug research.

As well as treating bacterial infections and tumour growth, interference with nucleic

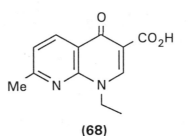

(68)

acid related enzymes represents the only therapeutic way currently available of treating viral infections. Viruses are particularly difficult to treat since they use little independent biochemistry of their own and proliferate by subverting the host mechanisms, eliminating the possibility of selective interference. However, some viruses, so-called retroviruses, are unique in that their genetic material is RNA rather than DNA. These viruses use an enzyme called reverse transcriptase which reverses the "normal" flow of genetic information to produce double-stranded DNA from retroviral single-stranded RNA. This enzyme is not needed in host organisms, so its inhibition presents an obvious selective target. The most important agent currently functioning by this mechanism is AZT **(69)** which is at present the only agent approved for the treatment of AIDS.

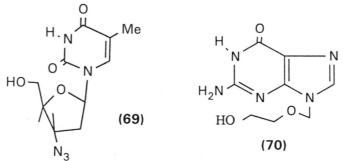

(69)   **(70)**

A more subtle selectivity is provided by the antiviral, acyclovir **(70)**. Thus it is first phosphorylated much more efficiently by thymidine kinase from viruses than from the host, and then the resultant triphosphate selectively inhibits DNA polymerase found in by virally infected cells to a much greater extent than it inhibits polymerase from non-infected cells.

A number of antitumour agents act by intercalating the DNA by inserting between the base pairs of DNA, unwinding the helix and thus preventing interaction with DNA and RNA polymerases. An example of this mechanism is actinomycin D **(71)**, an antitumour antibiotic, whilst netropsin **(22)** causes equivalent disruption without intercalating, both it and CC-1065 **(23)** binding into the minor groove in A-T rich regions.

4.11.8 Catalytic antibodies

In his perceptive writing on catalysis in the late 1940s Pauling contrasted the difference between enzymes and antibodies as arising from the fact that enzymes bind

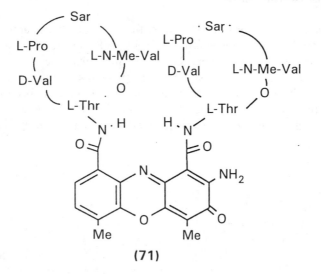

(71)

to parts of the substrate in the transition state whilst antibodies bind to parts of antigens in the ground state. Otherwise these macromolecular interactions had much in common. Antibodies are produced by B-cell lymphocytes in response to invasion of the body by foreign proteins or antigens, the versatility of the body in being able to produce on demand proteins capable of binding tightly with virtually any natural or synthetic molecule being truly amazing. In many cases the specificity of antibodies for antigens is greater than that of enzymes for their substrates. In 1975 Kohler and Milstein showed how it was possible to produce monoclonal antibodies, that is antibodies consisting of a single distinct molecular structure specific for a single antigen, this transformed much of immunology and biochemistry.

In the mid-1980s the separate Californian research groups of Lerner and Schultz mused on the connection between enzymes and antibodies and theorised that producing antibodies to a reaction transition state should give a catalytic antibody. Of course the major difficulty is that a normal transition state has too short a life to generate antibodies, but this could be overcome by the use of a stable transition state analogue as discussed earlier. The first successful examples of this theory were antibodies capable of catalysing acyl transfer reactions with rate accelerations of 10^3-10^4 compared with uncatalysed ones and which followed Michaelis–Menten kinetics. Subsequently, a wide range of reactions including carbonate, ester and amide hydrolysis, Claisen and Diels–Alder reactions, amide formation, lactonisation and redox reactions have been described. Not all of these are synthetically useful, but their existence promises much for the future in chemistry, biology, and medicine.

4.11.9 RNA as enzymes

Until the early 1980s it was a central dogma of biochemistry that all enzymes were proteins. The independent groups of Altman and Cech then showed conclusively that RNA could also function as an enzyme. Cech was studying the way in which ribosomal RNA, which is transcribed from DNA in a form much longer than required, undergoes cleavage to the active RNA. The answer was clearly that the RNA alone could adopt a three-dimensional structure that contained an active site able to recognise and bind to a specific site in the RNA and thus cleave it. Altman showed that the RNA subunit of an enzyme RNase-P which processes tRNA to produce a mature tRNA, acts as a true catalyst, whilst the protein subunit has no such activity. Such RNAs have been referred to as ribozymes and have now been found to have widespread activities, being capable of cleaving other RNA which may have great use in future in cleaving specifically sequences of viral RNA as potential antiviral treatments.

5

Drug discovery processes

5.1 INTRODUCTION

This section will outline current practice in the art and science of drug design. The basic elements of the drug discovery process remain much as they have been for many years and which have resulted in the many very significant modern medicines. There is a need for a hypothesis about the underlying cause of the disease state, for a prototype lead structure, and for an optimisation process which produces the molecule with the best profile of activity, as exemplified in section 5.3. The modern discovery process is outlined schematically in scheme 5.1 leading from an unfulfilled medical need through scientific evaluation of potential biological targets to the specific targets for chemical synthesis.

The knowledge of the mechanisms of disease states, the ability to determine the structure of molecular targets, and, thanks to progress in the power of computers and theoretical chemistry, the ability to model both small molecular weight ligands and their macromolecular targets and the energy of their interaction have progressed enormously in recent years. Together these offer the ultimate promise of genuine *de novo* drug design, where, armed with their own ingenuity and a computer, medicinal chemists will be able to design an entirely new drug to better treat the disease state. Already this is beginning to occur, and no doubt many more examples from research laboratories will soon be published.

The drug design process (scheme 5.2) begins with identification of a lead structure by the multidisciplinary teams implied in scheme 5.1, possessing some elements of the desired therapeutic profile or its hypothetical mechanism of action.

Three key strategies are shown in scheme 5.2. Databases, preferably three-dimensional ones which accurately reflect the true spatial relationships between functional groups, can be searched for new molecules similar to those of the lead structure. If the interaction with the target receptor can be modelled this can be used to rapidly screen large numbers of molecules and the results used to hypothesise the likely pharmacophore. Increasingly, computer-aided drug design (CADD) is used to

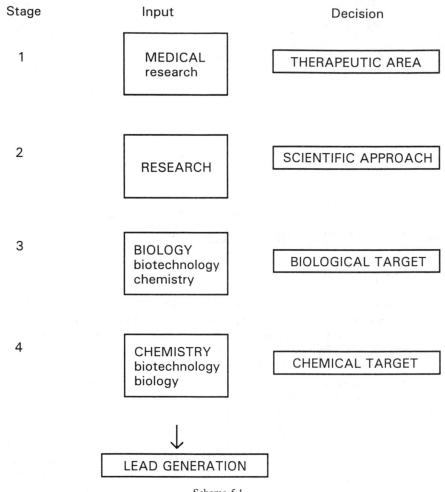

Stage	Input	Decision
1	MEDICAL research	THERAPEUTIC AREA
2	RESEARCH	SCIENTIFIC APPROACH
3	BIOLOGY biotechnology chemistry	BIOLOGICAL TARGET
4	CHEMISTRY biotechnology biology	CHEMICAL TARGET

LEAD GENERATION

Scheme 5.1.

design entirely novel structures either from that of the lead or the target. These processes will be discussed in detail in subsequent sections.

5.2 SOURCES OF LEAD STRUCTURES

There are four main sources of a lead structure, namely clinical or pharmacological side effects, random screening, natural products (known or newly discovered) and *de novo* rational design.

5.2.1 Clinical and pharmacological side effects

There are many examples of drugs being used in patients for one clinical indication showing an entirely unexpected side effect. For example, although it was originally shown in 1890 that gold–cyanide complexes were effective against the tuberculosis

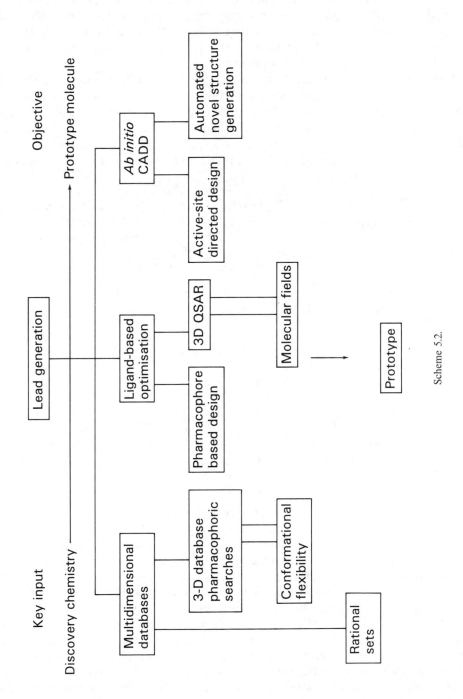

Scheme 5.2.

bacillus *in vitro* [in clinical trials] showed no antibacterial effect [some thirty years later], but did show significant relief of joint pain in arthritis. This led to the study of other gold compounds in this distressing disease and eventually to the clinical use of sodium aurothiomalate (**1**) and Auranofin (**2**). It should be noted that the mechanism of action of such agents is not clear, even today.

Isonicotinic acid hydrazide (**3**) was originally found to be a potent, and widely used, anti-tubercular drug, and amongst the analogues of (**3**) which were also marketed for anti-tubercular activity was the *iso*-propyl analogue (**4**), Iproniazid. This had pronounced central nervous system side effects and, in particular, the ability to alleviate the mood of severely depressed tubercular patients. This led to the use of Iproniazid in depression and to the synthesis and evaluation of many structural analogues.

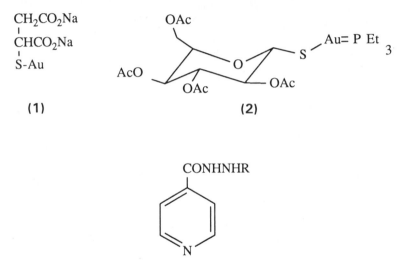

(3) R=H

(4) R=iPr

Even more remarkable was the discovery of the antimanic activity of lithium ions, which resulted from animal studies testing the hypothesis that manic depressives excrete in their urine a material directly related to their disease. In the event, concentrates of such urine were found to be more toxic to guinea pigs than those from normal individuals, and it was conjectured that excess uric acid was responsible for this toxicity. Only the lithium salt was sufficiently water soluble to test this hypothesis, when, surprisingly, it was found that this salt was actually protective against the effects of urea. Further work showed that the activity was in fact due entirely to the lithium ion. Subsequently, large-scale clinical trials of lithium salts showed their ability to treat manic-depressant illness prophylactically. For many years the mechanism of action of lithium was not understood, but it now appears that it affects an enzyme in the "second messenger" system, thus suggesting new targets for drug design.

The lesson from these and other similar examples is that clinicians and pharmacologists need to be always observant of unexpected pharmacological effects with new chemical substances.

5.2.2 Random screening

The random undirected testing of large numbers of diverse compounds in animal tests is time consuming, wasteful of materials and animals, and is of dubious efficacy and morality. However, such testing *in vitro* uses very much less material, is rapid, and forms part of all broadly based new drug research programmes.

As the receptors and enzymes which play key roles in diseases are progressively identified, they become the new targets for drug design. The biochemical techniques of enzyme inhibition and receptor binding (receptorology) have already been described in the previous chapter. To improve throughput and reproducibility of data, a number of these techniques have been automated, and commercial apparatus is increasingly available.

At a higher level of biological complexity cells can also be used as test systems. This is particularly true in the case of the immune system whose activity entails the interaction of separate cell types mediated by polypeptides and where candidate molecules can be tested by their modulation of the effect of natural mediators on particular cells.

The analogous studies of the effects of compounds on the growth of microorganisms and viruses have of course been a feature of medical research into new antibiotics and antiviral agents for many years.

Sources of the compounds used in random screening are many and varied. These include speculative chemistry carried out in pharmaceutical and academic laboratories and in the chemical libraries which all pharmaceutical companies have built up over many years. In addition, in recent years biological and chemical techniques have been developed which are capable of generating very large numbers of novel peptides. Combined with selective analytical techniques capable of detecting the activity of specific peptides these systems provide powerful new ways of generating novel minipeptide lead structures.

The use of randomly generated oligonucleotide fragments in gene expression systems is capable of generating very large numbers of unusual peptides, the principal problem being to identify those interesting ones and the system in which they arise. These systems can then be used as the source of sufficient amounts of the peptide for further evaluation. One such approach uses a filamentous phage as the vector. The phage carries a coat protein pIII which normally mediates the infection of a bacterium, e.g. *E. coli*, by fusing to the host cell. When the new DNA fragments are fused into the phage DNA in the region which codes for pIII, the coat protein is expressed carrying the new peptide. The phage retains its infectivity and the new peptides are thus susceptible to antibody formation operation. It is possible to use a specific antibody to identify the phages carrying peptides of interest. Normal cloning techniques then enable large quantities of the peptide of interest to be synthesised. The extension of this technique to finding novel peptides able to bind to receptors of pharmacological interest is extensively used.

Traditional chemical methods of synthesising rapidly large numbers of peptides and then analysing the binding of the products to selected antibodies and receptors are also used. Early techniques employed solid-state syntheses with the growing peptide fused to "pins" or "beads" and exposed to synthetic media containing mixtures of amino acids. More recently the Merrifield solid-state synthesis has been combined with the techniques of photolithography to generate the peptide fragments, using photolabile amino protecting groups in the peptide synthesis procedure (Figure 5.1).

A large array of initiating substrates is fixed to a solid support and the amino group of the substrate is protected by a photolabile nitroveratryloxycarbonyl group. A patterned mask is placed over the support and illuminated by light which results in deprotection only of those parts of the support exposed through holes in the mask. The whole surface is then treated with standard coupling reactions, coupling occurring only in those regions where deprotection took place (Figure 5.1). The reagents are removed, a different mask applied, and photoactivation repeated, and the whole process can be repeated over as many stages as required. It should be noted that photolithographic techniques are very precise, so it is possible to define the structures of the actual peptides in any region of the plate extremely accurately, and subsequent treatment of the plate with a receptor or antibody can be used to indicate peptides able to combine strongly with the selected receptor.

Dower and Fodor,[1] in an excellent review of this area, show how the above two techniques can be combined to give an extremely powerful insight into peptide structure–activity relationships. The recombinant technology was used to generate a hexapeptide ligand capable of binding to a specific antibody, and light–directed chemical synthesis was then used to rapidly generate 1024 derivatives of this peptide. From this collection only 15 compounds were still bound to the antibody, and the variation in the strength of this binding gave a very detailed picture of the structure–activity relationships.

5.2.3　Natural sources of drugs

Man, along with many other animals, has had a long history of using materials gathered from his surroundings to alleviate the ailments with which he is afflicted. Through the centuries the leaves, roots, stems, fruit, and exudates of plants have provided most of these treatments, but microbes and the sea have also become important sources of therapy in recent years.

5.2.3.1　*Plants*

Herbal remedies have been documented from earliest recorded times until the present day. Pharmacopoeia detailing such materia medica are amongst the earliest recorded writings from a number of civilisations such as the Egyptian Ebers papyrus of 1550 BC, the Chinese Huang Di Nei Jing of 300 BC, the Indian *Charaka Samhita* of 500– 200 BC and the Greek Dioscorides's *De Materia Medica* of the first century AD. All these texts, and, one may presume, many others that have been lost, together with verbal communications of generations of medical men have extolled the properties of many hundreds of plant preparations.

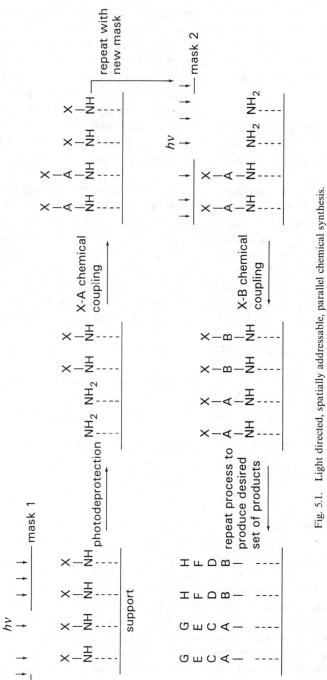

Fig. 5.1.   Light directed, spatially addressable, parallel chemical synthesis.

With the evolution of modern science, efforts were made to try to identify pure chemical substances responsible for the activity of these biological materials. The techniques thus developed to isolate such products,[2] to establish their chemical structures, and ultimately to synthesise the pure substances have provided the foundations of modern organic chemistry. Ultimately studies also led to the development of modern drugs but, to date, not to the exclusion of herbal remedies. These are still widely used in many developed countries throughout the world where, ironically, lower standards are demanded than are required for synthetic agents, and also in developing countries where local extracts administered by an appropriate authority may be the only available treatment. In fact, it is estimated that in some African countries more than 90% of the "medicines" used today are locally produced herbal remedies.

Amongst the notable therapeutic agents which have been derived from plants are the antimalarial quinine (cinchona bark), the diuretic theobromine (tea), the local anaesthetic cocaine (cocoa leaves), the cardiac stimulant digitalin (foxglove), the analgesic opiates (poppy), the antigout colchicine (crocus), the bronchospasmolytic ephedrine (Ma Huang, *Ephedra vulgaris*), the anticholinergic atropine (*Atropa belladonna*, deadly nightshade), the muscle relaxant curare (*Chododendron tomentosum*), and the hypotensive, antidepressant reserpine (*Rauwolfia serpentina*). All of these modern drugs were discovered by analysis of typical herbal remedies used by the indigenous populations from the localities where the plants commonly grow. This partial list gives some indication of the debt which modern therapy owes to plant sources for drugs, and there is every reason to believe that many more potentially useful agents await discovery.

Four main problems are to be confronted in isolating interesting molecules from any natural source, namely selecting the source to be investigated, isolating the active component and defining its structure, determining its pharmacological activity, and preparing sufficient quantities for testing.

There is an almost incalculable number of plants available in the world, each of which has constituents which vary from root to stem, from leaf to seed, and from season to season. It may never be possible to evaluate them all, but the legacy for future generations must be to ensure that the loss of species is minimised as tropical rain forests are eroded.

The more systematic alternative to random screening is *ethnopharmacology*, the detailed investigation of traditional folk medicines, which is how all the drugs listed above were discovered. The particular plant to be studied is thus selected from local usage when the next step is to separate the pharmacologically relevant compounds from the bulk of the plant constituents. This is, of course, an exercise well understood by organic chemists when all the usual chromatographic techniques including modern versions of countercurrent chromatography are used. Since the amounts of material initially isolated are so small, the biological tests used need to be extremely sensitive. Initial studies concentrate on detecting antimicrobial activity together with enzyme, receptor, and cell assays which greatly expand the range of pharmacological activities which can be discovered.

Preparing a pure active agent can pose major problems when the natural product has a complex structure. This is well illustrated by the case of Taxol **(5)**[3] which currently shows interesting activity in phase II clinical trials as an anticancer agent against solid tumours, particularly those of the breast and ovaries. Taxol was originally isolated from the bark of the Pacific Yew tree as part of a general search coordinated by the National Cancer Institute. The very promising clinical data stimulated a great demand for large supplies of the material. Unfortunately, these cannot be obtained from natural sources without destroying the whole tree, and total synthesis is extremely complex and not viable. This has sparked considerable efforts to isolate the drug or hemisynthetic analogues from renewable resources such as the leaf.

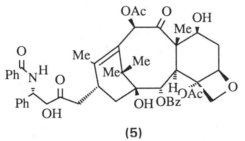

(5)

An imaginative approach to the discovery of the bioactive constituents from African plants is provided by Kostellmann and Martin,[4] who reasoned that such plants are subject to constant fungal attacks and those surviving must have evolved a natural defence mechanism. Thus extracts of these plants were eluted on tlc plates and the plates sprayed with fungal spores and incubated, when active fractions could then be readily identified from the zones of resistance. Similar approaches will certainly be more widely used in future.

5.2.3.2 Microbes

Diverse microbial products are amongst the most powerful antibiotics, antifungals, and immune suppressant agents available to medicine. It is a popular misunderstanding that the concept of microbes producing chemical agents which could kill other microbes arose from the work of Fleming and the initial discovery of penicillin. In fact the eminent French scientist Louis Pasteur showed in 1877 that the growth of anthrax bacilli in urine could be inhibited by the presence of other microbes, and other researchers subsequently extended the finding to typhoid bacilli. It was almost fifty years eventually before Dubos isolated a bactericidal protein-free extract from *Bacillus brevis* which was shown to include the antibiotic gramicidin **(6)**. Waksman postulated that soil should be expected to contain pathogenic bacteria resulting from animal excreta, the fact that such bacteria are rare being due to the presence of antibiotics produced by the ubiquitous soil bacteria. He studied a class of anaerobic bacteria, the actinomycetes, and demonstrated that they indeed do produce antibiotics, although none isolated were suitable for clinical use. At that time there was a great need for an effective antitubercular agent (as indeed there is again today), and Waksman cultured his soil samples in the presence of a nonpathogenic strain of the tuberculosis-causing bacterium hoping to induce the production of an appropriate antibiotic. This strategy led to the successful isolation of streptomycin (**7**).

Val-Gly-Ala-Leu-Ala-Val-Val-Val-Val-Trp-Leu-Trp-Leu-Trp-Leu-Trp

CHO

Leu

Trp

NHCH$_2$OH

(**6**) Gramicidin

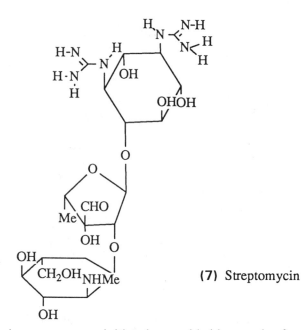

(**7**) Streptomycin

This pioneering programme initiated a worldwide search of soil samples which continues today. In rapid succession the important antibiotics chloramphenicol (**8**), tetracyclin (**9**), and erythromycin (**10**) were discovered and identified. Soil bacteria have also provided the antifungal griseofulvin (**11**) and the immunosuppressant cyclosporin A (**12**) which enabled transplant surgery to develop from an experimental procedure to a modern clinical technique with excellent prognosis. More recently, FK 506 (**13**), an even more powerful immunosuppressant, has been developed, while examination of marine bacteria extended the β-lactam class of antibiotics to include the cephalosporins (**14**).

The search for antibiotics in recent times has been fruitful, and by 1987 nearly 8000 such compounds had been isolated from microorganisms and a further 4000 from lichens, algae, and other microorganisms[5]. Bacteria are not solely a source of antibiotics, however, and a wide range of compounds with interesting biologically activity have also been isolated. Amongst these are compactin (**15**) which was isolated from *Penicillium citrinum* and originally shown to have antifungal activity. It was subsequently shown to be a potent inhibitor of the enzyme HMGCo-A reductase, a

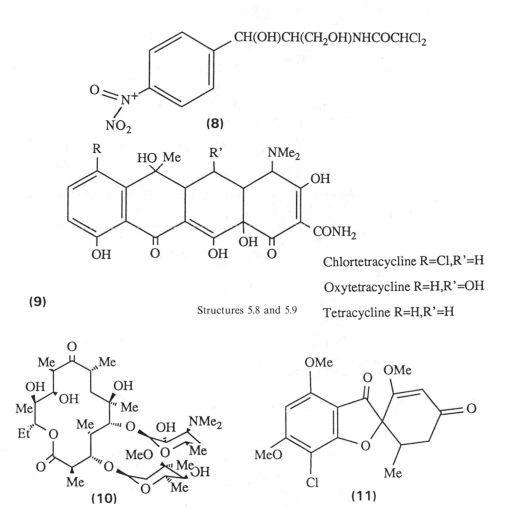

CH(OH)CH(CH₂OH)NHCOCHCl₂

(8)

Structures 5.8 and 5.9

Chlortetracycline R=Cl,R'=H

Oxytetracycline R=H,R'=OH

Tetracycline R=H,R'=H

(9)

(10)

(11)

key enzyme in the biosynthesis of cholesterol, and an effective hypocholesterolemic agent. Interestingly the chemically related mevinolin (16) was isolated from *Aspergillis terreus*, and found to be an even more potent inhibitor of this enzyme, and it is used to reduce blood cholesterol levels clinically.

Our understanding of the wide range of interesting microbial products, in addition to the antibiotics, is due to the extensive work of the Japanese chemist, Kamao Umezawa, who has isolated some hundreds of low molecular weight enzyme inhibitors from microorganisms.[6] The enzymes inhibited by these compounds include diverse proteases, glycosidases, hydrolases, oxido-reductases, transferases and lyases. Waksman originally hypothesised that soil microbes would produce their antibiotics as a means of survival or of gaining a competitive edge over other microbes, although the problem with this hypothesis is that such organisms do not seem to produce suffient antibiotics to be effective. The widespread presence of the enzyme inhibitors

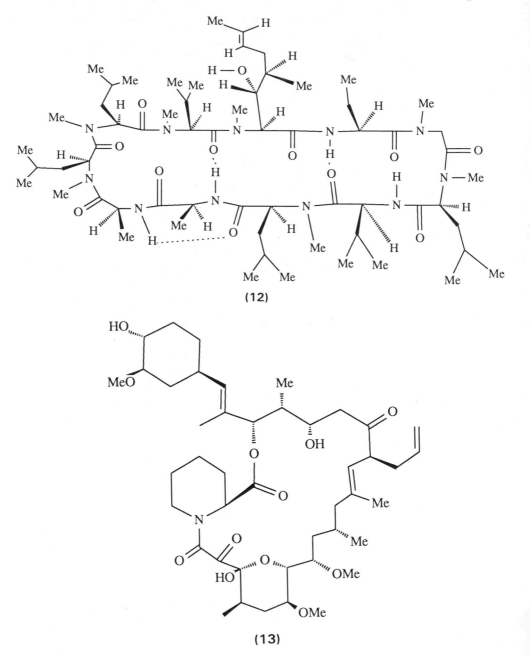

(12)

(13)

is even more perplexing since these natural products seem to have no function within the producing organism nor indeed have significant antibacterial activity. Regardless of their motivation, however, microbes are a rich source of diverse pharmacologically active molecules and will continue to provide interesting leads for research. In comparison with plants, microbes have a number of advantages as sources of natural

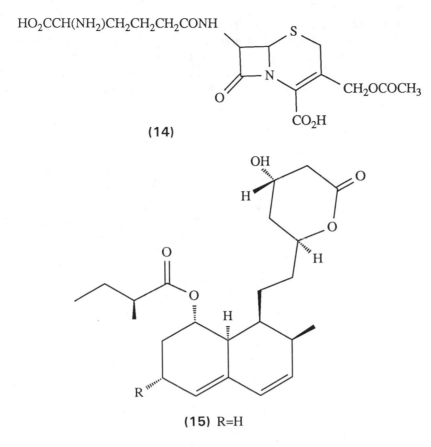

$HO_2CCH(NH_2)CH_2CH_2CH_2CONH$

CH_2OCOCH_3

CO_2H

(14)

(15) R=H

(16) R=Me

products. They are numerous, more easily collected and transported, and they can be more easily grown and cultivated. It is possible to induce their mutation, notably by X-rays or anticancer agents, to increase the yield or change the distribution of their by-products. Bördy,[5] however, has claimed that to date the screening of 100 000 microbes has led to only 5–50 useful new compounds so that the success of such research should not be overestimated. All of the compounds mentioned above have been modified extensively by synthetic chemistry in the search for more potent and selective agents.

5.2.3.3 Marine sources

The products of sponges, algae, shellfish, snakes, plants, and invertebrates are amongst the most complex and toxic natural products yet isolated.[7,8,9] Toxic constituents of fish have produced massive outbreaks of poisoning along the coastal regions of Central America and the widespread occurrence of the disease ciguatera, which is a combined disorder of the digestive, neurological, and cardiovascular systems.

Not all marine products are poisonous, and amongst the more useful agents discovered are the didemnins (**17**) which are found in Caribbean tunicates and have antiviral, antitumour and immunosuppressant activity. The antileukaemic bryostatins (**18**), also found in tunicates, the sponge product manoalide (**19**), a potent phospholipase A_2 inhibitor, and the antiviral eudistomins (**20**) are additional tunicate products.

Amongst the toxins so far identified are brevetoxin (**21**), a product of the Florida

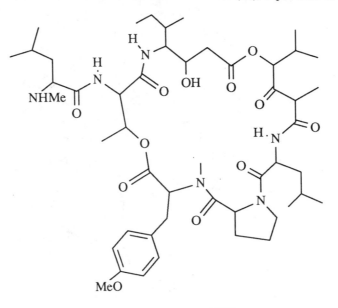

(**17**)

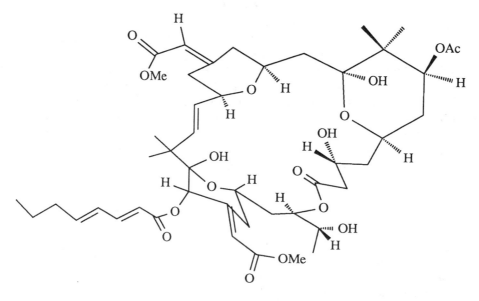

(**18**)

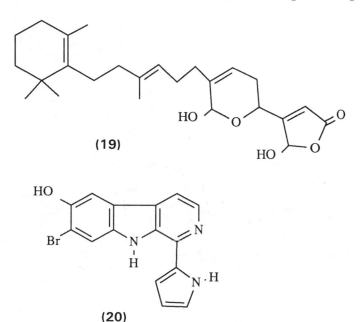

(19)

(20)

red tide organism *Gymnodinium breve*, which is a potent activator of sodium channels, the cholinesterase inhibitor anatoxin a (ANTX-A) (**22**), obtained from blue-green algae, and a number of peptidic venoms from sea snails and snakes. These venoms containing some 60–70 amino acids are neurotoxins of quite appalling toxicity (LD_{50} less than 0.1 μg/g in the mouse). The antiviral agent Ara-A (**23**) developed from the sponge product spongoihymidine (**24**) was first approved for clinical use in herpes infections of the eye some 35 years after the sponge was first collected. An insight into the range of structures produced by marine organisms and identified in a one-year period is given by Faulkner.[10]

This brief overview illustrates the debt medicinal chemistry owes to the natural world when clearly many molecules of both clinical and chemical interest have been derived from natural sources; predictably, many more will be in future. Automated assay procedures are sensitive, selective modern chromatographic techniques are able to separate increasingly complex mixtures, and current spectroscopic methods can resolve the most complex of structures.

5.3   MACROMOLECULAR TARGETS FOR DRUG DESIGN

The phase "rational drug design" used in modern medicinal chemistry should not imply that all previous methods of drug design were irrational and unsuccessful. Whilst it is true that some drug discoveries have indeed been serendipitous, the vast majority have entailed the structured and creative use of the best scientific procedures of the period to elaborate the molecules from which the new medicines were developed.

Today, however, many more macromolecules with defined receptor targets of established structure are known for which it is possible to design potential ligands.

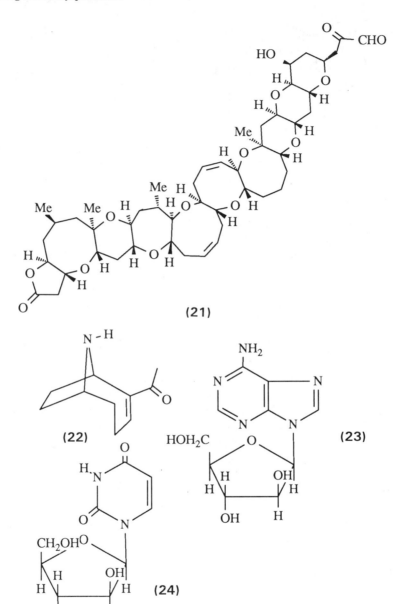

(21)

(22)   **(23)**

(24)

The modern procedures constituting today's rational drug design are described in the following sections.

5.3.1   Proteins as targets

Most drugs interact with proteins either via enzymes or proteinaceous receptors on membrane surfaces: nucleic acids and carbohydrates are secondary targets at least in numbers, if not in biological importance. This section will concentrate on the isolation and structure determination of proteins.

Proteins are so important to the structure and functioning of the living organism that considerable efforts have been made, and continue to be made, to establish their structures and to determine their chemical and biological properties. If a cell makes sufficient of a particular protein then it can be isolated by sophisticated chromatography, such as affinity chromatography. In this technique ligands which bind selectively to the protein of interest are chemically bound to the solid phase and thus preferentially separate the target protein from others of similar structures. The isolation of 100 mg of pure protein will enable it to be sequenced, to have some of its biological properties analysed, and for specific antibodies to it to be raised, thus enabling cellular distribution to be determined. As will be described later, nuclear magnetic resonance spectroscopy may be used to determine its partial structure, and, if the protein can be crystallised, X-ray crystallography will give its complete crystal structure.

5.3.1.1   Molecular biology and the production of proteins

However, these techniques can be used only when the cell produces enough protein, and this is, unfortunately, limited to a few proteins, notably haemoglobin, trypsin and the immunoglobulins. Many proteins of interest, including the receptors for neurotransmitters, are produced in only very small amounts in the living organism, and for these it is unlikely that any separation procedure will ever isolate sufficient material for detailed studies.

It is frequently necessary in these circumstances to enhance the production of the target protein, and this is where the potential of recombinant DNA technology comes into play[11,12]. Expressed very simply this technology involves isolating a gene or portion of DNA which codes for the protein under investigation, inserting this gene into the genome of a bacteria or yeast where it can be expressed, and growing the host on a sufficient scale to produce the required amount of protein product. Like many concepts relatively simple in theory, the practice is considerably more difficult than the outline.

A major problem resides in the fact that the gene for any protein does not exist as a separate entity in the living organism but as a segment of a very long DNA sequence. In fact in mammalian cells the situation is even more complex because the genes do not occur as discrete units but as fragments separated by stretches of non-coding DNA. Thus the identification of any required gene represents a major challenge for the technology.

The systemic cleavage of DNA molecules became reality only when a class of enzymes known as restriction nucleases was discovered in bacterial systems. It appears that such enzymes play a major role in protecting the bacterium from invasion by viruses, by cleaving the viral nucleic acid before it can be incorporated into that of the host. Restriction enzymes cleave DNA at specific sequences of four to eight nucleotides, and, as different bacteria produce different enzymes with different specifications, there are now available more than a hundred such enzymes. Many of these cleave double stranded DNA, leaving behind a stretch of single stranded DNA at the end of each cleaved fragment which can subsequently act as a template on which other strands of DNA may be attached. It is then possible to use these fragments of DNA to produce many copies, as described below. However, because much of the DNA does not code for meaningful proteins and because many genes are divided into subunits spread over a much greater region of DNA, this is normally a very inefficient process. Instead, it is better to use the knowledge that the cell's own mechanisms select out the genes when DNA is transcribed into messenger RNA (mRNA). If this material is isolated and then complementary DNA (cDNA) copies are made by incubating the mRNA with nucleotide bases in the presence of the enzyme reverse transcriptase, then fragments of DNA which correspond only to functioning genes are produced. In the first instance these are single-stranded DNA which are then converted to double-stranded molecules by another enzyme, DNA polymerase (Figure 5.2).

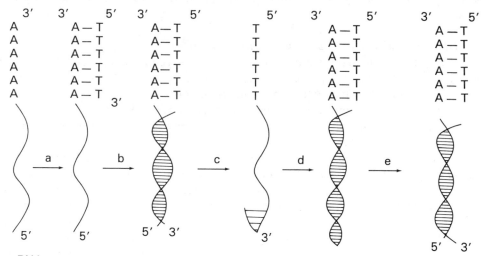

Fig. 5.2.   Generation of double stranded cDNA from mRNA. a. Anneal primer. b. Make DNA copy by the use of the enzyme reverse transcriptase. c. Treat with alkali to degrade RNA (note that the 3′ end of the cDNA forms hairpin loop). d. DNApolymerase uses the hairpin loop as a primer to synthesis complementary strand. e. The terminal loop is cleaved with the enzyme S1 nuclease to give a double stranded cDNA copy of the original mRNA.

The amount of DNA which can be isolated from a single cell is obviously limited, and thus an amplification process is consequently necessary. *In vivo* this is usually accomplished by expressing the appropriate DNA in either bacteria or yeasts after introducing the DNA into the organism by means of a vector such as a plasmid or virus. Plasmids are small circular double-stranded lengths of DNA which are found inside many bacteria in addition to their normal chromosomal DNA. In evolutionary terms, plasmids are possibly precursors of viruses before the latter obtained their outer proteinaceous coats, and they have survived in symbiotic relationship with their hosts by providing them with proteins essential to the well-being of the cell, particularly those conferring resistance to certain antibiotics and toxins. Plasmids are significantly smaller than chromosomal DNA and thus can be readily separated. Treatment of plasmids with restriction enzymes will cleave the strands, leaving single-strand fragments to which the fragment of cDNA can be annealed and covalently linked by means of the enzyme DNA ligase (Figure 5.3). Plasmid containing the insert can be reinserted into the bacterium which is then allowed to replicate. Each of the daughter cells will also contain replicated plasmid and, consequently, replicated DNA of interest. However, there will be many such plasmids of which only a few will contain the interesting DNA fragment, and the problem is to identify them. A screening technique which is often employed is to use a plasmid which also carries the gene for an antibiotic resistance and then to grow the bacterium in the presence of the appropriate antibiotic. This process ensures that only these bacteria carrying modified plasmids survive and these can be subsequently harvested and the plasmid isolated.

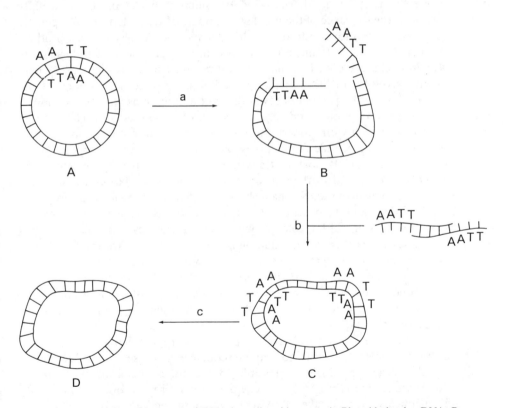

Fig. 5.3.   Fusion of fragment of DNA into plasmid vector. A. Plasmid circular DNA. B. Ring opened plasmid DNA. C. Fragment of required DNA joined in plasmid DNA by "sticky ends". D. Regenerated plasmid circular DNA containing new section of DNA. a. Clevage of circular DNA by restriction enzyme. b. Annealing of fragment of DNA produced by action of the same restriction nuclease on chromosomal DNA (use of same enzyme generates same sticky ends). c. Use of enzyme DNA ligase to produce new circular plasmid DNA.

The major problem still to be resolved is the detection of those plasmids carrying the DNA of interest. In very favourable cases the protein of interest may be a major product of the cell and the DNA fragment of interest is present in such abundance that it can be isolated. Alternatively, there may exist two very similar cell types producing very similar but not actually identical ranges of proteins. The first step in this case is to produce the total cDNA copies from the cell of interest and to hybridise these to the mRNA of the other cell. Since most of the protein products are identical, these cDNA will hybridise to the corresponding mRNA, but the unique cDNA will be left unbound as a single strand and can be readily separated. This technique has been successfully applied to the isolation of cDNA from T and B lymphocytes.

When sufficient protein of interest has previously been isolated to enable a monoclonal antibody to be produced this can be used to isolate the polyribosome on which the protein is being synthesised. This process enables the target mRNA to be separated to a very much greater level of purity than is possible when all the mRNA in the cell is isolated. Alternatively, 100 micrograms of protein is usually sufficient to allow the sequence of the first few amino acids to be derived. The genetic code can then be read in reverse to derive the DNA sequence necessary to produce this amino acid structure, but, unfortunately, because the genetic code is degenerate and most amino acids are coded by more than one triplet of nucleotide bases, there is not a unique sequence of DNA. Thus the technique is to select a segment from the known structure of the protein of seven or eight amino acids with the minimum possible variations in oligonucleotide sequences. All of these sequences can then be made by processes which with modern automated equipment, are not difficult.

Each of these oligonucleotide fragments is radio-labelled by the incorporation of radioactive phosphorus (^{32}P) so that trace amounts can be readily detected, and these fragments can be used in the following way. Colonies of bacteria containing the plasmids into which the cDNA have been inserted are grown on appropriate media in a petri dish, and absorbent cloth or filter paper is pressed against the gel and removed, taking some of the colonies with them. Treatment with alkali releases the DNA and separates it into individual single strands which are treated with a solution of the radioactive synthesised oligonucleotides. If the bacterial colonies contained any of the gene for the particular protein it will be detected by hybridisation with the oligonucleotide which can be readily detected by auto radiography. The appropriate bacterial cell colonies are thus identified and then grown on a large scale. Separation of the plasmids and cleavage by the original nuclease will liberate the cDNA, and further purification will give the pure gene (Figure 5.4).

A pure strand of DNA thus obtained can be sequenced and used to produce larger qualities of the target protein. It is possible to use either chemical or enzymatic methods to sequence the DNA.[13,14] The chemical method relies on the availability of specific chemicals which cleave DNA to leave chains ending in one of the four bases, adenosine, guanosine, cytidine, and thymidine. Thus if a strand of DNA is treated with the first of these it will be cleaved into a number of chains each of which has adenosine at its 3′ end and the number of chains will depend on how many times the base appears in the DNA.

The first step of the sequencing process is to label the 5′ end of the DNA chain

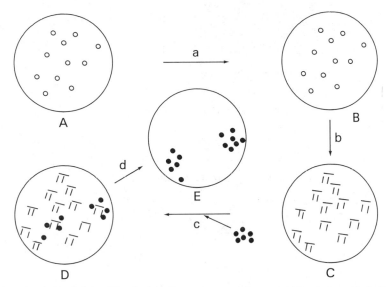

Fig. 5.4.   A. Petri dish with colonies of bacteria containing recombinant plasmids. B. Paper containing replicated bacteria. C. DNA bound to paper. D. Paper with colonies containing plasmids of interest now labelled with DNA probe. E. Position of desired plasmids now detected by autoradiography. a. Replication of colonies onto paper. b. Bacteria lysed and DNA denatured. c. Incubate with labelled DNA probe. d. Expose to photographic paper.

with a ^{32}P using the enzyme polynucleotide kinase and ^{32}P labelled ATP. Of course in a double helix strand of DNA both chains will be labelled, but subsequent cleavage with a nuclease will give a segment labelled solely in one chain. The double helix is then denatured by heating to give single stranded material, and this is separated into four equal batches. Each of the batches is treated with one, and only one, of the cleaving agents with the result that each batch will consist of a large number of chains of varying lengths each terminating at the 3′ end in a specific nucleotide each being radioactive by virtue of the ^{32}P carried on the 5′ end. Samples of each of the batches are then applied to the same gel and subjected to electrophoresis, and it is a simple matter to count sequential chain lengths and then deduce the whole structure of the DNA (Figure 5.5).

The alternative enzymatic method necessitates taking a single strand length of DNA to be sequenced, adding a labelled primer, and then growing the new chain with a supply of all four normal deoxyribonucleoside triphosphate precursors in the presence of DNA polymerase. Normally this would rapidly produce a complementary DNA chain. If, however, amongst the triphosphate precursors are added analogues lacking the 3′-OH group (dideoxyribonucleosides), whenever these are incorporated into the growing chain they will block its growth. The reaction is run in four separate batches, adding different dideoxy analogues when each batch will give a collection of chains terminating in each of the positions that this particular base appears in the DNA parent. Separation by gel electrophoresis readily allows the structure to be determined (Figure 5.6).

Experimentally it is usually easier to sequence the DNA than the protein, and, of

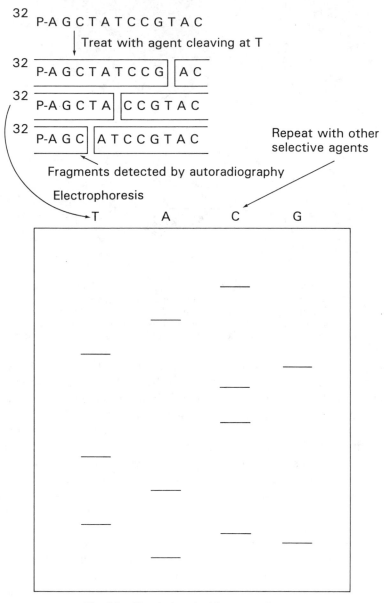

Fig. 5.5.   Chemical method for sequencing DNA.

course, the protein structure is readily derived from that of DNA. The reader is referred to the work of Dixon[15] on the mammalian β-adrenergic receptor which was previously mentioned to see the potential of this technology.

When the pure cDNA is now eventually available it may be used to produce quantities of the target protein. This is usually done by inserting the DNA into a bacterium or a yeast, incorporated into a plasmid or virus. In such circumstances

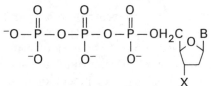

B = adenine, guanine, cytosine, thymine
X = OH; H (dideoxynucleotide)

4 separate pots each containing a mixture of all nucleosides and a limited quantity of a single dideoxynucleotide are treated with a single-strand DNA to be sequenced, a fluorescently labelled probe (different colour for each pot) and DNA polymerase. DNA chain growth continues until dideoxynucleotide is incorporated.

single-stranded DNA
to be sequenced   ⬜ T G A C G A A T A T G G C T A

primer with
fluorescent probe   ⬜ A C T G C T T A (X = H)
                                growing chain terminated by
                                incorporation of dideoxynucleotide

Each pot now contains a mixture of different lengths of DNA all terminating in the same dideoxynucleotide. The combined contents of all pots are separated by weight using gel electrophoresis. The colour of the fluorescence identifies each base and thus allows the sequence to be read and readily converted to that of the original DNA

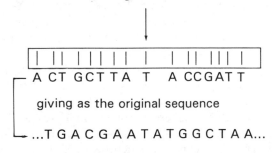

A CT GCT TA T A CCGAT T

giving as the original sequence

...T G A C G A A T A T G G C T A A...

Fig. 5.6.   Enzymatic method of determining DNA sequence.

the cDNA is usually closely associated with another length of DNA which acts as a promoter of gene expression so that the cell produces large quantities of the desired protein. The selection of the optimum conditions for the production of any particular protein is complex, but an increasing number of important proteins such as insulin, interleukin 2, and interferon-γ are being produced on an industrial scale.

It is also possible to reproduce stretches of DNA *in vitro* by means of the polymerase chain reaction (PCR, Figure 5.7),[16] an idea of elegant simplicity. The technique requires that small sections of DNA around the segment of DNA of interest are characterised such that oligonucleotide precursors can be synthesised corresponding to these sections. The length of double-stranded DNA is first heated to separate the two strands and then the two primers are annealed, one each to each chain and each capable of growing only from the 5' to the 3' ends. DNA polymerase and a supply of nucleotide triphosphates are added, and the chains grown across the region of interest, the reaction is stopped, the chain separated (again by heat), more primer added, and the chain elongation process repeated. The DNA in the media will now consist of the two original chains, four chains where length depends on how long the polymerisation process lasted and two identical chains ending in the primers and covering the region of interest. Repeating the cycle very rapidly builds up the short chain DNA covering the region of interest as this doubles with each cycle. Twenty to thirty cycles, which can be conducted automatically, usually gives the desired degree of amplification (Figure 5.7).

This has been a brief overview of a complicated and rapidly evolving subject, but it is hoped that it gives the reader the essence of the topic and its importance in advancing knowledge of many of the crucial structures of the living organisms.

5.3.1.2   Determination of protein structure

Having isolated a protein and established its total amino acid sequence either by the DNA techniques described previously or by classical means, the next challenge is the definition of secondary and tertiary structures. These may be determined by use of X-ray crystallography, nmr spectroscopy and theoretical calculations.

5.3.1.2.1   X-ray crystallography

Von Laue and W. L. Bragg showed in the early years of this century how the structures of crystals could be determined from the diffractions of X-rays. Subsequently, the technique has been applied to molecules of steadily increasing complexity.[17] Vast advances in the development of equipment, particularly computers, and in techniques have resulted in the availability of modern instruments which can generate the structures of simple molecules in a few hours, provided of course that suitable crystals can be prepared. The Cambridge Crystallographic Database now contains the structures of many thousands of molecules which have been determined by X-ray crystallography, and this database is an essential resource for scientists seeking information on precise bond lengths, angles and interatomic distances.

X-ray crystallography of complex structures such as proteins remains a challenge, but in the late 1950s Kendrew and Perutz reported the structures of sperm whale myoglobin and haemoglobin respectively, and, subsequently, the structures of several hundred proteins have been recorded and deposited in the Brookhaven Database. This database also serves as a very valuable source of information for drug design, providing defined targets for producing new compounds. Nonetheless the crystallisation of proteins remains a formidable challenge although a number of types

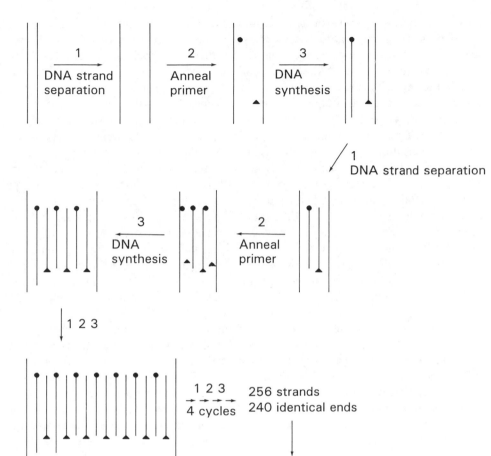

Fig. 5.7.   The polymerase chain reaction (PCR).

of automatic apparatus have been described to achieve this, and the interpretation of the diffraction patterns is not a trivial task. Many excellent textbooks are available[17] to describe this technique, and over the last decade remarkable new advances have emerged which offer the promise of a greatly expanded usefulness.

The increased power of X-ray crystallography in recent years results from the use of synchrotron radiation which is produced when charged particles are accelerated at relativistic velocities and are constrained to a curved trajectory by an external magnetic field. Typically, electrons are injected from a linear accelerator into a booster synchrotron and subsequently into a storage ring where they are kept at a fixed energy by constant magnetic fields for many hours. Power lost through radiation is replenished by radio frequency power generated by a klystron. The radiation produced is intense, tuneable, polarised and grouped into small bunches a few millimetres in length in bursts some 10 to 500 picoseconds long.[18] Compared with normal laboratory X-ray sources, the intensity is 10^4–10^6 times greater and the wavelengths range from hard X-rays to microwaves. Of course, this is not laboratory scale equipment, and today only some nine centres for synchrotron radiation exist around the world, although more are being planned.

It is the intensity and the polychromatic nature of synchrotron radiation which gives it the great advantage over conventional, less powerful monochromatic laboratory X-ray sources. Its intensity means that much smaller crystals are required for analysis, a great advantage since growing protein crystals is often the most difficult and time consuming part of the investigation. Secondly the polychromatic character of synchrotron radiation lends itself to a technique known as Laue diffraction.[19,20] This was in fact the method first used in 1912 to record an X-ray diffraction image from a crystal of copper sulphate but was subsequently abandoned owing to the difficulty in analysing the poor diffraction images which were produced. The very intense white radiation produced by synchrotrons results in a large number of lattice planes diffracting simultaneously as the Bragg condition ($\lambda = 2d \sin \phi$, where ϕ is the angle of incident beam, d is the interplanar distance and λ is the wavelength of the incident X-ray beam) is satisfied for each plane by at least one wavelength. Thus, in favourable circumstances, one single exposure is able to give the complete data set.

The contrast with conventional monochromatic X-ray diffraction is remarkable as in the latter situation only a small proportion of the lattice planes diffract at any particular orientation of the crystal and the crystal has to be rocked through 1–2° to record the full reflection. The crystal then has to be rotated to a new setting to bring other planes into the diffracting position, and the procedure is repeated with a new recording film. Such procedures not only take a great deal of researcher's time but expose the crystal to radiation for so long that radiation induced damage to the structure is a distinct possibility. Additionally, the detection of short-lived species is not feasible.

On the other hand, Laue spectroscopy is so much more rapid that not only is radiation induced damage minimal but also it holds the prospect of detecting transient species, such as substrates bound to the active site of an enzyme. It can be readily appreciated how much such structures can add to our knowledge of enzymatic reaction mechanisms. Thus the first reported use of Laue spectroscopy on a protein[20] analysed the enzyme glycogen phosphorylase b before, during, and after infusion with a solution of the oligosaccharide ligand, maltoheptose. Very high quality software and experimental technique are necessary to handle the derived information, but difference structures between those of the enzyme with and without the substrate do give good information on the binding of the substrate. Such "time resolved" X-ray crystallographic studies have been expanded to other systems including the oncogene product Ha-Ras p21 which complexes with guanosine triphosphate (GTP)[21] and hydrolyses it to guanosine diphosphate (GDP). It is possible to prepare p21 complexed with GTP which is protected from hydrolysis by a photolabile group. Photolysis releases GTP thus initiating hydrolysis, and details of the process can be seen in the generated diffraction patterns.

Laue spectroscopy has also been used to solve very complete structures, such as that of the animal virus, human rhino virus 14.[22] An excellent review of the work of the Oxford group of Johnson has been published[23] providing further insight into the potential of the method.

The third application of synchrotron radiation[24] uses the continuously intense spectral output to determine crystal structures directly from measurements of anomalous diffraction made at multiple wavelengths (multiwavelength anomalous diffraction, MAD). The central problem in crystal structure analysis is the determination of the phase of the diffracted waves, and for macromolecules this has usually been achieved by the method of isomorphous replacement with heavy atoms, where the positions of the heavy atoms are derived from differences in diffraction intensities from the derivative and native crystals. The MAD technique essentially uses the principles of physics, in the form of the resonant absorption of X-rays which is produced when the frequency of the incident radiation approaches the frequency of oscillation in a bound electronic orbital, rather than chemistry to generate *in situ* isomorphous replacements.

All these techniques are in the early stages of development but will clearly provide greater insights into protein structures in the future.

5.3.1.2.2   Nuclear magnetic resonance (nmr) spectroscopy
The drawbacks of using X-ray crystallography to determine the tertiary structures of proteins are: that the protein must first be crystallised, which is often a nontrivial problem; that the determined structure will be that for the crystal but not necessarily for the biological environment of the protein, and that it is difficult to examine the interaction of the protein with its ligands. In contrast, nmr studies do not require the availability of crystalline materials and may be carried out in aqueous solutions which may better approximate to the natural environment of the protein under investigation. In addition, nmr may now be used to determine the conformations of ligands whilst bound to their biological receptors.

Proteins are complex structures containing large numbers of protons, many of which will be in very similar magnetic environments, which leads to complex overlapping peaks in their spectra severely limiting the amount of information which can be obtained from a proton spectrum. Protein structure determination has become a reality only with three recent advances in technique, namely the introduction of very high field (>400 MHz) spectrometers, the development of computer controlled pulse sequence techniques giving 2D, 3D and 4D spectra which can resolve overlapping signals, and the writing of iterative computer programs which use all generated data to produce the structures.[25, 26, 27]

It is not the intention here to give a detailed account of these techniques, for which the reader is referred to any of the specialist texts now available, but to try to outline the way in which nmr has been used to generate structures of ever increasing complexity.

By the use of coupling constants nmr can, in general, detect protons coupled to one another via covalent bonds and, from nuclear overhauser effects (NOEs), can detect protons which are in close proximity but are not directly bonded. Such information covers only short distances amounting, in the case of bonded atoms, to three bonds, whilst NOEs are proportional to the inverse of the sixth power of the distance between the atoms. Whilst this information allows a maximum interatomic separation of 5 Å it is highly accurate and well able to determine such separations within an accuracy of 0.2 Å.

It has only become possible to contemplate the use of nmr spectroscopy to determine protein structures since 2D techniques were introduced. Normal Fourier transform nmr spectra necessitate exciting all nuclei of the sample simultaneously with a strong radio frequency pulse, resulting in free induction decays which can be collected at given time intervals. Fourier transform analysis of the overlapping decays provides the usual spectra. In the 2D spectroscopy techniques two pulses and two time intervals are used, with the time between the pulses being regularly increased, and two successive Fourier transforms are thus required to produce the 2D spectrum, which is usually displayed as a frequency–frequency contour map. The two most commonly used techniques have the acronyms COSY and NOESY with the former detecting these protons directly coupled to one another whilst the latter detects those atoms close enough to show nuclear overhauser effects. In both techniques the resulting spectrum has the appearance of that shown in the highly simplified form in Figure 5.8. All such spectra consist of two types of peaks, typically A, B and C, where F_1 is equal to F_2 resulting in peaks lying along the diagonal and cross peaks represented here by D and D'. The existence of the cross peaks shows that, in this example, A and C but not B are interacting. In a COSY spectrum A and C will be coupled, whilst in a NOESY spectrum they will be within the distance over which NOE effects operate.

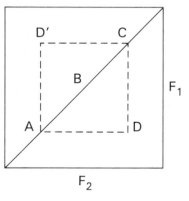

Fig. 5.8.

Protein structure determination using 2D nmr spectroscopy uses what is known as the sequential resonance assignment technique[25] which requires the use of COSY spectra to identify strongly coupled proteins, namely those on the same amino acids, and NOESY spectra to identify adjacent residues. Since NOE give accurate interatomic distances these can be used to generate the three-dimensional structure of proteins.[28] This can now be achieved with the aid of the third development, the use of interactive molecular dynamics programs which use the normal range of bonding and nonbonding forces, but also include energy terms from the NOE distances. Proteins, however, are dynamic structures in solution, and the result of these calculations will be a range of structures differing slightly in energy. By using computer graphics these different states may be portrayed in different colours, giving a very good representation behaviour of the protein. 2D spectroscopy has been used to determine the structure of complement factor (C5a), a 74 amino acid protein of molecular weight 8000, which is critically involved in a number of inflammatory processes. The upper limit of structures which can be solved by this method, however, appears to be of the order of 100 amino acid residues. Two reasons account for this. Firstly, such a large number of protons means that the cross peaks merge with one another and cannot be resolved, and, secondly, the line widths of the peaks become greater than the couplings because of the increasing rotational time of these large molecules.

The solution to these problems has been to stretch the technique into 3D and 4D spectra. If one imagines all the information in a multivolume work process being condensed into one line it is obviously unintelligible, which is equivalent to the "normal" proton spectrum of a large protein. Expanding this information over a single page (2D spectrum) still results in massive overlap, whilst further expansion to a book (3D) and ultimately to several books (4D) allows all information to be readily available.[29]

Such futuristic techniques entail modifying the pulse sequences into two linked 2D pulses (3D) and three pulses (4D), leaving out the detection phase of the first process and the preparation pulse of the second. The selection of appropriate pulses and the actual 2D experiments to be combined are not trivial exercises, and the interpretation of the results is also difficult. Homonuclear 3D spectra are inevitably more complicated to interpret than the analogous 2D spectra. However, heteronuclear 3D and 4D spectra in which the protein is enriched in ^{13}C or ^{15}N provide massive increases in information. The preparation of such labelled materials is relatively easy, at least for proteins expressed in bacteria, since the bacteria can be grown in a mixture suitably enriched in $[^{13}C_6]$ glucose and/or $^{15}NH_4Cl$. This technique conveniently uses the large heteronuclear couplings to further spread out and resolve peaks which overlap in a 2D spectrum. Its potential value is demonstrated by a recent report of the determination of the structure of the 153 amino acid, 17.4 kDa protein, interleukin $1\beta^{30}$, to which the reader is referred for further details. This structure appears, at the time of writing, to be that of the largest protein whose structure has been determined by nmr spectroscopy. There is little doubt that the technique will be applied to much larger proteins in the future. The precision of the resulting structure, the fact that it is determined in solution, and the avoidance of the technically complex, tedious and time consuming task of protein crystallisation, make this a highly valuable method of structural determination.

The techniques described above have also been used to determine the conformation of ligands directly bonded to their receptors. As will be discussed in the later section on drug design, the ultimate goal of drug research is to design, de novo, molecules from the structure of the receptor. In the meantime the practice of designing drugs from the conformation adopted by a molecule in interacting with its receptor remains the best approach available. Until now the active conformation of a target molecule has had to be implied from its uncomplexed, unbound structure in solution, or from theoretical calculations. Clearly, if the exact conformation adopted by an active molecule on binding to its receptor were known, the model on which subsequent drug design could be based would be that much better. Modern nmr techniques offer the possibility of achieving this, with the actual approach used depending on the strength of the ligand binding in the process being investigated.

For weakly bound ligands that are exchanging rapidly the transferred NOE due to these interactions can be measured. Negative NOEs resulting from the bound state are observed on the free, or averaged, signals of the ligand and these are narrower than those due to the receptor and, consequently, readily distinguished. Such measurements then allow the conformation of the ligand to be determined and provide the basis for drug analogue modelling.

For more strongly bound ligands where transferred NOEs are not applicable, another approach is to use the detection of protons attached to isotopically labelled nuclei. Thus, for instance, a ligand can be labelled with either or both ^{13}C and ^{15}N. Such an isotope-edited spectrum only detects signals due to the ligand and not to the macromolecular receptor. 2D spectroscopy in this isotope-edited mode is also possible, and the resultant NOE can be used both to determine the conformation of the ligand and interaction with the receptor. A quite remarkable example of the power of this technique is provided by the study of the immune suppressant cyclosporin (12), which is known to actively bind to an intracellular 17 kDa, 165 amino acid protein, cyclophilin. The structure of cyclosporin in both the crystal and in solution has been well established, having a *cis* 9,10 peptide bond. However, when cyclosporin was synthesised with the 9,10 methyl leucine residues labelled with ^{13}C and the ^{13}C-edited and two-dimensional NOE spectrum of cyclosporin bound to cyclophilin measured, it was shown that binding to the macromolecule causes rotation of this bond to give the 9,10 *trans* amide bond. As might be appreciated, this results in a very significant change in the complete conformation of the backbone ring of cyclosporin, and questions, at least in this case, any drug design study based on the solution structure (Figure 5.9).[31]

These findings were further supported by studies of the binding of uniformly labelled 13C cyclosporin to cyclophilin using heteronuclear 3D NOE experiments, which not only established the total conformation of cyclosporin, but also identified the binding regions of the cyclophilin. Clearly this is a powerful technique whose usefulness is only just becoming apparent; as more receptors are cloned, and become available in significant numbers, many such investigations will give the medicinal chemist precise, physically based evidence concerning the active conformations of biologically interesting molecules.

5.3.1.2.3   *The prediction of secondary and tertiary structures of proteins from their amino acid sequences*

Determination of the amino acid sequences of proteins is now much less technically complex than the determination of the ultimate secondary and tertiary structures. Consequently the number of known primary sequences may be measured in the thousands, whilst 3D structures are exemplified only in the hundreds.[32] The attraction

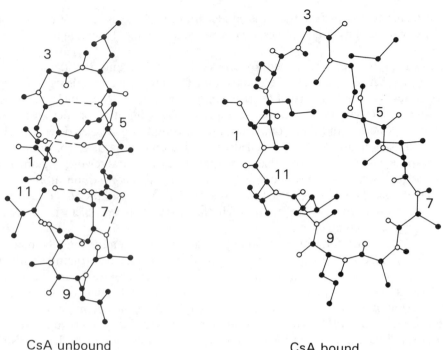

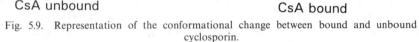

Fig. 5.9. Representation of the conformational change between bound and unbound cyclosporin.

of being able to determine a primary sequence and calculate its secondary and tertiary structures according to a set of rules is therefore obvious. Unfortunately, the fundamental problem in protein folding, namely the ability to accurately and reliably predict the three-dimensional structure of a collection of amino acids, remains unsolved. Nevertheless considerable progress has been made towards this goal.

The most successful approach to date is that of homology modelling, namely relating the span of a new protein to a similar span in another protein whose structure is known. This approach requires computer programs[33] which can rapidly search databases and relate segments of the new protein to any search where structures have already been described. This homology will rarely be exact, so these programs also quantify the degree of similarity. Such a procedure will usually identify highly defined secondary structures, notably α-helices, β-sheets, or strands. That these factors are seen so regularly in large numbers of proteins of differing primary sequences shows how tolerant proteins are to amino acid changes underpinning the assumption that homology modelling can be used when sequence agreements are less than perfect.

When marked secondary characteristics have been identified the problem then remains to model the linking regions between them which are usually loop regions and typically the most variable sections of any protein. Blundell[34] has elucidated an approach which entails first identifying the loop length, selecting a conformer from the literature on the basis of the sequence and finally testing the conformer by least-square fitting to the β-strands of the model framework. This is an area in which computer calculations and graphics are essential in arriving at meaningful structural determinations.[34]

As more structures are solved by physical methods, and the data bank of relationships between primary, secondary and tertiary structures also grows, then the accuracy and applicability of these techniques will grow. Nevertheless it is now possible to appreciate the power of the approach by using it to predict an already established structure and then comparing the measured and predicted results. Thus porcine phospholipase A_2 was modelled on bovine and rattlesnake enzymes which have respectively 87% and 47% sequence identities in a framework region of 88 amino acids.[35] The root mean square deviation for all the α-carbon atoms in the main chain was 1.46 Å which fell to a value of 0.63 Å if residues 56–66 in a loop region were excluded, and the authors felt that part of this problem lay in X-ray error or crystal packing effects.

For those proteins for which no homology is evident, attempts must be made to predict the three-dimensional structure. The prediction of tertiary structures with any degree of accuracy is, currently, impossible owing to limitations in the energy calculations needed in predictions. Such calculations are dependent on both the parameterisation of the force fields and the complexity of the energy minima which are not well sampled in the available computer times. It is likely, however, that these problems will be overcome with increasing access to supercomputers. It is possible, however, to predict secondary structures with greater confidence. The methods used depend on the generation of computer algorithms many of which are based on the assumption that short similar sequences of amino acids have similar secondary structures.[36] However, the methods will fail if a significant amount of local secondary structure is controlled by the tertiary structure imposed by the whole protein.

Despite these problems it is possible to build up the structure of a protein from the combination of identifiable sections. Nevertheless, the goal of total prediction of protein structure has still to be achieved, and, until then, physical methods of structure determination will be crucial to the further understanding of protein function.

5.3.2   DNA as a macromolecular target

The other major macromolecular receptor important for drug action is, of course, DNA. This is the site of action of numerous carcinogens, anticancer agents and antibacterials but, to date, has not been the subject of a large amount of targeted research. Progress and opportunities in the area have recently been well reviewed by Hurley.[37]

It should be noted that DNA is a somewhat different type of target from the proteins which have just been discussed, since structural variations are restricted to arrangements of the four basic nucleotides and so are more limited. Mammalian DNA is associated with strongly bound proteins (histones) and so may only become susceptible to binding during active transcription processes. Furthermore, the cell possesses many repair mechanisms which can overcome the effects of any drug much more rapidly than is possible with proteins. It should not be forgotten that the cell possesses mitochondrial DNA in addition to the nuclear material, which is much less protected by membranes, proteins and by repair mechanisms, and so may preferentially interact with an exogenous agent.

Before significant progress can be made in this area, four major concerns remain to be addressed. Firstly, a clearer understanding of the mechanisms of action for those agents which are already known to interact with DNA is required and, secondly, strategies are required to improve the selectivity of such agents. Thirdly, better mechanism-based assays for measurement of DNA interference are needed, and related mechanisms, e.g. enzyme inhibitors and histone displacement, which could lead to DNA inhibition, need to be investigated.

Compounds acting on DNA have been differentiated into four major classes, notably alkylating agents, e.g. cisplatin (**25**) and mitomycin (**26**), DNA strand breaking agents such as bleomycin (**27**), intercalating compounds such as actinomycin D (**28**) and a group which includes CC-1065 (**29**) which bind to the minor groove of DNA.

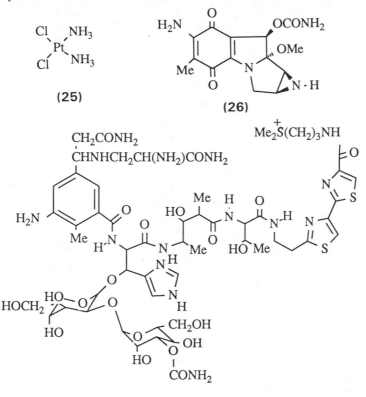

Some very important drugs are included in the first three categories of compounds, but, to date, the clinical utility of the last series has not been defined.

Despite the large number of compounds available which do interact with DNA it has proved to be an enormously difficult task to identify the crucial biologically important interaction. This is partly because of the complexity of the human genome and partly because most agents are not selective. However, the use of oligonucleotides

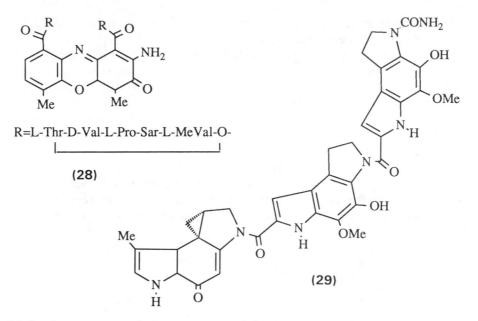

R=L-Thr-D-Val-L-Pro-Sar-L-MeVal-O-

(28)

(29)

of defined structure, restriction enzymes to define breaks, and plasmids for appropriate *in vivo* experiments is slowly providing more information. It has been found, for instance, that bleomycin cleaves preferentially in regions of DNA that are actively transcribed following glucocorticoid induction.

It has been known for a considerable time that relatively flat heterocycles intercalate into DNA, and X-ray structural analysis has confirmed the same phenomenon for actinomcycin D (**28**). Existing structure–activity relationships do not strongly support this mechanism as the cause of the cytotoxicity of molecules and their antitumour activity indicating that other effects are operative.

As has been continually stressed in this book, the essential determinent of any agent is its mechanistic selectivity, and this also applies to all molecules acting on DNA. Such selectivity in DNA is, however, likely to be achieved by relatively lengthy stretches of base pairs. The human genome, for example, is so long that nominal target sites of 10, 11, or 12 base pairs could occur on average 2080, 1024, and 528 times whilst sites of 15 or 16 pairs may occur only once.[38] That highly ordered, selective and strong binding is possible is exemplified by the histones which bind into the major groove of the DNA helix. To date, no drugs have been identified to act in this area, but a number of anti tumour agents, e.g. CC-1065, do bind to the minor groove. Since the minor groove is "information-poor" compared with the major one, results from compounds like this give an indication as to what might be achieved by targeting the richer areas.

A third necessity for constructive drug design in this area is the availability of appropriate *in vitro* models. Most of the known agents were discovered by their effects in cytotoxic screens involving the L-1210 leukaemia cell line. Whilst this has been very successful in identifying interesting compounds, to date these have shown little *in vivo* selectivity. Recent progress has widened the choice of screens to include a great many more cell lines derived from human tumours, but no clear progress has been demonstrated so far. Other screens developed include the ability to induce DNA repair mechanisms in the expression of B-galactosidase by a lambda promoter fused to a lac Z gene in *E. coli*; the detection of DNA breaks in covalently closed circular DNA by gel electrophoresis and the effects of candidates on the growth of yeast mutants. Together these new tests represent a very substantial array of methods for detecting agents which could interfere with the functioning of DNA by a number of mechanisms. The future development of the field necessitates a better understanding of the complex interrelationships between DNA, histones and enzymes, and the interference with such interactions will provide another array of potential targets.

It must be concluded that these are very early days in the design of drugs acting on DNA, but with increased knowledge of the functioning of DNA, its related proteins, and the availability of suitable screens, this will become a successful area of research.

5.3.2.1 *"Anti-sense" oligonucleotides*

One aspect of drug design involving DNA which has evolved recently is that of "anti-sense" oligonucleotides, which owes more to molecular biology rather than medicinal chemistry and so will only be discussed briefly here.

It is becoming increasingly clear that many illnesses arise because of inappropriate signalling from malfunctioning genes, and a possible therapy could be gene insertion, namely adding a normal healthy gene to the system in order that correct gene products are subsequently produced. Another possibility is to block the functioning of the malign gene by combination with an "antisense" oligonucleotide, in which case the concept is extremely simple. A section of DNA or mRNA encoding for a disease-causing protein is identified and the appropriate complementary DNA sequence is designed which will bind to the sequence and consequently inactivate it. As was noted above, a 15 or 16 base pair segment of DNA is probably unique, the complementary binding to it will be extremely strong, and thus the antisense molecule will be highly specific. The base pairs of such a molecule are, of course, dictated by the sequences in the target gene, but considerable variation in the phosphate, sugar bridge is possible to increase the stability of the agent to enzymatic attack or to increase its penetration into the cell.

To date most reported studies in this area have concentrated on anticancer and antiviral compounds. In certain types of Burkitt's lymphomas specific translocations involving the c-myc oncogene are seen, and the effect of these translocations is to create abnormal RNAs in which noncoding intron sequences which are normally spliced out from pre-mRNA persist in the mature mRNA. Agents targeted to these sequences have shown selective inhibition of cell growth and reduced c-myc protein production. Antisense DNA oligonucleotides have also been devised to selectively inhibit the production of HIV-encoded p15 and p24 proteins in cells infected with the AIDS virus. Reference 39 provides an interesting account of the problems and potential of the technique which certainly has enormous promise.

Assuming that the three-dimensional structure of a target protein has now been determined, the key question is how to design drugs to fit the active site. The following section will be concerned with the computational methods which are increasingly being developed and applied to this problem.

5.4   COMPUTATIONAL CHEMISTRY

Most organic chemists have little intuitive feel for theoretical chemistry and thus have good reason to be grateful for introductory texts such as that of Richards.[40,41] There are three major techniques which have been applied to molecular pharmacology, quantum mechanics, molecular mechanics, and molecular dynamics. Of these, the most fundamental is quantum mechanics, but its complexity is such that, even with approximations, it can be applied only to relatively small molecules.

5.4.1   Quantum mechanics[42]
The basis of quantum mechanics is the Schroedinger equation (equation (1)).

$$H\Psi = E\Psi \tag{1}$$

where H is a mathematical operator
Ψ is a wave function
and E is the energy of the system.

Solving this equation exactly for the hydrogen atom gives the familiar series of electronic orbitals, and similar solutions can be obtained for all atoms if it is assumed that each electron can be treated individually with its own orbital. Life becomes much more complicated when molecules are examined, and the Schroedinger equation can be solved exactly only for the hydrogen molecule ion. The first approximation to be used is that of Born and Oppenheimer, which recognises the great difference in mass between the nuclei and the electrons and treats the Schroedinger equation as being a product of a function due to the electrons and another due to the nuclei. Solution of the electronic equation for a fixed geometry gives the electron distribution for that configuration. Then energy gradient optimisation procedures which allow the nuclei to be moved can be added, thus giving, at the expense of much computing time, optimal geometries.

However, solving the electronic equation itself requires approximations and compromises, the nature and extent of which will affect the reliability of the derived solution.

The commonest procedure used is the Hartree–Fock self-consistent field (SCF) method in which each electron is treated independently and each is assumed to move in the average field of all the other electrons. The spatial distribution of a single electron is described by a set of atomic orbitals and the total energy of the system is minimised by the iterative solution of the Schroedinger equation until the electron distribution, or total internal energy, converges to a predetermined level of variation between cycles. The main problem here is the very large number of one and two electron integrals which must be evaluated and stored, and much effort has been extended to find ways of reducing the computer power needed to solve such equations.

From these studies two main, and qualitatively different, approaches have emerged, *ab initio* and *semi-empirical*, differing essentially in whether all electrons are involved (*ab initio*) or only the valence electrons (*semi-empirical*). Both types of approach are greatly affected by the factor that is used to describe the electronic spatial distribution. This is usually done by assuming that the electron exists in a molecular orbital (MO) comprising a linear combination of atomic orbitals (LCAO) based on each nucleus. The actual shapes of atomic orbitals were devised by Slater and are known as Slater-type orbitals (STOs) and the task is then to calculate all the molecular integrals of these orbitals.

This is a mammoth task since there are two sets of integrals. Overlap integrals record the amount of overlap between two separate orbitals, and coulombic integrals monitor the interaction between the differently charged entities in the molecule. This comprises four separate terms: repulsive nuclear–nuclear energies, attractive nuclear–electronic forces, repulsive electron–electron interactions, and the exchange integral resulting from the fact that the latter force is further modified by the spins of the two electrons. A few moments, thought will convince the reader that in any molecule all these interactions will add up to a potentially formidable sum of calculations. Nevertheless, *ab initio* calculations using no assumptions can be conducted on sufficiently powerful computers for molecules with up to 40 atoms. The program Gaussian 80 obtainable from the Quantum Chemical Programme Exchange enables such calculations to be performed.

For circumstances where the molecule of interest is larger, or the computer power available insufficient, recourse must be made to semi-empirical methods, which include directly only the valency electrons. Further, some of the complicating integrals are neglected and others approximated by parameters gained from experiment. The types of semi-empirical methods differ in the way in which they handle these approximations, and the choice between them depends on the nature and size of the system under investigation, the properties to be described, the reliability of a particular technique for these properties, and the type and amount of computer time available.

The simplest, Huckel approach considers π electrons only, ignores overlap altogether, and generalises coulombic integrals to nearest neighbours only. This technique and the more refined iterative extended Huckel method (IEHT) have been used to calculate atomic charges, spin densities, dipole and higher moments, polarisabilities, electron field gradients, magnetic moments, and magnetic field energies, but they are not appropriate if the geometry is not known or total molecular energies are required.

More complicated, and of more value to graphics and computer calculations, are methods which use the general zero differential overlap (ZDO) methods of approximation. This is the simplest all-valence electron method which includes electron repulsion integrals, and is capable of giving total state energies with optimised geometry. Variations of this approach include the complete neglect of differential overlap (CNDO) which applies empirical values to most of the integrals and ignores many electron repulsions, intermediate neglect of differential overlap (INDO), modified INDO (MINDO), and modified neglect of differential overlap (MNDO). Of these, MNDO contains the fewest approximations and, in the right circumstances, is capable of giving answers very similar to those from *ab initio* calculations using only 10% of the computer time. It can predict bond angles, the stabilities of double and triple bonds, and can handle lone pair repulsions. Overall MNDO is the best semi-empirical quantum mechanical method for large organic molecules containing only atoms from the first, second and third rows of the periodic table. A modified version of MNDO, MOPAC, is available from the Quantum Chemical Programme Exchange (QCPE) and readily integrates to commercial graphics programs, as will be discussed later.

Another semi-empirical method differs from those above by considering bonding orbitals to be mainly localised to given bonds rather than delocalised over the whole molecule. This is the perturbative configuration interaction using localised orbitals (PCILO) method which, as the name suggests, is a perturbative rather than an interactive method needing many fewer calculations. Because of this it can be used to calculate energy conformation profiles for large molecules such as proteins and nucleotides. It is thus suitable for use to survey a large number of conformations of flexible molecules to define possible energy minima before using MNDO or *ab initio* methods to refine the calculations.

Using the quantum mechanical programs which are now available, it is possible to calculate minimum energy conformations and the energy barriers to exchange between conformations, charge distributions, and molecular electrostatic potentials. The application of these findings to the study of biological systems is described in the references.

Despite the approximations and the increases in computer power, quantum mechanical methods are restricted to molecules of around 100 atoms. For larger systems molecular mechanical techniques are more appropriate.

5.4.2   Molecular mechanics[43]
Molecular mechanics assumes that the energy of molecules can be described by the sum of the energies of their various mechanical and electrical interactions. It calculates the potential energy of a system in terms of its nuclear coordinates and is very much less demanding of computer time than quantum mechanical methods. This has two major consequences for the drug designer since it can be applied to much larger molecules, including proteins, and energy calculations can be performed within the time frame of real-time computer modelling.

The method follows from the realisation that any change in a bond length from its predefined resting state will result in an increase in the energy of the system, and, further, that such an increase will follow some simple mechanical law. The difference of this approach is reflected in the information which must be supplied to complete a molecular mechanics study compared with that for a quantum mechanics calculation. The latter requires only the nuclear and net charge, quantum mechanical state multiplicity, and appropriate basis functions. Molecular mechanics, however, needs all the atoms classified into distinct types, the bonding topology to be specified, equilibrium values and force constants for all valency terms, nonbonded interaction parameters for all atoms, atomic partial charges, and bond dipoles. The outcome of a molecular mechanics calculation is a molecular mechanical force field which is a description of the potential energy surface of the molecule and which is unique to that molecule. However, this force field can, at a good approximation, be broken down into components which are transposable to other molecules. There are different ways of calculating the force field, and the result is a number of programs which are suited to specific types of molecules. Thus small molecules are best handled by the program MM2, originally developed for hydrocarbons but now expanded to a wider range of molecules, and AMBER and CHARMm™ for macromolecules.

A typical force field equation (e.g. equation (2)) has terms due to bond stretch, angle bending, torsions, van der Waals, interactions and coulombic interactions.

$$E_{total} = E_{bond} + E_{angle} + E_{torsion} + E_{vdW} + E_{coulomb} \qquad (2)$$

It is also possible to add items for hydrogen bonding, for out-of-plane distortion of sp^2 centres, and for changes in bond force constants as angles are deformed. Clearly one can treat small molecules in a much more elaborate manner than macromolecules.

Energy increases due to deviations from equilibrium bond length (E_{bond}) are given by equation (3) in which k is the stretch force constant and Δl is the difference between actual and equilibrium bond length.

$$E_{bond} = k/2 \, (\Delta l)^2 \qquad (3)$$

These are commonly around $300 \, kcal \, mol^{-1} \, A^{-2}$.

For distortions of bond angles, equation (4) is used where k is now the bending force constant and $\Delta\phi$ is the difference between actual and equilibrium bond angles. Energy increases due to these deviations are about $0.1 \, kcal \, mol^{-1} \, degree^{-2}$.

$$E_{angle} = k/2 \, (\Delta\phi)^2 \qquad (4)$$

The changes in energy due to rotation of torsion angles are given by (5) where V is the barrier to rotation and W is the torsion angle

$$E_{torsion} = V/2(1 + \cos W) \qquad (5)$$

The calculation of van der Waals' interaction energies is perhaps the most difficult in this approach. At close range the interaction potential between two nonbonded atoms is steeply repulsive, but at longer ranges the potential becomes attractive. One possible, and widely used, equation is due to Buckingham (6), where c and d are constants and r the interatomic distance.

$$E_{vdW} = ce^{d/r} - d/r^6 \qquad (6)$$

Finally, the coulombic energy is given by (7) where q is the partial charge, r the distance between the atoms, and D the dielectric constant.

$$E_{coulombic} = q_1 q_2 / D.r \qquad (7)$$

The choice of a value for D is extraordinarily difficult, especially in proteins where it is likely to vary with the precise structure of parts of the molecule.

To use equations (2–7), it is necessary to have access to databases from which the necessary coefficients for each atom in each environment can be obtained. Clearly a shortcoming of the method lies in these values, their origins and the appropriateness with which they may be applied to the problem in hand.

Nevertheless, experience shows that if you use a minimum of five energy contributions and a comprehensive set of generalised force fields, a reasonable three-dimensional structure can be predicted. To determine the structure of a low-energy conformation an initial conformation is subjected to a full geometry optimisation. All parameters defining the structure are modified slightly until the overall energy reaches a local minimum. A major problem arises from the difficulty experienced in determining whether or not this is the global minimum or merely a local one.

5.4.3   Molecular dynamics

The interaction of a ligand with its receptor is a dynamic one, and thus we need a procedure to model small-scale motion. Two techniques to achieve this are currently used, molecular dynamics and Brownian dynamics. Molecular dynamics follows the motions of atoms in a molecule over a short period (typically 1–100 ps) by using Newton's equations of motion. The forces on the atoms are derived from the same kind of potential energy functions described in the above section on molecular mechanics. To complete a molecular dynamics simulation we must define the geometry of the system (possibly using dimensions derived from X-ray or nmr measurements) and the potential energy function to be used to describe interatomic interactions. The system must then be equilibrated with great care being taken to remove any large interatomic forces. Then the atoms can be moved according to Newton's equations and the resulting trajectories analysed.

A particularly important use of the molecular dynamics approach is as part of the thermodynamic cycle-perturbation method which seeks, *inter alia*, to discover the effects of small changes in structure of either a ligand or the receptor on their interaction. In considering the comparative interaction of, say X and X^1 with Y, the thermodynamic cycle can be constructed:

$$X + Y \longrightarrow XY \qquad\qquad (8)$$
$$\downarrow \qquad\qquad\quad \downarrow$$
$$X^1 + Y \longrightarrow X^1Y$$

This is constructed from two processes, (9) and (10), with the latter being a non-physical one.

$$
\begin{aligned}
X + Y &\longrightarrow XY & \Delta G_1 \\
X^1 + Y &\longrightarrow X^1Y & \Delta G_2
\end{aligned}
\qquad (9)
$$

$$
\begin{aligned}
X + Y &\longrightarrow X^1 + Y & \Delta G_3 \\
XY &\longrightarrow X^1Y & \Delta G_4
\end{aligned}
\qquad (10)
$$

The relative free energy change, $\Delta \Delta G$, is equal to both $\Delta G_2 - \Delta G_1$ and $\Delta G_4 - \Delta G_3$, and the latter difference can be calculated by molecular dynamics. Because the changes represented by equation (10) are smaller and more localised than those in (9) the molecular dynamics calculations are simpler and more accurate. Full details of how this can be done and its application to the binding of substituted benzamidines to the enzyme trypsin are given in reference 44. It is expected that these types of approaches will be especially useful in designing new inhibitors for enzymes which have mutated, for example, in building up drug resistance.

Brownian dynamics differs from molecular dynamics in that the solvent molecules are now no longer treated explicitly but rather their effects are implicitly included by modifying the equations of motion. The diffusional motions of solvent molecules in a liquid are treated in Brownian dynamics by generating trajectories derived from certain basic equations. The method can be used to simulate diffusion phenomena, and in drug research has been used to determine the effects of electrostatic interactions on the rates of protein–ligand or protein–protein binding. Again the interested reader is referred to the original reference and the further references contained therein.

5.5a COMPUTER GRAPHICS[45]

Van't Hoff showed in 1874 that the carbon atom has a tetrahedral shape, but the fullest consequences of this for the chemical and physical properties of organic molecules do not seem to have been greatly considered until Barton introduced the concept of conformational analysis in 1953. It was then recognised that two-dimensional line drawings of organic structures were inadequate and three-dimensional models began to appear. The first of these were the stick models introduced by Dreiding, but these gave little impression of bulk and so space-filling CPK (Corey–Pauling–Koltun) models, which represented atoms as globes, also appeared. While CPK models give a much better representation of molecular bulk, they are very inflexible, and it is not uncommon to be unable to model a crowded molecule which actually exists.

Whilst these models were being accepted by organic chemists, X-ray crystallographers, who were now beginning to determine the structure of proteins, were faced with the difficulty of visualising these structures. These they did with complex wire structures supported by a network of rigid rods which took months to build as every atom had to be precisely placed in space and every bond and angle had to be accurate. Once finished these models could not be adjusted, and, over time, were prone to distortion through sagging.

As well as the above problems, these models suffer from two other drawbacks. They are inflexible in that the bond lengths of Dreiding models and atomic radii of CPK models are average values, and it is almost impossible to adjust these to fit a particular circumstance. Even more importantly, it is impossible to show electronic distributions and charges which govern the reactivity of the molecules under study.

All these problems can be addressed by the use of computer-generated graphical displays. Thus the representation can be made specific to the molecule of interest, especially if bond lengths and angles are known from physical measurements. Even when these are not known, it may be possible to find such measurements from suitable analogous molecules whose structures are known. The energy of particular conformations, especially the lowest one, can be calculated by using quantum or molecular mechanics and electronic distributions calculated and displayed. Also molecular structures can be deliberately changed and the effect on the overall energy of the system calculated. The interaction between molecules can be observed, as can the degree of similarity between different molecules. Finally, even complex structures such as those of proteins, can be rapidly generated, manipulated and stored.

Computer representation of molecular structures has benefited greatly from the rapid evolution of computer power throughout the 1980s. Thus the very earliest systems used black and white screens, and required the computer power of mini-mainframe machines such as those pioneered for scientific use by the Digital company. Today, colour graphics are the norm and very significant studies can be performed on desktop personal computers, although dedicated workstations such as the Silicon Graphics Personal Iris seem to offer the best compromise between performance and cost.

Two types of display technology, vector and raster, are used to produce the images. Raster displays work in a manner very similar to that of a television screen, with a series of interlaced lines (rasters) traced on the phosphor of a cathode ray tube. Each line is composed of a number of points, picture elements or pixels. Manipulation of the electron beam by the output of the computer produces the required colours and shades at each pixel. Raster displays readily produce CPK model-like images, but the great demands on computer power needed to manipulate complex structures in real time mean that it is only recently that such displays have become commonplace.

Vector graphics draw lines from one point to another very much as an X-Y plotter would and the computer output is used to drive the X-Y plots on the cathode ray tube. In this case the program does not have to fill in the background information and thus it is much easier to manipulate large structures in real time. Despite this advantage, the greater realism of raster displays means that they now have a dominant position.

The requirements for modern computer software essentially are that it should allow the user to build any molecule, to define a surface and compare those of different structures, to define the low-energy conformations, to communicate with molecular mechanics and quantum mechanical programs and display their outcomes. It is possible with all programs to display stick models (with cueing to give a three-dimensional effect), CPK-like models (with different colours for different atoms), surfaces defined by dots so that a stick model skeleton can be seen underneath, a "solvent accessible" surface, and electron distribution over the molecular surfaces.

To see how this is achieved, it is perhaps instructive to consider a typical product QUANTA™ which is marketed by Polygen (Polygen Corporation, 200 Fifth Avenue, Waltham, Massachusetts 02254, USA). This program can model all sizes of molecule and readily interfaces with either the company's own molecular mechanics software (CHARMm™) or the QCPE programs CNDO and AMPAC. In addition, it accepts coordinates from the Brookhaven Protein Structure Database or the Cambridge Crystallographic database for small molecules. If such structures are not known, the program will convert a two-dimensional representation of a structure into a three-dimensional one. Use of any of the supported calculation programs then allows the molecule under investigation to be energy minimised and its election distribution calculated and depicted. The surface of any molecule can be depicted in a number of formats, e.g. CPK or dot surface, as required. The consequences on energy of bond rotations or conformational change can be readily calculated. Structural comparisons, docking of two molecules, and protein modelling are all possible. QUANTA is but one of a number of similar programs from a range of software houses which all perform basic manipulations, but with individual features of greater or less importance to the user.

Whilst QUANTA is a program capable of modelling structures of virtually all sizes, it needs a reasonably substantial workstation to function. In contrast, the program ALCHEMY™ from Tripos (Tripos Associates Inc, 1699 South Hanby Road, Suite 303, St Louis, Missouri 63144, USA) is specifically designed for IBM PC, AT, XT, PS/2 or compatible desktop personal computers. Nevertheless, it will build electronic Dreiding models, minimise energies for molecules in the range of 130–170 atoms using molecular mechanics and visually compare, and superimpose molecules.

The ease of use of these programs depends greatly on the computer literacy of the user, but both are accessible to the practising medicinal chemist with only moderate levels of training.

The above text has referred to two features which warrant further discussion. The problem of how to determine the "true" surface of a molecule, particularly a protein, is a difficult one. The concept of solvent-accessible area was introduced and defined by Connolly[46] as the area traced out by the centre of a probe sphere representing a solvent molecule as it is rolled over the surface of the molecule of interest. He showed how it was possible to calculate a surface which is partly composed of the van der Waals' surface of those atoms which are accessible to solvent molecules connected by a network of concave and saddle-shaped surfaces and which, which smooths over the gaps and pits between the atoms. Within this surface any solvent molecule would experience van der Waals' repulsions, and it is generally felt that these representations give an overall picture of the molecule.

A second feature of computer graphics is the ability to compare structures. One of the constant features of drug design through the years has been that of bioisosterism, the idea that different functional groups can confer similar biological activities to a parent molecule and thus be interchangeable. In the past the identification of bioisosteres has been totally dependent on the intuition of the medicinal chemist, whereas today the appropriate computer software can establish the concept on a much more solid theoretical basis, by performing detailed comparisons of the electronic potential distribution around parts, or indeed the whole of the molecule. Notably the program ASP™ from Oxford Molecular (Oxford Molecular Ltd, The Magdalene Centre, Oxford Science Park, Sandford on Thames, Oxford, OX4 4GA, UK) provides a quantifiable comparison of the similarity between two molecules based on their molecular electrostatic potentials and fields.

A recent review[47] has critically examined currently available software and methods for molecular modelling, and the interested reader is referred to this for further information.

5.6 MODELLING DRUG-RECEPTOR INTERACTIONS

Modelling receptor and ligand molecules as described above is obviously extremely valuable, but the whole foundation of medicinal chemistry is the positioning of these molecules in the putative biological interaction, such that these models can be used for future drug design. However, the problems of the calculations, described above for individual molecules, are increased by an order of magnitude when additional interactive forces are added to the equations, and the solvent effects are consequently more important and difficult to calculate. It will be appreciated that *de novo* drug design remains the major challenge for the medicinal chemist.

A complete calculation of binding processes would produce the free energy of binding, broken down into enthalpy and entropy terms, and it would account for attractive and repulsive interactions which depend on the shape and electrostatic potential surfaces of the molecules. The forces which have to be considered include ion–ion, ion–dipole, hydrogen bonding, polarisation, charge transfer, van der Waals' dispersion and repulsion, loss of rotational and translational entropy, and hydrophobic interactions. The relative importance of these forces will, of course, depend on the nature of the interacting species. Thus in nonionised but polar molecules the dipole–dipole forces are the most important, with significant contributions from polarisation and charge transfer. In nonpolar molecules or nonpolar sections of polar molecules, hydrophobic effects[48] can become dominant.

Attempts to calculate these interactions by using quantum and molecular mechanics have been made (see, for example, Reference 45). No doubt the value and accuracy of such efforts will improve in the near future with improvements in techniques and computer power. However, a recent series of articles have shown how a different concept, the free energy perturbation (FEP)[49] method, can be used to calculate some remarkably accurate values for differences in binding energies of similar compounds to the same receptor. This is, of course, exactly the sort of information needed to predict whether a change in a lead structure is likely to be advantageous. The basic concept is depicted in equation (11), in which L and L^1 are the related ligands and E is the receptor

$$
\begin{array}{ccc}
 & \Delta G_1 & \\
L + E & \longrightarrow & E{:}L \\
\Big\downarrow \Delta G_2 & & \Big\downarrow \Delta G_4 \\
L^1 + E & \longrightarrow & E{:}L^1 \\
 & \Delta G_3 &
\end{array}
\qquad (11)
$$

The problem is to measure the differences in binding energies between L and L^1, ΔG_1 ΔG_3, but, as indicated above, the direct calculation of ΔG_1 and ΔG_3 is at best extremely difficult or impossible. Because the free energy is a *state* function this binding energy difference is also given by $\Delta G_2 - \Delta G_4$, and these are nonphysical processes much more amenable to calculation. This entails calculating the energy change when converting L to L^1 in solution to give ΔG_2 and also bound to the receptor to give ΔG_4, using either *ab initio* or molecular dynamic methods, depending on the particular system.

In an example of the method Kollman[50] calculated that the difference in binding energy of two closely related inhibitors of the enzyme thermolysin, phosphoramidate and phosphonate esters, was 4.21 ± 0.54 kilocalories per mole. This should be compared with the measured value of 4.1 kcal/mol. The difference between the two inhibitors is the replacement of the NH group of the amidate by an oxygen in the ester, and the method therefore requires calculating the effect of these changes on the overall energy of the inhibition. Other studies have given equally remarkable results, and it must be concluded that this method holds enormous promise.

5.7 DRUG DESIGN METHODS

In this section three recently described drug design methods will be discussed, namely receptor fitting, Goodford's GRID program, and Dean's site-directed methodology, and a detailed drug design study outlined which incorporates many of the features presented earlier in this chapter.

5.7.1 Receptor fitting[51]
Once the structure of a receptor has been determined, then the most straightforward method of drug design should be to devise a structure which fits the atomic constraints of the receptor site and interacts positively with the electronic distribution around that site. This sounds logical, natural, and even obvious, but in reality the number of studies which have been based on this approach is surprisingly limited. Four such studies have, however, been selected to illustrate the approach.

5.7.1.1   Haemoglobin[52]
The first two examples deal with the binding of small molecules to macromolecules in systems which were chosen as models for drug–receptor interactions. The haemoglobin study was the first to describe a systematic attempt to design a molecule to fit a site of defined structure in a macromolecule, and, as such, stands as a seminal paper in drug design. The molecular structure of haemoglobin was established by Perutz and co-workers in the 1960s as part of the work which proved that X-ray crystallography could be used to determine the structure of complex, biologically important macromolecules.

This showed that the haemoglobin molecule consisted of two α and two β subunits, each of which was a polypeptide chain. It was known that 2.3-diphosphoglycerate (DPG), (30) exists in erythrocytes (red blood cells) where it catalyses the phosphoglycer-omutase reaction and combines with haemoglobin, stabilising the deoxy conformation, thus releasing oxygen. It is thus possible to envisage this system as a model of a drug–receptor interaction in which the drug is DPG, the receptor is haemoglobin, and the biological response is release of oxygen. As a further aid, the structure of deoxyhaemoglobin plus DPG had also been established by the use of X-ray crystallography. This (Figure 5.10) clearly indicated that the phosphate group hydrogen bonds to histidine 2 and 143 in each β_1 and β_2 submit and the N-terminal amine group of both chains. In addition, the carboxylic acid forms a salt bridge with the 82-lysine of one chain. Through a gradual structural evolution, the authors eventually arrived at the bisulphite addition structure (31) in which the masked aldehyde can covalently bond to the terminal amino groups, the sulphite can hydrogen bond to 2, 2^1, 143 and 143^1 histidines, and the carboxylic acid forms a salt bridge to 82-lysine (Figure 5.11). The 1,2 biphenyl ethane framework was selected on geometrical grounds as being suitable to cover the interatomic distances in the molecule.

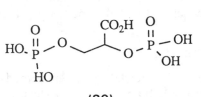

(30)

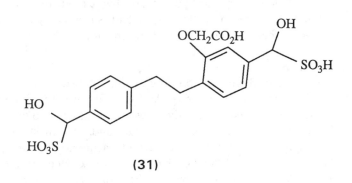

(31)

Gratifyingly, the compound (**31**) was as potent as DPG in releasing oxygen, and the activities of other analogues also fitted into the assumptions underlying the hypothesis. It is very difficult to imagine that structure (**31**) could have been derived from DPG by conventional molecular manipulation, and this approach, consequently, provided a new series of compounds. Subsequent work supported the predicted bonding interactions for these compounds. Finally, it should be noted that this work predated the current use of computer graphics by some time and was essentially completed by using wire models.

5.7.1.2   *Thyroid hormone-prealbumin interactions*[53]

Some years after the haemoglobin programme, Blaney and co-workers investigated another challenging model system, but were now able to use computer graphics rather than wire models to visualise the active site. The group chose to work on the

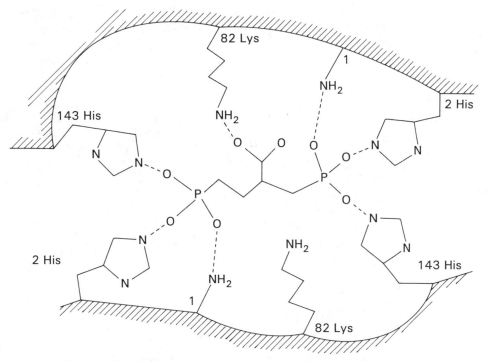

Fig. 5.10.   The binding of 2,3-diphosphoglycerate at the proposed binding site.

interaction of the thyroid hormone thyroxine (32) with the protein, prealbumin, as a model for the interaction of thyroid hormones with the nuclear thyroid hormone receptor. Again, the model is not a true representative drug–receptor interaction since prealbumin acts only as a carrier protein; the binding is specific, however, and there is a well-defined binding site. The structure of the complex had been determined by X-ray crystallography, but these authors were able to visualise and examine the data by using molecular graphics. This was not only a simpler process but also indicated many relationships between the hormone and the protein which would not have been apparent in simple wire models. As well as the obvious ion pair groupings between the amino acid of thyroxine and lysine-15 and glutamine-54, it was established that there are six pockets capable of binding the large iodine atoms. As there are only four iodine atoms this must leave two unoccupied pockets potentially available for extra binding. One apparently contains a well-defined water molecule, but the other is essentially empty. From this insight the authors designed a series of naphthyl derivatives such as (33) and were able to predict their relative binding efficiencies. It is highly unlikely that these naphthyl derivatives could have been logically designed from thyroxine without the use of computer graphics.

5.7.1.3   Inhibition of phospholipase A_2[54]
The enzyme phospholipase A_2 (PLA$_2$) catalyses the release of arachidonic acid (34) from its membranal phosphilipid stores (Scheme 5.3). Subsequent enzymatic

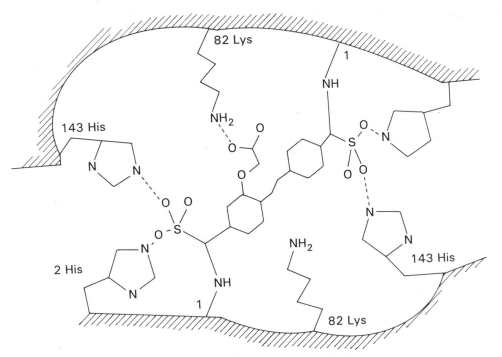

Fig. 5.11.   The binding of 31 to the proposed binding site.

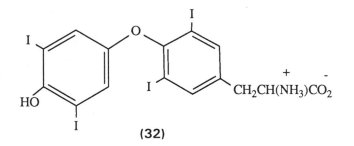

(32)

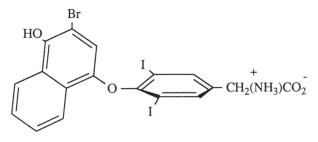

(33)

transformations of arachidonic acid lead to the prostaglandin and leukotriene mediators involved in many aspects of the inflammatory process. Suitable PLA_2 inhibitors could be novel anti-inflammatory agents. A collection of kinetic and X-ray studies had already established a reasonably complete picture of the active site and mechanism of action of the enzyme (Scheme 5.4). A number of potential inhibitors based on this mechanism have been developed, and such an approach was described in Chapter 4.

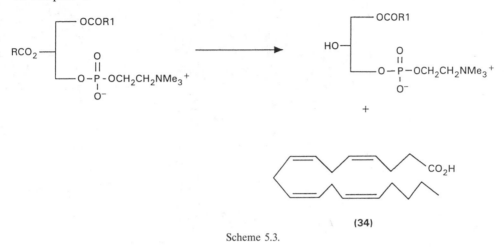

(34)

Scheme 5.3.

Ripka, however, based his approach on the structure of the active site as determined by crystallography and by a molecular modelling tool known as distance geometry. This method plots the total conformational space available to a natural substrate and showed the existence of a hydrophobic slot between residues leucine-2 and tyrosine 69. The group conjectured that a flat rigid naphthalene ring could fit into this slot and act as a framework or template on to which other groups could be situated to interact specifically with appropriate amino acid residues lining the active site. After much further model building the acenaphthalene derivative (35) was generated and found to have a satisfactory level of inhibitory activity. In this example the novelty of the final structure is perhaps even more marked than in the two previous examples, and it is very difficult indeed to see how such structures could have been arrived at conceptually simply with the known structure of the natural substrate of the enzyme.

5.7.1.4   The inhibition of dihydrofolate reductase[55]
The brilliant research of Hitchings and Elion on nucleic acid biosynthesis led to a number of valuable therapeutic agents including the antibacterial trimethoprim (36). Only subsequently was it discovered that the antileukemic methotrexate (37) worked by inhibiting the enzyme dihydrofolate reductase which catalyses a crucial step in the conversion of the vitamin folic acid to its tetrahydro derivative, which acts as a "carrier" of essential one-carbon units in the synthesis of precursors of purine and pyrimidine intermediate of the nucleic acids.

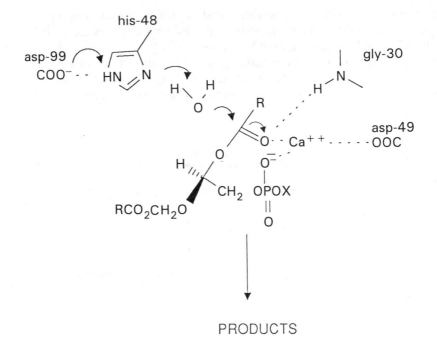

Scheme 5.4.

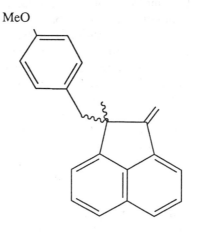

(35)

The crystal structures of both inhibitors bound to DHFR's from a variety of mammalian and bacterial sources have been described, and selective antibacterial activity is attributed to structural differences in the enzymes. By comparing putative active sites in the structures of (**36**) and (**37**) it became apparent that there was

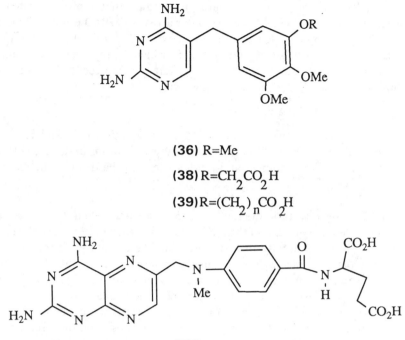

(36) R=Me

(38) R=CH$_2$CO$_2$H

(39) R=(CH$_2$)$_n$CO$_2$H

(37)

additional scope for suitable groups in trimethoprim in order to increase its binding. One such compound was (**38**) in which the extra carboxylic acid group can bind with the arginine 57 residue.

The new derivative was found to be more active in binding to the enzyme, although its *in vitro* antibacterial activity was less, possibly owing to difficulty in penetrating the bacterial cell wall. As well as this reminder that there are other factors in biological activity, the modelling procedure was not able to rationalise the affinity of DHFR derived from chicken liver for these components. Clearly any use of these techniques has to bear in mind that there may well be other factors in the mechanisms being considered.

5.7.2   Grid

Goodford[56] has described a method for determining energetically favourable binding sites on macromolecules by calculating the energies of interaction between the macromolecule and a series of probes at a number of points around the protein. The probes he used included water, methyl, amine nitrogen, carboxy oxygen, and hydroxyl.

When water is used as the probe it is treated as an electrically neutral group with no dipole but with the ability to accept or donate up to two hydrogen bonds. The first stage in the calculation is to obtain the atomic coordinates of the atoms in the macromolecule, most conveniently from the Brookhaven Protein Data Bank. A table entitled GRUB lists the energy parameters for all the nonbonding, electrostatic and hydrogen bonding interactions for the probes and the atoms of the protein, whilst the program GRIN attaches these to the atomic co-ordinates of the protein. The central program GRID then establishes a regular array of "GRID points" throughout and around the protein and calculates an energy value E_{xyz} for all these points. The energy is calculated according to equation (12) in which E_{1j} represents the Lennard–Jones function for nonbonding interactions where E_{el} represent the electrostatic interactions and E_{hb} the hydrogen bonding effects.

$$E_{xyz} = \Sigma E_{1j} + \Sigma E_{el} + \Sigma E_{nb} \qquad (12)$$

The Lennard–Jones potential is calculated from equation (13) and is a highly repulsive value for small values of the distance between the atoms under consideration; d is attractive for medium distances and tends to zero as the distance increases.

$$E_{1j} = A/d^{12} - B/d^6 \qquad (13)$$

The term for the electrostatic interaction is complex and attempts to account for changes in the dielectric constant of the medium as the probe moves from the medium closer and closer and eventually into the protein. The calculation process actually treats each $x-y$ plane in turn at given values of z moving from outside the protein and through it, and the separation between the planes can be adjusted, depending on the particular circumstances and the computer time available.

Amongst the applications of the method exemplified was the probe of the enzyme phospholipase A_2 with water. This approach demonstrated a binding region within 0.3 Å of the position found in an X-ray structure as well as defining several others on the surface of the protein. The region around trimethoprim (**36**) bound to the enzyme dihydrofolate reductase was also probed by the ammonium group. This approach suggested the presence of slightly different areas which could be examined, and further studies using the carboxylate oxygen showed the presence of the binding region in which the carboxylic acid derivative (**39**) fits.

The method may also work for macromolecule–macromolecule interactions, exemplified by the use of the methyl group as a probe to examine the binding areas between insulin chains involved in producing stable dimers.

The examples cited led Goodford to propose that the method could have significant merit despite its neglect of entropy and changes incurred in macromolecular structure on binding and other difficulties relating to the additivity of separate probe interactions and the state of ionisation of amino and carboxy groups.

5.7.3   Automated site-directed drug design
The ultimate drug design package would take into account the structure of a target, identify potential binding regions, define the angles and distances for optimum binding to these regions, and then generate for the operator the appropriate structure. Unfortunately, or fortunately perhaps for the peace of mind of medicinal chemists, such programs are not yet available, although Dean has recently[57-60] begun describing an approach to such a system.

Dean begins from the viewpoint that logical design is essentially a problem in three-dimensional construction in which the geometry of the site controls the atomic constants, whilst the atoms comprising the site determine the type of molecular interaction. Of course this is the process by which drugs have been designed for many years, empirically, by the medicinal chemist albeit aided latterly by the computer technology described in this chapter. The aim of Dean, however, is more ambitious, being a computing strategy that goes beyond normal computer-aided ligand design, moving towards a fully automated artificial intelligence system.

The first stage in his process[57] is a program HSITE for the computation of hydrogen bonding regions from the atomic coordinates of any protein. Such regions can be both donor and acceptor and, as hydrogen bonds have favoured orientations, the program constructs the regions in space situated above the protein for optimum binding to the appropriate atoms or groups. The output from the program is a graphic representation, colour-coded according to the probability of finding a suitable hydrogen bonding site. The method was tested[58] by comparing his calculated results with the actual positions of water molecules in myoglobin and plastocyanin, with the hydrogen bonded atoms in dihydrofolate reductase crystallised with methotrexate and NADPH, and with amidinophenylpyruvate crystallised with trypsin. Overall, the calculated results were in good agreement with experimental findings although a number of complicating features were noted in interpreting the findings in the hydrated proteins. These features were essentially due to the large amount of water in such systems and the fact that only the oxygen atoms are defined in X-ray crystallography.

Dean then examined the next stage of the process, namely the design of three-dimensional ligands to fit those bonding regions previously defined. This process necessitates identifying the positions in space at which the appropriate atoms should sit to maximise various interaction energies and then fitting these into a meaningful framework. In fact the process is broken down into two parts, namely primary structure generation, which is a geometric process to create a molecular graph to fit the designated ligand points, and a secondary process to convert this structure into a real molecule. To date only approaches to the first process have been published.

The primary structure is generated by means of a series of "spacer skeletons" which arise from the realisation that many biologically active structures contain rings and that all planar ring systems can be modelled by a group of about 20 spacer skeletons. Molecular templates are subsets of spacer skeletons from which can be derived actual compounds. Figure 5.12 shows how a putative quinazoline ligand can be generated from an appropriate molecular template, itself generated from the spacer skeleton comprised solely of hexagons. Other spacer skeletons could contain different-sized ring structures and various orientations of the rings. The bond lengths and angles for the ring fragments which form the spacer skeletons were derived from actual crystallographic data contained in the Cambridge Crystallographic Database, and an interactive program MNET is used to construct spacer skeletons to verify deviation from planarity with any resultant distortions.

Having generated a suitable collection of spacer skeletons the next stage is to attempt to manoeuvre into the ligand binding region an appropriate skeleton whose vertices match as closely as possible the points for optimum binding. The spacer skeleton can then be "clipped" to remove unwanted groups or those which would interfere with the protein, thus providing a molecular template from which a tangible

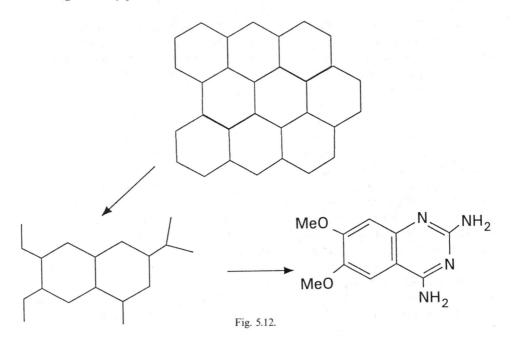

Fig. 5.12.

molecule can be generated. This is a complex process with many possible spacer skeletons to be investigated, albeit into two dimensions, although, of course, eventually an extension to three dimensions will be necessary. The programs DMSEARCH and OPTIMUS are used to define and refine the derived molecular templates.

The actual application of the technique to the enzyme dihydrofolate reductase is discussed in detail,[60] the molecular templates generated by the method suggesting a number of possible structures which could bind to the active site of the enzyme, including the pteridine ring found in methotrexate itself.

This approach is still in its infancy but clearly the initial procedures are already producing tangible results and, undoubtedly, this method must provide the basis for future rational *de novo* drug design.

5.8   APPLICATIONS OF DRUG DESIGN TECHNIQUES

Many papers have been published describing applications of one or more of the techniques described above, but a recent paper by Appelt and colleagues at Agouron[61] is particularly noteworthy for the range of techniques applied. The work concerned the design of inhibitors of the enzyme thymidylate synthetase which mediates the methylation of deoxyuridylate to thymidylate using 5,10-methylenetetrahydrofolate as a cofactor. As this is the rate-limiting step in the *de novo* pathway to thymidine nucleotides such inhibitors could be novel antifolate antitumour agents and thus be of clinical value. A number of inhibitors of the enzyme, notably **(40)**, have been described, but a clinically useful lipophilic inhibitor does not exist and was a target of the work.

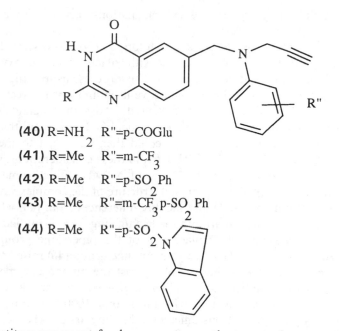

(40) R=NH$_2$　　R"=p-COGlu

(41) R=Me　　R"=m-CF$_3$

(42) R=Me　　R"=p-SO$_2$Ph

(43) R=Me　　R"=m-CF$_3$ p-SO$_2$Ph

(44) R=Me　　R"=p-SO$_2$

Since an antitumour agent for human use was the target, the appropriate target enzyme was of human origin. However, the enzyme was conveniently available from *E. coli.* in gram quantities and readily gave X-ray diffraction quality crystals. Moreover, the primary sequence of the *E. coli.* enzyme has high homology (46%) with the human sequence, and the active site residues around the binding site are 75% identical. Most of the design work, consequently, was concentrated on the bacterial enzyme, although human enzyme has been cloned and the crystallographic structure of the enzyme–inhibitor complex is being determined.

The first design approach led to elaboration of structure (**40**) in an attempt to increase the lipophilicity. It was noted that the X-ray structure suggested a possible hydrophobic binding site around the meta region of the phenyl ring and, accordingly, the 3-trifluoromethyl derivative (**41**) was prepared and its crystal structure complexed into the enzyme determined. Gratifyingly, the trifluoromethyl group fitted the expected pocket, but, unfortunately, the activity was rather less than expected. In a search for increased hydrophobicity the phenyl ring was substituted by *p*-phenylsulphonyl (**42**) after a molecular mechanics energy minimisation process had indicated that the low-energy conformers could be accommodated within the active site.

The new molecule was more active, but the activity was again reduced in the m-CF$_3$ p-SO$_2$Ph derivative (**43**), although calculation indicated that the two groups should have little effect on each other. X-ray crystallography, however, showed that the presence of the CF$_3$ in the active site caused an unfavourable displacement of the sulphonyl group. Further examination of the amino acids in the active site suggested that the available space would accommodate a larger group than a phenyl, and the indole derivatives (**44**), were consequently prepared. These were again active and more work to improve their activity continues. Thus the appropriate combination of X-ray crystallography and theoretical calculations has lead to a potent lead structure with scope for optimisation.

At this point the group also began a search for *de novo* prototypes. Their starting point was the crystal structure of the enzyme with cofactor 5-flurodeoxyuridylate but from which inhibitor (**40**) had been removed. This process ensured that the structure of the enzyme being used was that of the active itself and not the resting state. The GRID program described above was then used to design a ligand. A site which would interact favourably with a CH probe was identified and a naphthalene skeleton inserted into the position; further groups could then be added to the skeleton to accept binding groups identified by GRID. From these considerations, structure (**45**) was synthesised and found to have significant activity, albeit some 3 orders of magnitude less than that of (**40**). The crystal structure of the complex was determined to verify the actual binding mode and identify differences from (**40**) when problems in the hydrogen bonding region around the lactam ring were identified as one cause of the lower activity observed. Replacement of the piperazine group by a more lipophilic phenyl ring and the lactam by an amidine group (**46**) raised the activity of the molecule to about 50% of that of (**40**) against the human enzyme. The crystal structure confirmed the anticipated binding to *E. coli.* enzyme but corresponding data with the human enzyme, against which it is some 1000-fold more active, is not yet available. It is possible that this differential binding arises because a tryptophan residue in *E. coli* enzyme is converted to an asparagine molecule in the human enzyme and this would better accommodate the bulky naphthalene group.

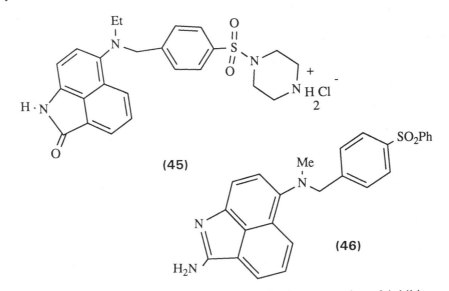

(**45**)

(**46**)

Not content with having designed one completely new series of inhibitors the authors re-examined the binding site and synthesised (**47**). Quantum mechanical calculations on the low-energy conformation of (**47**) showed that it was possible to fit this into the active site, and further structural modifications led to structure (**48**) which was also about 50% as active as (**40**) against the human enzyme.

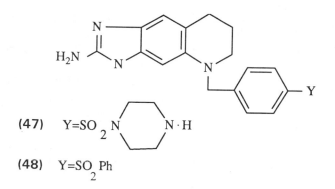

(47)   Y=SO$_2$ N⌒N·H

(48)   Y=SO$_2$Ph

Thus by a very systematic study of the crystal structures of enzymes and their putative ligands an interesting series has been developed and two entirely novel active series designed. This paper may be considered a landmark in drug design which will be followed by many others.

5.9   OPTIMISATION OF LEAD STRUCTURES

Over the years much research effort and creativity has been devoted to the problem of optimising a lead structure, whatever its origin, and to understanding the structural features responsible for its activity. A number of techniques have been applied, and these are most conveniently grouped as Hansch and discriminant analyses.

5.9.1   Historical[62]

The concept that the biological activity of a compound could be related to its structure was first proposed by Crum-Brown and Fraser in 1868.[63] They showed that the paralysing activity of a series of quarternised strychnine derivatives depended on the quaternary substituents. When it is considered how little was known about chemical structure and biological activity at that time it will be appreciated just how revolutionary was this proposal. In fact, so original was the concept, and so difficult was it to test with the knowledge then available, that it was over thirty years before any experimental verification appeared. Then, Meyer and Overton, working independently, verified some earlier work by Richet and showed that the narcotic action of a wide range of compounds on tadpoles in a tank was related to their oil–water partition coefficients.

The partition coefficient, of course, measures the relative affinity of the compound for the two liquids, but the fact that the narcotic activity of the compounds studied by Meyer and Overton could be related to this parameter led to some interesting conclusions. Since the compound was added to the water in which the tadpole was swimming, it must distribute itself simply as if the tadpole were a drop of oil. The precise mechanisms of narcosis are still the subject of much debate, but the fact that chemically inert gases such as xenon can act as anaesthetics is a powerful argument that in some circumstances it may be the result of a bulk dissolution effect disrupting a gross structural feature. In this situation narcosis is induced solely when the concentration of the compound reaches a certain level. Such agents are referred to as *structurally nonspecific drugs* in contrast to the *structurally specific drugs* which act at a defined site and are the major subject matter of medicinal chemistry.

Subsequent studies similar to those of Meyer and Overton led, *inter alia*, to correlations between insecticidal activity and boiling points and narcotic activity with surface tension. Each of these properties is based on an equilibrium process and, subsequently, the observed effect of the drug. Such depressant activity is rapidly achieved and maintained while a drug reservoir exists and activity is reversed when the supply of drug is removed. In all cases these studies used nonspecific drugs and they were rationalised by Ferguson who derived equation (14):

$$C_i = KA_jm \tag{14}$$

where C_i = concentration of the ith member of a series producing an equivalent response, K,m = constants for a given system, and A_j = a physicochemical distribution constant, e.g. solubility, partition coefficient, vapour pressure or a parameter related to these constants.

The only circumstance where the thermodynamic arguments of Ferguson appear to have led to the discovery of a chemically useful agent was that of the gaseous anaesthetic halothane. Normally they do not apply to structurally specific drugs acting in humans, or living organisms, where such equilibria that do exist are less important than kinetic processes. In these circumstances a somewhat different approach was necessary.

During the 1930s and 1940s physical organic chemistry was firmly established largely through the efforts of the groups lead by Hammett and Ingold. Nowadays chemists are acclimatised to thinking of chemistry in terms of quantifiable substituent effects where an atom or group of atoms can be regarded as exerting electronic and steric effects which can be measured in one molecular system and then extrapolated to others. This predictivity of effects rationalises much otherwise unconnected data and enables the properties of a new molecule to be predicted even before it has been synthesised. The basic Hammett equation (equation (15)) was first proposed in 1937 to correlate the effect of meta and para substituents on the reactivity of substituted benzene derivatives.

$$\log K_x/K_h = p\sigma_x \tag{15}$$

where K_x = rate or equilibrium constant for substituent group x, K_h = rate or equilibrium constant for unsubstituted benzene, σ_x = a constant characteristic of the electronic effect of x, and p = constant characteristic of the reaction being investigated

Equation (15) can be used to derive σ constants for a range of x substituents acting on a particular reaction centre Y, and the same values can then be used for different reaction centres thus giving the valuable elements of predictability and extensive applicability. Equation (15) is an example of a linear free energy relationship (LFER).

The Hammett equation correlating chemical reactivity for a homologous series of compounds with electronic factors was, of course, developed by organic chemists considering *in vitro* conditions, and early attempts to apply the approach to biological systems, *in vivo*, were discouraging. Indeed Jaffe in a review of the Hammett equation in 1953 said he had not been able to find any series of compounds where *biological* action had followed such a relationship, though he did not consider such an occurrence inconceivable!

The reasons for the failure of these early attempts appear to be that researchers concentrated on trying to find single parameter equations following linear relationships. However, in 1962 the situation changed as Corwin Hansch published the first of a series of papers which essentially established the field of multiparameter quantitative structure–activity relationships. Hansch had been working with a botanist, Muir, for some 15 years trying to develop structure–activity relationships for plant growth regulators. From a series of phenoxyacetic acids it became apparent that there was a dependence on lipophilicity, and so Hansch and Fujita revived the idea of Meyer and Overton and began to measure partition coefficients as a measure of this.[64] In place of oil, Hansch used *n*-octanol as the organic phase.

The measurement of partition coefficients will be discussed later with hydrophobic substituent constants in the manner of the Hammett equation defined by equation (16).

$$\log \left\langle \frac{p_X}{P_H} \right\rangle = \Pi_X \tag{16}$$

where P_x is the partition coefficient for benzene substituted with X, P_H that for the unsubstituted case, and Π_X is the hydrophobic substituent constant

Fujita then suggested that an approach used by Taft should be adopted where he had shown how the original Hammett δ constants could be factored into inductive and resonance components and then be recombined into a linear relationship. Fujita reasoned that biological activity could be due to a combination of lipophilic and electronic effects, which led to equation (17) in which the linear free energy relationship (LFER) formalism is assumed by defining the biological response in a logarithmic form.

$$\log (1/c) = k_1 \Pi + k_2\sigma + k_3 \tag{17}$$

where c is the molar concentration of a compound producing a standard response in a constant time interval, k_1, k_2, k_3 are constants, and Π and σ as defined above.

This equation fitted well a number of situations but it required further insights by Hansch to be developed further. Considering the question of lipophilicity he well appreciated that an "ideal" lipophilic value would have to be a compromise for the following reasons. If a compound were too water-soluble it would never cross the many biological membranes which it would encounter in its passage from the point of entry into the living organism to its ultimate target site. On the other hand, if it were too lipid-soluble, then it would be likely to remain in the first lipid layer it encountered. These arguments suggested that the dependence of activity on lipophilicity should be parabolic in nature and led to the essential, and seminal, Hansch equation:

$$\log (1/c) = k_1 (\log P) - k_2 (\log P)^2 + k_3\sigma + k_4 \tag{18}$$

In this equation log P is the octanol–water partition coefficient, σ the Hammett constant, and k_1, k_2, k_3 and k_4 are constants. Many variations on equation (18) in which σ has been replaced by a variety of other physicochemical parameters have been reported and will be discussed later.

It should be pointed out that the Hansch equation as defined is intended to fit series of homologous compounds with changes in a few defined substituents. To generate the equation and solve it for the necessary values of the constants requires that a substantial number of compounds have been synthesised and their biological activity measured. Its great utility is to define what values of the substituent constants are likely to give maximum values of biological activity and thus guide new syntheses.

5.9.2   Linear free energy relationships

5.9.2.1   *Partition coefficients*

The partition coefficient log P is defined as the ratio of solubility of the substance in water to that in a solvent:

$$\log P = C_1/C_2 \tag{19}$$

Since this essential component of the Hansch equation is meant to represent the interaction of the drug with the biological membranes it encounters in the body, the solvents chosen to determine P should represent these membranes as closely as possible. The very earliest solvent to be studied was olive oil followed by a number of other systems until Collander and then Hansch finally established n-octanol as the medium of choice. n-Octanol contains a saturated fatty alkyl chain, hydroxyl groups for hydrogen bonding, and is soluble in water giving at saturation a 1.7 M water solution. Thus partitioning in this case is not being measured between water and an anhydrous organic phase, but between water and a waterlogged organic phase. This system of lipophilic chains, hydrophilic hydroxyl groups, and water molecules appears to give n-octanol properties very close to those of natural membranes and macromolecules. However, it is not ideal and a variety of other solvents have been proposed. Amongst these is the diester propylene glycol dipelargonate (PGDP) which, it has been suggested, more closely resembles the lipid end of a typical phospholipid whereas octanol is a better model for the more amphiprotic regions of a typical membrane. It is theoretically possible that selectivity of action could be achieved, resulting solely from differential partitioning between the membranes containing the same receptors responsible for both desired and unwanted pharmacological effects. Thus an attempt has been made to use differences in partitioning between water and octanol and water and cyclohexane to model compounds for brain penetration, and no doubt more such studies will be reported. Taylor, in his excellent, thorough review states "the proper choice of solvent system is more open now than at any time in the last 50 years". Whilst further progress will be made, it should also be noted that the simple log P (octanol/water) has worked outstandingly as a model for the complex variety of structures constituting biological membranes.

The actual measurement of log P values is, in theory, straightforward, but, in practice, much more problematic. The simplest method is to dissolve the material in one solvent, add the second, shake for long enough to establish equilibrium, allow the phases to separate, and then measure the concentrations of the solute in each layer. In practice, both the phases must be presaturated, shaking must be vigorous, and centrifugation is usually essential to permit complete separation. Analysis of the layers can then be by any convenient accurate method. This method is most accurate for P values around 1, with errors appearing with values much less or greater than this.

A second method uses counter-current chromatography, or a close variation, with octanol and water as the two phases. This method, however, appears to have been even less widely used than is counter-current chromatography for other organic separations.

A more successful application of chromatography uses liquid chromatography in which octanol is absorbed on a hyflo-supercel diatomaceous earth solid support. In essence, the system is calibrated by measuring the retention times of a series of compounds of known log P value, plotting a graph, measuring the retention of a new compound, and reading off the log P. This appears to be the most convenient and accurate method currently available.[65]

In view of the importance of partition coefficients in medicinal chemistry, efforts have been made to determine them theoretically so that values could be deduced for unknown and unmeasurable compounds.[66,67] Early approaches considered log P to be an additive-constitutive property in which it was possible to regard the value of a substituted compound as being the sum of the log P value for the parent and a "substituent partition coefficient Π" for the substituent replacing a hydrogen atom:

$$\Pi(X) = \log P(RX) - \log P(RH) \tag{20}$$

Clearly, with a sufficiently large collection of Π values, and provided that there exists at least one member of a homologous series with a measured log P value, the value for the rest of the series can be calculated. The fact that at least one experimental measurement is required renders this approach somewhat limited, and thus a more fundamental method is needed. This has been provided by Rekker's "fragmental" approach,[68] which assigns values to a large number of atoms and small groups of atoms, which are obtained by statistical analysis of a comprehensive collection of measured partition coefficients.

At first this method was applied manually, but subsequently computerised methods have been developed, notably by the Hansch group. Their program CLOGP will take any molecule, divide it into appropriate fragments, obtain the appropriate constants from its database, and calculate the log P value. The program appears to be very powerful, and the more it is used, the more its accuracy is improving. In addition, the program, by breaking down the molecule into fragments and investigating how these fragments interact with their surroundings and combine to give an overall result, should provide a greater insight into the property of partition. Thus, as Leo has stated, "it is more important, perhaps, to keep in mind that log P values are not just numbers to be used as parameters in a regression equation. Being aware of why each value is what it is—that is what correction factors come into play in that particular structure, what solvation forces are competing in the transfer between lipid membrane and serum or cell plasma—this knowledge could give additional insights into pharmacology and drug design".

A major complication in predicting partitioning effects arises with compounds which can ionise at physiologically meaningful pH. Partitioning of ions into nonaqueous medium is disfavoured, thus any partition coefficient measured under these conditions will greatly underestimate the P value for the neutral species. Equations (21) and (22) show how the measured distribution ratio, D, relates to P for acids or bases respectively.

$$\log D = \log P - \log [1 + \text{antilog} (pH - pK_a)] \tag{21}$$

$$\log D = \log P - \log [1 + \text{antilog} (pK_a - pH)] \tag{22}$$

Many ionic species can, of course, be extracted into organic layers as ion pairs, and in this case an empirical extraction coefficient, E, can be defined, which represents the total concentration of ion in the organic phase divided by its concentration in water. An ion pair partition coefficient P_{ip} and an ion pair association constant K_{ip} for the aqueous phase can be defined, leading to the equation (23) where X is the counter ion.

$$E = P_{ip} K_{ip} [X^-] \tag{23}$$

There have been a number of reports of correlations of biological activity simply with log P. Thus the toxicities of a series of alcohols to the red spider were related to their log P by value of equation (24), and the effect of phenols on the conversion of P450 to P420 cytochromes was given by equation (25)

$$\log (1/c) = 0.69 \ (\pm 0.09) \log P + 0.16 \ (\pm 0.08) \tag{24}$$
$$N = 14, r = 0.979, s = 0.087$$

$$\log (1/c) = 0.57 \ (\pm 0.08) \log P + 0.36 \ (\pm 0.19) \tag{25}$$
$$N = 13, r = 0.979, s = 0.132$$

A parabolic relationship was observed for the ability of a series of barbiturates to induce hypnosis in the mouse:

$$\log (1/c) = -0.44 \ (\log P)^2 + 1.58 \log P + 1.93(0 \pm 0.24) \tag{26}$$
$$n = 13, r = 0.969, s = 0.098$$

The parabolic dependence of activity to log P leads to the realisation that there must be an optimum value of log P, log P_0, for biological activity in any chemical series. Indeed Hansch has shown that there is an optimum value of log P_0 for a large number of nonspecific hypnotics, i.e. barbiturates, alcohols, amides, of approximately 2. He concluded that virtually any compound which was not metabolised or excreted, with a log P value of 2, would show general hypnotic properties. This common log P_0 value implies that the rate-limiting process for nonspecific hypnotic activity is the membrane transport relevant to the site of action.

Whereas the concept of partitioning and the log P are important in drug research, only relatively nonspecific therapeutic agents would be expected to show biological activity which was solely dependent on this parameter. For the vast majority of drugs concomitant dependence on electronic and steric factors is equally important.

5.9.2.2 Electronic effects[69]

It is evident that electronic effects must be present in the binding of specific drugs to their binding sites, and this was recognised by equation (17) which included a term containing σ:

$$\log (1/c) = k_1 \, \Pi + k_2 \, \sigma + k_3 \tag{17}$$

Since σ was first introduced by Hammett its precise meaning has been the subject of considerable detailed, and increasingly sophisticated, analysis. The result of this work has been the derivation of a plethora of terms applicable in appropriate circumstances (Table 5.1). Whilst the relative importance of these parameters is still the subject of debate there is general agreement that the major influences can be attributed to localised effects, notably the field and inductive effects, and delocalized resonance effects. Thus Swain and Lupton proposed that electronic substituent effects could be separated into a field constant, F, and a resonance constant, R, related by:

Table 5.1 Electronic parameters

Parameters	Comments
σ_m	Hammett constant for meta substituent derived from ionisation of benzoic acid.
σ_p	Hammett constant for para substituent derived from ionisation of benzoic acid.
σ_p^-	Hammett constant used when there is direct conjugation between substituent and reaction centre; derived from anilines and phenols.
σ_p^+	H. C. Brown constant derived from solvolysis of dimethylphenylcarbinyl chlorides.
σ_I	Constant describing solely polar effects.
σ_R	Constant describing solely mesomeric effects.
σ^*	Taft's polar substituent constant derived from hydrolysis of aliphatic esters.
$q^\cdot$	Homolytic constant for substituent interacting with a free radical reaction.
$F \ R$	Field and resonance components derived from linear combinations of σ_m and σ_o values

$$\sigma = fF + rR \tag{27}$$

In this equation f and r are field and resonance weighting scales. The scale was set up on two assumptions, firstly, that the effect of 4-substituents on the ionisation of bicyclo [2,2,2] octane-1-carboxylic acids (49) is entirely due to a field effect and, secondly, that for the substituent NMe_3^+ no resonance is possible and $R = 0$. The first assumption allows a scale of F values to be set up, using the 14 known values of this system (equation 27) and the second allows equation (27) to be solved for the para σ value of any substituent and gives f as 0.56. Using this gives a constant set of 42 values derived from meta and para σ values.

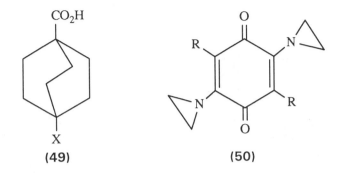

(49)   **(50)**

$$F = 1.369\sigma_m - 0.373\sigma_p - 0.009 \tag{28}$$
$$n = 14, r = 0.992, s = 0.042$$

Whilst the accuracy and applicability of the approach of Swain and Lupton are still being debated, it does appear to be a useful procedure and is widely used by scientists for QSAR. Its convenience is the fact that no assumptions are needed regarding the positional influence of substituents, that it is independent of measurements of the field and resonance susceptibilities, and that data from biological studies which are much less accurate than those obtained from *in vitro* measurements of equilibrium constants or reaction rates limits the precision achievable. The method was used to correlate the activity of a series of benzoquinones (50) against the tumour LI210 in the mouse:

$$\log(1/\text{med}) = -3.95(\pm1.05)F - 1.49(\pm0.49)\,R$$
$$-0.49\,(\pm0.09)\Sigma\Pi_{1,2} + 5.30(\pm0.20) \tag{29}$$
$$n = 35, r = 0.9l0, s = 0.29$$

(MED = minimum effective dose)

However, if the appropriate data are available it is possible to use any of the Hammett values, σ_m, σ_p, σ^+_p, σ^-_p and σ^0_p, where the existence of a dependence on one particular constant can provide an insight into the possible mechanism of action for the drug with its target site. Thus, for example, in the analysis of the adrenergic blocking activity of β-halo-β-arylethylamines (51), the first results led to equation (30) which was re-analysed to give (31) in which r_p is the van der Waals' radius for para substituents.

$$\log(1/\text{ED}_{50}) = 1.221\,\Sigma\pi - 1.5876\,\Sigma\sigma^- + 7.888 \tag{30}$$
$$n = 22, r = 0.918\ s = 0.238$$

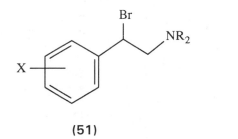

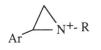

(51) (52)

$$\log(1/ED_{50}) = 0.747\ (\pm 0.123)\ \pi_m - 0.911\ (\pm 0.249)\ \sigma_m$$
$$+ 1.666(\pm 0.124)r_p + 5.769 \tag{31}$$

$$n = 22,\ r = 0.961\ s = 0.168$$

This had the effect of reducing the standard deviation and increasing the correlation coefficient, but could be criticised since it requires an electronic effect solely from meta substituents contrary to the usual findings from physical organic chemistry. The equation (32) was consequently derived in which the use of σ^+ could be more appropriate if (51) reacts via the carbonium ion (52).

$$\log\ (I/ED_{50}) = 0.82(\pm 0.27)\Sigma\pi - 1.02(\pm 0.45)\Sigma\sigma^+ \tag{32}$$
$$+ 0.62(\pm 0.43)\ r_p + 7.06(\pm 0.55)$$
$$n = 22,\ r = 0.96\ s = 0.164$$

The moral here is clearly that practitioners of QSAR should not ignore the lessons of their basic organic chemistry. A number of compilations of substituents and their electronic parameters have now been published for the use of medicinal chemists. One of the most recent is given in Table 5.2 which comes from the review of Bowden.[69]

5.9.2.3 Steric effects

Since the interaction of a drug with its sites of action necessitates the close approach of two molecules, steric effects must be a consideration in any attempt to derive a comprehensive correlation of drug structure and activity, but, unfortunately, steric effects are those which are the most difficult to quantify. One commonly used parameter, however, is the Taft E_s function derived from the acid hydrolysis of aliphatic esters by:

$$\log\ (K/K_0) = E_s \tag{33}$$

where K is the rate of acid hydrolysis of substituted ester and K_0 is the rate of acid hydrolysis of parent ester.

Other steric parameters which have been used are derived from physical descriptions such as the van der Waals' volume, polar refractivity, the parachor, molecular weight and geometric descriptions based on van der Waals' radii. The major problem with attempting to define steric effects is their directional qualities which can vary in different environments. A truly spherical shape as found in individual atoms presents

Table 5.2   Electronic substituent constants

Substituent	σ_m	σ_p	σ_p^+	σ_p^-	σ_p^0	σ_I	F	R	Aromatic μ (Debye)	Aliphatic μ (Debye)
Br	0.39	0.23	0.15	b	0.30	0.46	0.44	-0.17	-0.57	-1.97
CF$_3$	0.43	0.54	b	0.68	[0.53]a	0.42	0.38	0.19	-2.61	-1.94
CN	0.56	0.66	b	0.96	0.71	0.57	0.51	0.19	-4.08	-3.63
CO$_2^-$	-0.10	0.00	b	0.30	[-0.14]	-0.17	-0.15	0.13		
CHO	0.35	0.42	b	1.02	[0.47]	[0.25]	0.31	-3.02	-3.02	-2.58
CO$_2$H	0.37	0.45	b	0.78	[0.44]	[0.32]	0.33	0.15	-1.30	-1.65
CH$_2$Cl	0.10	0.12	-0.01	b		0.15	0.10	0.03	-1.83	-1.93
CONH$_2$	0.28	0.36	b	0.62		0.27	0.24	0.14	-3.42	-3.73
CH$_3$	-0.17	-0.31	b	-0.12	-0.12	-0.04	-0.04	-0.13	0.36	0.0
CH$_2$OH	0.00	0.00	0.01	b		0.05	0.00	0.00	1.73	
C≡CH	0.21	0.23	0.18	0.52	[0.22]	0.35	0.19	0.05	-0.77	-0.78
CH$_2$CN	0.16	0.01	0.12	b	[0.18]	0.18	0.21	-0.18	-3.60	
CH = CH$_2$	0.05	-0.02			-[0.01]	0.09	0.07	-0.08	0.20	-0.40
COCH$_3$	0.38	0.50	b	0.83	[0.47]	0.29	0.32	0.20	-2.90	-2.77
CO$_2$CH$_3$	0.37	0.45	b	0.69	[0.44]	0.34	0.33	0.15	-1.92	-1.75
CH$_2$CH$_3$	-0.07	-0.15	-0.3	b	-0.13	-0.03	-0.05	-0.10	0.39	0.0
c-C$_3$H$_5$	-0.07	-0.13	-0.4	-0.1	-[0.22]	0.01	-0.06	-0.08	0.51	-0.14
n-Pr	-0.07	-0.13		b		-0.02	-0.06	-0.08		0.08
i-Pr	-0.07	-0.15	-0.28	b	-0.15	-0.03	-0.05	-0.10	0.40	0.08
2-Thienyl	0.09	0.05	-0.3	0.19		[0.21]	0.10	0.04	0.81	
n-Bu	-0.08	-0.16		b	-0.16	-0.04	-0.06	-0.11		0.08
C(CH$_3$)$_3$	-0.10	-0.20	-0.26	b	-0.17	-0.07	-0.07	-0.13	0.52	
C$_5$F$_5$	0.34	0.41	0.26		[0.27]	0.31	0.30	0.13		
C$_6$H$_5$	0.06	-0.01	-0.2	0.09	0.04	0.12	0.08	-0.08	0.00	-0.38
2-Benzoxazolyl	0.30	0.33		0.68			0.28	0.07	-1.22	
2-Benzothiazolyl	0.27	0.29		0.65			0.25	0.06	-0.94	
COC$_6$H$_5$	0.34	0.43		0.88	[0.46]	[0.27]	0.30	0.16	-3.04	-2.90
Benzyl	-0.08	-0.25	-0.25	b	[-0.06]	0.03	-0.08	-0.01	0.36	-0.39
Ferrocenyl	-0.15	-0.18	-0.7	-0.04		-0.15	-0.04			
Adamantyl	-0.12	-0.13	-0.27	b	[-0.13]		-0.12	-0.02		
Cl	0.37	0.23	0.11	b	0.28	0.47	0.41	-0.15	-1.59	-1.93
F	0.34	0.06	-0.07	b	0.20	0.54	0.43	0.34	1.43	-1.90
H	0.00	0.00	0.00	0.00	0.00	0.00	0.00	0.00	0.03	
I	0.35	0.18	0.13	b	[0.27]	0.39	0.40	-0.19	-1.36	-1.79
IO$_2$	0.68	0.78	b				0.63	0.20		
NO$_2$	0.71	0.78	b	1.25	0.82	0.76	0.67	0.16	-4.13	-3.59
N$_2^+$	1.76	1.91		3.24	[2.18]		1.69	0.36		
N$_3$	0.27	0.15		[.08]		0.42	0.30	-0.13	-1.56	-2.17
NH$_2$	-0.16	-0.66	-1.4	b	[-0.30]	[0.12]	0.02	-0.68	1.53	-1.35
NH$_3$	0.86	0.60		0.56			0.60	0.94	-0.27	
NCO	0.27	0.19			[0.19]	[0.36]	0.23	-0.08	-3.93	-2.81
NCS	0.48	0.38		0.34	[0.35]	[0.42]	0.29	-0.09	-2.91	
I-Tetrazol	0.52	0.50		0.57		[0.54]	0.50	0.02		

continued

no problems, whereas cone-shaped polyatomic groups have quite different volumes in different orientations. None of the above cited parameters adequately account for

Table 5.2 *continued*

Substituent	σ_m	σ_p	σ_p^+	σ_p^-	σ_p^0	σ_I	F	R	Aromatic μ (Debye)	Aliphatic μ (Debye)
$NHCONH_2$	−0.03	0.24	b			0.21	0.04	−0.28		
$NHCSNH_2$	0.22	0.16	b	[0.16]	[0.29]	0.23	−0.05	−5.16	−0.16	
$NHCH_3$	−0.30	−0.84	b	−0.46	[0.18]	−0.11	−0.74	1.69	−1.01	
$N(CF_3)_2$	0.40	0.53	b		[0.49]	0.34	0.22			
NHAc	0.21	0.00	−0.65	b	[0.14]	0.26	0.28	−0.26	−3.65	−3.81
$N(CH_3)_2$	−0.15	−0.83	−0.62	b	−0.32	[0.06]	0.10	−0.92	1.61	−1.26
$N(CH_3)_3^+$	0.88	0.82	b	b	[0.88]	0.73	0.89	0.00		
$N=NPh$	0.32	0.39	−0.15	0.65		[0.19]	0.28	0.13		
O^-	−0.47	−0.81	−2.3	b	−0.77	−0.16	−0.35	−0.49		
OH	0.12	−0.37	−0.9	b	−0.12	0.22	0.29	−0.64	−1.59	−1.66
OCF_3	0.38	0.35	b			[0.55]	0.38	0.00	−2.36	
OCH_3	0.12	−0.27	−0.78	b	−0.15	0.29	0.26	−0.51	−1.30	−1.27
$OCOCH_3$	0.39	0.31	b			[0.36]	0.41	−0.07	−1.72	−1.81
OEt	0.10	−0.24	−0.8	b	−0.14	0.27	0.22	−0.44	−1.38	−1.27
OC_6H_5	0.25	−0.03	−0.52	b	−0.05	0.42	0.34	−0.35	1.16	−1.38
$PO(OMe)_2$	0.42	0.53	[0.54]	0.80	[0.43]	[0.24]	0.37	0.19		
SO_2F	0.80	0.91	b	[1.32]		[0.75]	0.75	0.22	−4.59	−3.39
SF_5	0.61	0.68		0.77		0.57	0.57	0.15	−3.44	
SO_3^-	0.05	0.09			0.52	[0.30]	0.13	0.03	0.07	
SH	0.25	0.15	b	[0.06]		0.26	0.28	−0.11	−1.33	−1.51
SO_2NH_2	0.46	0.57	b	0.92	[0.58]	[0.44]	0.41	0.19		−4.60
$SOCF_3$	0.63	0.69	b			0.69	0.60	0.14		
SO_2CF_2	0.79	0.93	b	1.49		0.72	0.73	0.26		
SCF_3	0.40	0.50		0.61		0.44	0.35	0.18	−2.50	
SCN	0.41	0.52		0.60	[0.58]	0.58	0.36	0.19	−3.01	−3.89
$SOCH_3$	0.52	0.49	b	0.73	0.57	[0.50]	0.52	0.01	−3.98	−3.88
SO_2CH_3	0.60	0.72	b	1.05	0.75	0.59	0.54	0.22	−4.75	−4.26
SCH_3	0.15	0.00	−0.6	[0.13]	0.05	0.25	0.20	−0.18	−1.34	−1.45
$S(CH_3)_2^+$	1.00	0.90		1.16	[1.06]	[0.89]	1.02	−0.04		
$SeCF_3$	0.32	0.38	b			[0.42]		0.29	0.12	−2.48
$Si(CH_3)_3$	−0.04	−0.07	0.02	0.08			−0.13	−0.04	−0.04	

[a] Values given in brackets are considered to be less certain.
[b] Use of σ_p is considered permissible.

this but Verloop has produced a computer program STERIMOL which provides different parameters for different calculations. This program simulates three-dimensional model building of molecules or molecular groups using the Corey–Pauling–Koltun (CPK) space filling models and four width parameters, B, B_2, B_3 and B_4 are defined and determined by rotation of the substituents around the x-axis. In practice large numbers of substituents and active molecules need to be examined statistically to derive correlations with these steric parameters.

5.9.3 Use of the Hansch approach

What is the value of the Hansch approach for the practising medicinal chemist? Is it an essential tool for design, or a retrospective confirmation that the scientists had selected the optimum compound, long after synthesis has finished? The current situation is somewhere in the middle, and the recent coupling of the QSAR technique with modern graphics has underlined the essential value of the methodology.

Errors in the methodology have arisen because of the number of electronic parameters which may be chosen for a correlation analysis, with some interrelations being solely chance. Moreover, many of the parameters are related and thus are not independent variables. To better produce a meaningful correlation, Hansch has devised a set of criteria which should be considered before a "best correlation equation" for a set of congeners can be confidently derived. The first, and probably most important step, is to select independent variables, and the widest possible number of independent variables must be considered including σ, π, E_s, MR, other steric and molecular orbital parameters. In some cases indicator variables, set to have a value of 1 if a substituent is present and 0 if there is only a hydrogen atom in the same place, are also needed.

The selected parameters should be as independent of each other as possible, and having produced a correlation, the choice of the independent variables must be justified by stringent statistical analysis. To avoid chance correlations at least five or six data points should be chosen per variable. The resultant correlation should be as simple to derive as possible but must also make "chemical sense".

The work of Yoshimoto[70] on a series of 4-anilino-pyrimidines (**53**) which showed moderately potent antidepressant activities is an excellent example of modern QSAR. The activity of compounds was measured as the percentage of inhibition (A) of ptosis caused by reserpine in mice at the same dose level (p.o.). A number of compounds were available from a previous fungicide project, and 59 active compounds were used to seek correlations. Equation (34) was the outcome of the first investigation.

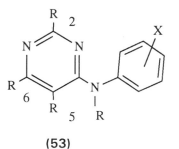

(**53**)

$$\text{Log} (A/(100-A)) = -1.38 \ (\pm 0.75)\pi_s + 1.51(\pm 1.45) \ \sigma_p - 1.40(\pm 0.68)\text{I-1} \quad (34)$$
$$+ 1.37 \ (\pm 0.62) \ \text{I-4} + 2.39 \ (\pm 0.76) \ \text{I-5} - 0.76(\pm 0.68)\text{I-6}$$
$$+ 1.50 \ (\pm 0.58) \ \text{I-7} - 0.68 \ (\pm 0.56)$$
$$n = 59, \ r = 0.837, \ s = 0.810$$

I-1 etc. are indicator variables with I-1 referring to the unsubstituted aniline moiety and I-4, I-5 to p-halogen and p-alkyl substitutions on the aniline. I-6 applies if R_5 is halogen and I-7 for structures bridged through $(CH_2)_3$ between R_5 and R_6. π_5 is the hydrophobicity parameter for the R_5 substituents with the $\Sigma\pi$ value of bridged compounds being assigned equally to R_5 and R_6. σ_p is the Hammett constant of X substituents located at the *para* position, but no statistical significance accrued to substituents in the *ortho* and *meta* positions.

Examination of equation (34) leads to some interesting insights. The fact that the I-1 term is negative indicates that any substituent on the aniline ring is detrimental to activity, but that halogen and alkyl groups at the *para* positions will cancel this (I-4 and I-5 positive). The combination of I-1, I-4 and I-5 suggests that *meta* substitution is unfavourable for activity. The conclusion from equation (34) was that compounds of general structures (54) should be active (X = CN, SO_2, NO_2) and indeed they were, and the best compound (54, X − *p*-CN) had an ED_{50} of 6.7 mg/kg p.o. with few side effects.

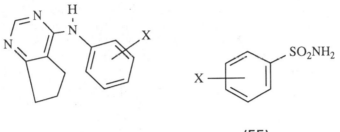

(54)   (55)

Whether compound (54) could have been designed without the use of Hansch analysis is questionable, but what is not is the fact that use of the Hansch approach obliges the medicinal chemist to seriously consider the effect of any proposed substitutions in real, measurable terms. This is perhaps the great legacy of the Hansch approach to QSAR.

Modern computer graphics have now provided a direct means of verifying some of the predictions of Hansch analysis.[71] The enzyme carbonic anhydrase, which governs the hydration of carbon dioxide to bicarbonate, has been studied by both techniques. The importance of this enzyme in medicinal chemistry lies in the fact that its inhibitors may have use as diuretics, antiepileptics, and anti glaucoma agents.

The series of sulphonamides (55) gave:

$$\log K = 1.55 \ (\pm 0.38)\sigma + 0.64 \ (\pm 0.08) \log P - 2.07(\pm 0.22) \ I_1 - \tag{35}$$
$$3.28 \ (\pm 0.23) \ I_2 + 6.94 \ (\pm 0.18)$$
$$n = 29, \ r = 0.991 \ s = 0.204$$

Here K is the binding constant and I_1 and I_2 are indicator variables where I_1 is 1 for *meta* substituents and I_2 is 1 for *ortho* substituents, and in this series all ortho and meta substituents are of the type $-CO_2R$ where R is an alkyl group. The large negative coefficient with I_2 suggests a steric effect with *ortho* substituents much less active than their *meta* equivalents. A computer graphic study of the binding site suggested that *ortho* interaction with Pro-201 was responsible for this effect. The positive coefficient with σ shows that electron withdrawing groups promote binding which would be expected to increase the stability of the anionic form of $-SO_2NH_2$ and the graphics study indicated that such complexation of the zinc atoms via the sulphamido nitrogen is possible with the 4-substituent falling on a large, slightly concave hydrophobic surface as suggested by the dependence on log P. There is thus good agreement between the two approaches, and a number of similar studies have also been reported.

The derivation of a significant Hansch equation can require the use of considerable computer time and sophisticated statistics to solve the generated regression equations. Such exercises are not in the domain of the organic chemist and, as an aid in the use of the principles of Hansch analysis in drug design, Topliss has proposed a "decision tree" approach.

5.9.3.1 Topliss approach[72,73]

In the early 1970s, Topliss suggested a nonmathematical, nonstatistical and non-computerised protocol for the use of basic Hansch principles in the most efficient optimisation of activity in a new chemical series. The only assumption of this technique was that the lead structure should contain a nonfused benzene ring. At that time this constraint in fact applied to some 40% of all organic molecules and 50% of new patents. The decision tree of general applicability which is then followed is shown in Figure 5.13. The first derivative to be synthesised is the o-chloro, and subsequent synthesis decisions depend on the relative activity of this compound. The subsequent course of action to be followed for the case where the compound is found to be more active is detailed in Figure 5.14. Since both π and σ values for a chlorine atom are positive, the simplest interpretation of the increased activity is that it results from the increase in π and σ values and, therefore, the next logical substitution should be to increase them still further. Such a result is achieved with the 3, 4-dichloro derivative (compound III), and, if the observed activity is increased yet again, further increases in π and σ should be achieved by the synthesis of the 4-Cl, $3CF_3$ (compound IV) and 4-NO_2, $3CF_3$ (compound V) derivatives. At this point both π and σ have been increased maximally, and V may indeed be the optimum compound in the series.

The procedural steps to be followed if the 4-chloro substitution results in a compound which is less or equiactive to the unsubstituted compound are shown in Figure 5.13 and left to the reader to elaborate the appropriate reasoning.

However, it must be stressed that this simple analysis has been based purely on π and σ values, and if other factors, notably steric, are important, the resultant analysis will be invalid. Reports of the failure of the Topliss approach are probably due to situations in which factors other than those considered by Topliss are important.

Topliss also extended his approach to the study of side chain alkyl groups typically found in esters, ketones, amines and amides. In this case, the reasoning regarding the effects of changes in substitution is conducted in terms of π, σ and E_s (Table 5.3). However, the approach is the same, with the introduction of predictable changes in these parameters, classification of the biological activity, and interpretation of the results by simple deduction. With the retrospective analysis of published S/A case histories using detailed Hansch analysis, Topliss was able to demonstrate that his approach could generate some of the most active molecules from the full analysis within the first few molecules from his scheme.

Thus the Topliss scheme provides an excellent guide to the medicinal chemist

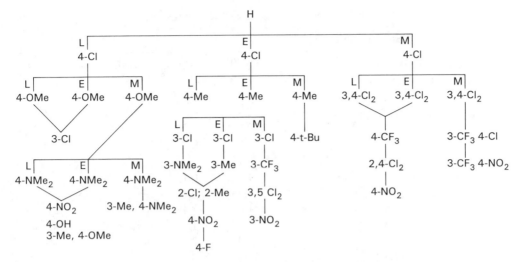

Fig. 5.13.   Operational scheme for aromatic substitution.

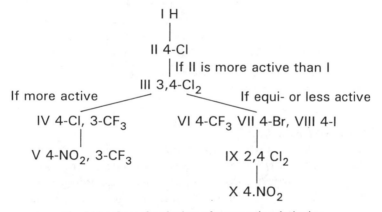

Fig. 5.14.   Operational scheme for aromatic substitution.

seeking to optimise the activity of a recently discovered compound. The scheme is simple to follow, uses the type of substituents usually investigated by the chemist, but structures their application in a logical and consistent manner such that the activities of the products can be more appropriately interrelated. The method does not require the use of computers, statistics, or of regression analysis, although if sufficient compounds have been synthesised there is no reason why the empirical analysis should not be refined by the Hansch analysis. Whilst this approach has been described in terms of π, σ, E_s and σ^* parameters, there is no reason why other suitable parameters, especially electronic and steric, could not be used as alternatives. Perhaps the major failing of this method is its very simplicity since it is very difficult to extend the method to account simultaneously for changes in more parameters than π and σ, and attempts to extend the method to account for other parameters complicates its application with the use of computers.

Table 5.3. Side chain substituent parameters

Substituent	π	σ	E_s
CH_3	0.50	0.00	0.00
$i\text{-}C_3H_7$	1.30	-0.19	-0.47
$cyclo\text{-}C_5H_9$	2.14	-0.20	-0.51
$cyclo\text{-}C_6H_{11}$	2.51	-0.15	-0.79
$CH_2C_6H_5$	2.63	0.22	-0.38
$cyclo\text{-}C_4H_7$	1.80	-0.20	-0.06
$CH_2CH_2C_6H_5$	3.13	0.08	-0.38
$CH_2\text{-}cyclo\text{-}C_3H_5$	1.80	-0.13	
$tert\text{-}C_4H_9$	1.98	-0.30	-1.54
C_2H_5	1.00	-0.10	-0.07
$CHCl_2$	1.15	1.92	-1.54
CF_3	1.07	2.76	-1.16
CH_2CF_3	1.57	0.92	
CH_2SCH_3	0.77	0.44	-0.34
C_6H_5	2.13	0.60	
H	0.00	0.49	1.24
CH_2OCH_3	0.02	0.64	-0.19
$CH_2SO_2CH_3$	-0.76	1.32	

From J. G. Topliss, *J. Med. Chem.* (1972), 15, 1009, reproduced with the permission of the copyright owner, the American Chemical Society.

5.9.3.2 *Batch selection methods*

Hansch[74] has produced an alternative method of logically directing the synthesis of a new congeneric series. He took the physicochemical properties of some 90 substituents, σ, π^2 F, R, MR and MW and clustered these into groups, as shown in Table 5.4. In each cluster all the groups have similar combinations of these properties, and this table can be used in two stages. Firstly, one substituent is chosen from each group so that an initial batch of 8–10 compounds will have the greatest possible range of physical values. A clear assignment of interesting activity in just one or two of the groups will then direct the system towards the other member of the group. An advantage of this method is that it can be followed from the published data of Hansch. A more interactive approach available to those with access to computers was described by Norrington[75]. This approach uses a more restrictive set of substituents than that of Hansch, and one begins by "telling" the computer the analogues already synthesised. The computer is programmed to respond by giving the next analogue which differs from the starting compound by more than a specified amount, and if this analogue is synthesised it is included in the data set and the next analogue is chosen according to the established criteria. If this is not accessible then the computer selects a suitable replacement. The process continues until all of the data space has been scanned. Of course, after using both the above approaches a regression analysis can subsequently be performed on the analogues to determine any structure–activity relationship and consequently suggest further derivatives. The great value of both approaches is that the initial batch of analogues selected for synthesis has the widest possible range of noninterrelated parameters.

Table 5.4.   Typical members of clusters based σ, π^2, F, R, MR and MW

Typical members

Me,H,3,4-(OCH$_2$O),CH$_2$CH$_2$COOH, CH=CH$_2$, Et, CH$_2$OH

CH=CHCOOH

CN, NO$_2$, CHO, COOH, COMe

C≡CH, CH$_2$Cl.,Cl,NNN,SH,SMe,CH=NOH,CH$_2$CN,OCOMe,
   SCOMe COOMe, SCN

CONH$_2$, CONHMe, SO$_2$NH$_2$, SO$_2$Me, SOMe

NHCHO, NHCOMe, NHCONH$_2$. NHCSNH$_2$. NHSO$_2$Me

F,OMc,NH$_2$,NHNH$_2$,OH,NHMe,NHEt,NMe$_2$

Br, OCF$_3$. CF$_3$, NCS,I,SF$_5$,SO$_2$F

CH$_2$,Br,SMe,NHCO$_2$Et,SO$_2$Ph,OSO$_2$Me

NHCOPh,NHSO$_2$Ph,OSO$_2$Ph,COPh,N=NPh,OCOPh,PO$_2$Ph

3 4(CH$_2$)$_3$,3,4-(CH$_2$)$_4$Pr,i-Pr,3,4-(CH$_2$)$_4$,NHBu,Ph,CH$_2$Ph,t-Bu,OPh

Ferrocenyl, adamantyl

So what is the value of Hansch correlation analysis today? It is probably fair to say that there are medicinal chemists who are committed, those who reject it, and those who are impartial and await spectacular successes. It is certainly true to say that visualisation and manipulation of target structures and candidate molecules by computer graphics is more appealing to the pragmatic synthetic chemist. The most logical approach to new drug design is probably the systemic use of graphics throughout the project phases with the introduction of Hansch-type QSAR at the point when sufficient compounds have been synthesised to focus the remainder of the chemistry programme.

5.9.4   The Free-Wilson method[76]

In 1964, Free and Wilson proposed a method of analysing the activity of a congeneric series of compounds in terms of the contributions of the different substituents contained in the different members of the series. Equation (36) expresses this in the simplest form:

$$\text{Activity} = \Sigma_{a_i} + \mu \tag{36}$$

where a_i is the activity contribution of each substituent and μ is the biological activity value of the unsubstituted parent molecule in the series. The Free–Wilson approach is a genuine structure–activity model because fragment contributions are derived from biological activity values by linear multiple regression analysis. In a Hansch analysis, on the other hand, properties rather than structural elements are correlated to the biological data. However, the numbers derived for a_i are meaningless outside the particular series under investigation, and, unlike the Hansch approach, inevitably cannot lead to a better understanding of drug action at the molecular level.

To use the Free–Wilson approach, a series has to be designed containing sufficient compounds to provide statistically significant results. Thus for a series with J different positions of structural variation with n_i different substituents in each position, equation (37) gives a minimum number of compounds needed and equation (38) the maximum.

$$N_{min} = \sum_j (n_i - 1) + 1 \tag{37}$$

$$N_{max} = n_1 . n_2 . \qquad n_j - 1; n_{;j} \tag{38}$$

Thus for a series with three positions of substitution and five different groups in each position, the minimum number of analyses necessary is 13 and the maximum 125. The actual number of compounds prepared will, of course, depend on ease of synthesis and the time available. The method can mix data from substitutions in different positions, unlike the Hansch approach where different values of the various parameters would probably have to be used for different positions. As an example, we can consider the antiadrenergic activities of a series of N,N-dimethyl-α-bromo-phenethylamines (56). Twenty-two compounds with X, $= Y = $ H, F, Cl, Br, I and Me in various combinations were prepared and their biological activities measured. In this case μ would be the activity of the parent (X $=$ Y $=$ H) molecule, and the activity of the other 21 compounds is given by:

$$\log (1/c)_x = a_{1k}[X_1] + a_{2k}[Y_1] + \mu \tag{39}$$

where a_{1k} is the activity coefficient for a substitution in position 1. There are thus 22 equations which can readily be solved by linear multiple regression analysis to give:

$$\begin{aligned}
\log (1/c) = & -0.301(\pm 0.50)[m\text{-F}] + 0.207(\pm 0.27)[mCl] \\
& + 0.434(+0.27)[m\text{-Br}] + 0.579(\pm 0.50)[m\text{-I}] + 0.454(\pm 0.27)[m\text{-Me}] \\
& + 0.34(\pm 0.30)[p\text{-F}] + 0.768(\pm 0.30)[p\text{-Cl}] + 1.020(\pm 0.30)[p\text{-Br}] \\
& + 1.429(\pm 0.50)[p\text{-I}] + 1.256(\pm 0.33)[p\text{-Me}] + 7.821(\pm 0.27) \\
& n = 22, r = 0.969, s = 0.194
\end{aligned} \tag{40}$$

This would appear to be quite a complex equation, but it does of course calculate the effect of any of the given substituents on the overall biological activity and enables the activity of further combinations to be calculated.

While the Hansch and Free–Wilson approaches may be different in the appropriate situation the two become equivalent. Thus the Hansch equation has to be linear and all physiochemical parameters, Φ, to be additive constitutive properties, as is the case with π, MR, σ and E_s:

$$\log (1/c = k_1\Phi_1 + k_2\Phi_2 \dots k_n\Phi + c \tag{41}$$
$$= \Sigma K_j\Phi_j + c$$

Then

$$a; j = \Sigma k_j\Phi_{ij} \tag{42}$$

where Φ_{ij} are the physicochemical properties Φ_j of the substituent X_i. The Hansch equations (43–45) have been devised for the bromophenylethylamines (56) in an attempt to fit the experimental results.

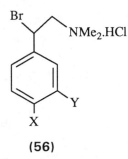

(56)

$$\log (1/c) = 1.26(\pm 0.19)\pi - 1.46(+0.34)\sigma^+ + 0.21(\pm 0.17)E_s\text{meta} + 7.62 \quad (43)$$
$$n = 22, r = 0.959, s = 0.173$$

$$\log (1/c) = 1.15(\pm 0.19)\pi - 1.47(\pm 0.38)\sigma^+ + 7.82 \quad (44)$$
$$n = 22, r = 0.944, s = 0.197$$

$$\log (1/c) = 0.83(\pm 0.21)\pi_\text{meta} + 1.33(\pm 0.20)\pi_\text{para} - 0.92(\pm 0.50)\sigma^+{}_\text{meta} - \quad (45)$$
$$1.89(\pm 0.57)\sigma^+{}_\text{para} + 7.80$$
$$n = 22, r = 0.966, s = 0.164$$

The differences between these perhaps indicates the difficulties of drawing physical conclusions from such studies. However, equation (42) could then be applied to each of these equations (43-45) to give activity contribution a_i values for each position (e.g. equation (46) gives a_i for meta) which show remarkable consistency.

$$a_i, \text{meta} = 1.15\pi_\text{meta} - 1.47\pi\sigma^+{}_\text{meta} \quad (46)$$

The two approaches may be further combined (equation (47)), and this is particularly valuable for a series in which there is sufficient variation at one point for Hansch analysis but not at another.

$$\log (1/c) = \Sigma\sigma_i + \Sigma k_j\Phi_j + c \quad (47)$$

As an example, consider the mesylamides and benzamides (**57,58**) and their binding to papain. The mesylamides give equation (48), the benzamides equation (49), and a combination which now includes the Free–Wilson parameter I ($I = 1$ for mesylamides) (equation (50)). The regression coefficient of I is the activity contribution of a mesyl group based on the benzoyl group as a reference substituent.

$$\log 1/K_m = 0.53(\pm 0.23)\text{MR} + 0.37(\pm 0.20)\sigma + 1.88(0.13) \quad (48)$$
$$n = 13, r = 0.935, s = 0.105$$

$$\log 1/K_m = 0.72(+0.67)\text{MR} + 0.73(+0.37)\sigma + 3.62(\pm 0.34) \quad (49)$$
$$n = 7, r = 0.971, s = 0.148$$

$$\log 1/K_m = 0.57(+0.26)\text{MR} + 0.56(+0.19)\sigma^-$$
$$- 1.92(\pm 0.15)\text{I} + 3.74(\pm 0.17) \quad (50)$$
$$n = 20, r = 0.990 \ s = 0.148$$

Equation (50) now accounts for all compounds and provides a very good value

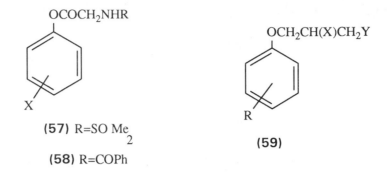

(57) R=SO$_2$Me

(58) R=COPh

(59)

for the regression coefficients, and such combined approaches have been helpful in improving Hansch analysis. Thus the antifungal activities of phenyl ethers **(59)** were originally fitted by equation (51).

$$\log 1/c = 0.691(\pm 0.14) \log P + 0.428(\pm 0.51)\sigma + 1.213 \tag{51}$$
$$n = 26, \; r = 0.911, \; s = 0.216$$

A Free–Wilson analysis showed significant difference for some substituents, especially for ortho substitutions and the para methyl group. This indicated that electronic properties of these do not contribute and that steric hindrance by *ortho* substituents may be responsible for their lower activities. This led to equation (52) which better fits the data.

$$\log (1/c) = 0.741(\pm 0.11) \log P + 0.214(\pm 0.08) \, E_s \text{ortho} + 0.846 \tag{52}$$
$$n = 28, \; r = 0.942, \; s = 0.170$$

It is fair to conclude that the Free–Wilson approach has much to offer in the statistical analysis of the results from biological testing of reasonably sized groups of congeneric molecules.

5.9.5   Selected pattern recognition techniques

5.9.5.1   *Statistical methods*
Over recent years a number of sophisticated statistical techniques have been applied to series of compounds for which the data available are not quantitative enough for either Hansch or Free–Wilson analysis. In particular, it is common for physical parameters for series of compounds to be available, where the activity is expressed crudely as "active" or "inactive" or, even, as " + + + ". If k physical properties are listed for each of the molecules, these can be represented as one element of k-dimensional space, and the methodology entails separating this space into regions. Ideally one region will contain all the inactive compounds and another all the active ones, and the corresponding values of the parameters can be used to predict further compounds.

One such method is linear discriminant analysis (LDA) where a simple plane is used to separate the different regions in space. The use of LDA requires computers, but good statistics programs, such as SAS, can handle the calculations. As with much of statistics, the methodology is complex and full of pitfalls for the unwary. In the first documented use of the technique in medicinal chemistry, Martin[77] was able to analyse a group of aminotetralins and aminoindans (**60**) which had shown unexpected monoamine oxidase inhibitory activity. The physical parameters used for the analysis were π, π^2, E_s^c, an indicator variable (X) which was set at 1 if the substituent was in the X-position and 0 if it was in the Y-position, and another indicator variable with a value of 1 for indans and 0 for tetralins. The program was able to classify accurately the largest number of molecules when π, E_s^c and X were used as the physical parameters, and this insight suggested future compounds to be prepared.

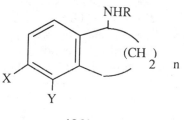

(60)

Another statistical analysis technique used is cluster significance analysis which seeks statistically significant groupings of points in space. The technique has not been used to a great extent in medical chemistry, but McFarland and Gans[78] give some examples.

Other techniques which have been applied include the linear learning machine, k-nearest-neighbour method, ALLOC and SIMCA, where the reader is referred to the original literature.[79]

5.9.5.2   Distance mapping

The final technique to be mentioned is that of "distance geometry" proposed primarily by Crippen[80] which starts from the premise that an understanding of the structure of a receptor can be gained from the structures of the molecules that bind to it. Crippen regards the method as falling between Hansch QSAR and the advanced theoretical design technique using a defined crystal structure of the receptor to design a new ligand. Thus three-dimensional structures of ligands in energetically allowed conformations are compared to deduce the optimum geometrical arrangements of atoms for a best fit; the method can be further refined by including electrostatic effects.

In the initial steps low-energy conformations of a series of active molecules are determined and the minimum and maximum distances between the atoms in the ligands are calculated. Thus if two molecules a and b bind to the same receptor, then the atoms a_i and a_j of molecule a and b_i and b_j of molecule b will occupy the same regions of the active site. It is probable that these atoms will not be in exactly the same position but that the differences between the positions of the ith and jth atoms in the two molecules will be small. From a large number of molecules it should be possible to reduce the uncertainties in the positions of those atoms to very small values indeed, and at this point the binding region of the receptor will be defined.

The method will fail of course if a major change in conformation of ligand or receptor occurs between the molecules used for the analysis. The use of statistical techniques on a reasonable number of ligands helps to reduce the possibility of these effects, and a number of ways of directing the search for interatomic distances to generate a novel structure have been described, all, however, requiring considerable computer input.

In one application of the method, the binding of twenty-five pyrimidines and fourteen triazines to dihydrofolate reductase obtained from *E.coli* was used to generate a model of the binding site. This showed nineteen site pockets of nine different types, and because this enzyme has been extensively studied, it was possible to compare the model with the known crystal structure. Gratifyingly, it showed that the preferred site pockets were sterically accessible and not overlapping with the receptor site atoms, that three sites identified as hydrogen bonding, sites were indeed surrounded by groups capable of hydrogen bonding and that pockets which showed high correlation with the hydrophobic properties of ligands were indeed surrounded by various hydrophobic groups. Once a structure has been proposed for the binding region, then binding to available conformations of ligands can be calculated and the information used to aid future drug design.

References

CHAPTER 3

1. C. R., Gardner, *Biomaterials* 1985 **6** 153
2. N. Bodor, *Med. Res. Rev.* 1984 **4** 449
3. E. C. Miller & J. A. Miller, *Pharmacol. Rev.* 1966, **18** 805

CHAPTER 5

1. W. J. Dower & S. P. A. Fodor, *Ann. Rep. Med. Chem.* **26** 271 (1991)
2. McAlpine & J. E. Hochlowski in *Natural Products Isolation* ed. G. H. Wayman and R. Cooper, Elsevier, New York 1989, p1
3. *Chemical and Engineering News,* 2nd September, 1991
4. K. Hostettmann and A. Marston in *Studies in Natural Product Chemistry* Vol. 7, ed. Atta-Ur-Rahman, Elsevier, New York 1990 p. 405
5. J. Bérdy in *Chemistry and Biotechnology of Biologically Active Natural Products* ed C. Szántay, Akádemiai Kiadó, Budapest 1988 p. 269
6. H. Umezawa in ref. 5 p. 481
7. J. S. Myndene, L. W. Crandall & J. H. Cordellina in ref. 5 p. 377
8. *Marine Toxins* ed. S. Hall & G. Strichartz, American Chemical Society, Washington, 1990
9. P. J. Scheuer, *Med. Res. Rev.* **9** 535 (1989)
10. D. Faulkner, *Natural Products Report* **3**, 1 (1986)
11. B. Alberts, D. Bray, J. Lewis, M. Roff, K. Roberts & J. D. Watson *Molecular Biology of the Cell* 2nd edn Garland Publishing Inc., New York 1989
12. K. Drlica in *Comprehensive Medicinal Chemistry* Vol. 1 ed. P. D. Kennewell, Pergamon Press, Oxford 1990 p. 361
13. F. Sanger, *Science* **214** 1205 (1981)
14. W. Gilbert, *Science* **214** 1305 (1981)
15. R. A. F. Dixon *et al. Nature* **321**, 25 (1986)

16. K. B. Mullis *Scientific American* April 1990 p. 36
17. C. J. de Ranter in *X-ray Crystallography and Drug Action* ed. A. S. Horn & C. J. de Ranter, Oxford University Press, Oxford 1984 p.1
18. C. R. A. Cotton & E. N. Greaves *Chemistry in Britain,* 805 (1986)
19. K. Moffat, D. Szebenyis & O. Bilderbank, *Science* **223** 1423 (1984)
20. J. Hajdu *et al. Nature* **329** 178 (1987)
21. R. S. Goudy *et al. Nature* **345** 309 (1990)
22. M. S. Rismann *et al. Nature* **317** 145 (1985)
23. J. Hajdu & L. N. Johnson *Biochemistry* **29** 1669 (1990)
24. W. A. Hendrickson *Science* **254** 51 (1991)
25. K. Wuthrich, *Science* **243** 45 (1989)
26. K. Wuthrich, *NMR of Proteins and Nucleic Acids* John Wiley, New York 1988
27. G. M. Clore, M. Nilges & A. M. Gronenborn in *Computer-Aided Molecular Design* ed. W. G. Richards, IBC Technical Services, London 1989 p. 203
28. M. P. Williamson, *Chemistry in Britain* April 1991 p. 335
29. G. M. Clore & A. M. Gronenenborn, *Science* **242** 1290 (1991)
30. G. M. Clore, P. T. Wingfield & A. M. Gronenborn, *Biochemistry* **30** 2315 (1991)
31. S. W. Fesik *J. Med. Chem.* **34** 2937 (1991)
32. *Protein Structure, Prediction and Design* ed. J. Kay, G. Lunt & D. Osguthorpe, The Biochemical Society, London 1990
33. *Cameleon* from Oxford Molecular Ltd 1990
34. T. L. Blundell, B. L. Sibandra, M. J. E. Sternberg & J. M. Thornton *Nature* **326** 347 (1987)
35. C. M. Topham *et al.* in ref. 32 p. 1
36. J. Garnier *et al.* in ref. 32 p. 11
37. L. H. Hurley, *J. Med. Chem.* **32** 2027 (1989)
38. L. H. Hurley & F. L. Boyd, *TIPS* **9** 402 (1988)
39. S. Akhtar & R. J. Julians *The Pharm. Journal* 20th July 1991 p. 89
40. W. G. Richards, *Quantum Pharmacology* 2nd edn. Butterworths, London 1983
41. J. G. Vinter in *Topics in Molecular Pharmacology* Vol. 3 *Molecular Graphics and Drug Design* ed. A. S. V. Burgen, G. C. K. Roberts & M. S. Tute, Elsevier, Amsterdam 1986 p. 15
42. G. K. Loew & S. K. Burt in *Comprehensive Medicinal Chemistry* ed. C. Hansch, P. G. Sammes & J. B. Taylor; Pergamon Press, Oxford 1990, Vol. 4 ed. C.A. Ramsden, p. 105
43. G. L. Siebel & P. A. Kollman in ref. 42 p. 125
44. J. A. McCannon in ref. 42 p. 139
45. R. Langridge & T. E. Klein in ref. 42 p. 413
46. M. L. Connolly, *Science* **221** 709 (1983)
47. N. C. Cohen, J. M. Blaney, C. Humblet, P. Gund & D. C.Barry, *J. Med. Chem.* **33** 883 (1990)
48. B. M. Pettitt & M. Karplus in ref. 41 p. 75
49. C. A. Reynolds & P. M. King in ref. 27 p. 51
50. P. A. Bach, U. C. Singh, F. K. Brown, R. Langridge & P. A. Kollman, *Science* **235** 574 (1987)

51. P. J. Goodford, *J. Med. Chem.* **27** 558 (1984)
52. C. R. Beddell, P. J. Goodford, F. E. Norrington, S. Wilkinson & R. Wootton, *British Journal Pharmacology* **57** 201 (1976)
53. J. M. Blaney, E. C. Jorgensen, M. L. Connolly, T. E. Ferrin, R. Langridge, S. J. Oatley, J. M. Burridge & C. C. F. Blak, *J. Med. Chem.* **25** 785 (1982)
54. W. C. Ripka, W. J. Sipio & J. M. Blaney, *Lecture in Heterocyclic Chemistry*, **IX** 95 (1987)
55. L. F. Kuyper, B. Roth, D. P. Baccanari, R. Ferone, C. R. Beddell, J. N. Champness, D. K. Stainnes, J. G. Darin, F. E. Norrington, D. J. Baker and P. J. Goodford, *J. Med. Chem.* **28** 303 (1985)
56. P. J. Goodford, *J. Med. Chem.* **28** 849 (1985)
57. D. J. Danziger & P. M. Dean. *Proc. R. Society London B* **236** 101 (1989)
58. D. J. Danziger & P. M. Dean. *Proc. R. Society London B* **236** 115 (1989)
59. R. A. Lewis & P. M. Dean *Proc. R. Society London B* **236** 125 (1989)
60. R. A. Lewis & P. M. Dean *Proc. R. Society London B* **236** 141 (1989)
61. K. Appelt *et al. J. Med. Chem.* **34** 1925 (1991)
62. M. S. Tute in ref. 42 p. 1
63. A. Crum-Brown & T. R. Fraser, *Trans. Royal Society Edinburgh* **25** 151 (1868)
64. C. Hansch, P. P. Moloney, T. Fujita & R. M. Muir, *Nature (London)* **194** 178 (1962)
65. P. A. J. Taylor in ref. 42 p. 241
66. C. Hansch & A. J. Leo *Substituent Constants for Correlation Analysis in Chemistry and Biology*, John Wiley, New York 1979
67. A. J. Leo in ref. 42, p. 295
68. R. F. Rikker, *The Hydrophobic Fragmental Constant*, Elsevier, New York 1977.
69. K Bowden in ref. 42 p. 205
70. H. Watanabe, S. Muyamoto, M. Yoshimoto, T. Kamuka, I. Nakayama, T. Kobayaclin & T. Hinda, *Chem. Pharm. Bulletin* **35** 1452 (1987)
71. J. M. Blaney & C. Hansch in ref. 42 p. 459
72. J. G. Topliss, *J. Med. Chem.* **15** 1006 (1977)
73. J. G. Topliss, *J. Med. Chem.* **20** 463 (1977)
74. C. Hansch, S. H. Unger & A. B. Forsythe, *J. Med. Chem.* **16** 1217 (1973)
75. F. E. Norrington, R. M. Hyde, S. G. Williams & R. Wootton, *J. Med. Chem.* **18** 604 (1975)
76. S. M. Free & J. W. Wilson, *J. Med. Chem.* **7** 395 (1964)
77. Y. C. Martin, J. B. Holland, C. H., Jarboe & N. Plotnikoff *J. Med. Chem.* **17** 409 (1974)
78. J. W. McFarland & D. J. Gans in ref. 42 p. 667
79. W. J. Dunn & S. Wold in ref. 42 p. 691
80. A. K. Ghose & G. M. Crippen in ref. 42 p.715.

Selected Bibliography

ENZYMES

L. Pauling, *Chemical & Engineering News* **24** 1375 (1946)

J. Kraut, *Science* **242** 533 (1988)

G. S. Adair, *J. Biol. Chem.* **63** 529 (1925)

J. Monod, J. Wyman & J. P. Changeux, *J. Molex. Biol.* **12** 88 (1965)

D. E. Koshland, G. Nemethy & D. Filmer, *Biochemistry* **5** 365 (1966)

M. F. Perutz, *Quart. Rev. Biophys.* **22** 139 (1989)

P. A. Ballett & W. B. Kezer, *JACS* **106** 4282 (1984)

W. Yuan, R. Berman & M. H. Gelb, *JACS* **109** 8071 (1987)

D. E. Tronrud, H. M. Holden & B. W. Matthews, *Science* **235** 571 (1987)

G. B. Elion, *Angew. Chem. Ind. Eng.* **28** 870 (1989)

G. H. Hitchings *Angew. Chem. Ind. Eng.* **28** 879 (1989)

H. Mitsuya, R. Yarchoan, S. Broder *Science* **249** 1537 (1990)

T. Blundell, R. Lapalto, A. Wilderspin, A. Hemmings, P. Hobart, D. Danley &
P. Whittle *TIBS* **15** 425 (1990)

N. Roberts *et al. Science* **248** 358 (1990)

R. A. Lerner, S. J. Benhovic & P. G. Schultz *Science* **252** 659 (1991)

T. R. Cech *Sci. Am.* 76 (1990)

J. A. Lather & T. R. Cech, *Science* **245** 276 (1989)

RECEPTORS

Receptors in Pharmacology ed. J. R. Smythies & R. J. Bradley, Marcel Dekker, New
York 1978

R. F. Furchgott in *Advances in Drug Research* Vol. 3 ed. N. J. Harper & A. B.
Simmonds Academic Press, London 1966 p. 21

W. D. M. Paton & H. P. Rang in *Advances in Drug Research* Vol. 3 ed. N. J. Harper
& A. B Simmonds, Academic Press, London 1967 p. 57

B. Albert, D. Bray, J. Lewis, M. Raff, K. Roberts & J. D. Watson, *Molecular Biology of the Cell*, 2nd edn Garland Publishing, New York 1989

M. Williams & S. J. Emma in *Annual Reports in Medicinal Chemistry* Vol. 21 ed. D. M. Bailey, Academic Press, New York 1986 p. 211

J. N. Langley, *J. Physiol. (London)* **33** 374 (1905)

E. Baumler, *Paul Ehrlich : Scientist for Life*, Holmes & Meier New York 1984

D. E. Koshland Jr, G. Némethy & D. Filmer, *Biochemistry* **5** 365 (1966)

J. Monod, J. Wyman & J.-P. Changeux, *J. Mol. Biol.* **12** 88 (1965)

L. T. Williams & R. J. Lefkowitz, *Receptor Binding Studies in Adrenergic Pharmacology* Raven Press, New York 1978

M. Williams & D. C. U'Pritchard in *Advances in Medicinal Chemistry* Vol. 19, ed. D. M. Bailey, Academic Press, New York 1984, p. 283

I. Creese, D. R. Burt & S. N. Snyder, *Science* **194** 546 (1977)

J. C. Venter & L. C. Harrison (Eds), *Receptor Biochemistry and Methodology* Vol. 1 *Membranes, Detergents and Receptor Solubilisation* Alan R. Liss, New York 1984

R. A. F. Dixon, B. K. Kobilha, D. J. Strader, J. L. Bluovic, H. E. Dohlman, T. Frielle M. A. Bolanouski, C. D. Bennett, E. Rouds, R. Diehl, R. Maniford, E. Stuter, C. S. Sigal, M. G. Caran, R. J. Lefkowitz & C. D. Strader, *Nature* **321** 75 (1986)

R. A. F. Dixon, C. D. Strader & I. S. Sigal in *Annual Reports in Medicinal Chemistry* Vol. 23 ed. R. C. Allen, 1988 p. 221

A. M. Spiegel in *Annual Reports in Medicinal Chemistry* Vol. 23, ed. R. C. Allen 1988 p. 235

M. J. Berridge & R. F. Irvine, *Nature* **341** 197 (1989)

L. H. Hurley, *J. Med. Chem.* **32** 2022 (1989)

A. D. Strosberg (Ed.), *The Molecular Biology of Receptors* Ellis Horwood, Chichester 1987

Index